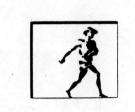

Books by Nancy Burstein

30 DAYS TO A FLATTER STOMACH FOR WOMEN
30 DAYS TO A FLATTER STOMACH FOR MEN (coauthor Roy Matthews)

The
EXECUTIVE
BODY

*A Working Woman's Guide to
Life Style and Total Fitness*

NANCY BURSTEIN

SIMON AND SCHUSTER
NEW YORK

Published by Simon and Schuster
A Division of Simon & Schuster, Inc.

Simon & Schuster Building
Rockefeller Center
1230 Avenue of the Americas
New York, New York 10020

SIMON AND SCHUSTER and colophon are registered trademarks of
Simon & Schuster, Inc.

Designed by Jennie Nichols

Manufactured in the United States of America

10 9 8 7 6 5 4 3 2 1

Library of Congress Cataloging in Publication Data

BT 16.45/9.41   3/85

Burstein, Nancy.
   The executive body.
   1. Exercise for women.   2. Women in the
professions—United States—Nutrition.
3. Stress (Psychology)—Prevention.   I. Title.
GV482.B87   1984   613.7'045   84-5507

ISBN-0-671-49437-6

613.7045
Burstein

Note:

Before starting any new exercise program, it is important that you consult your physician. This is a must if you have any serious medical conditions or if you are taking medication. Get your doctor's consent before you begin.

Photographs by Ron Contarsy
Drawings by Elaine Yabroudy

Acknowledgments:

Many thanks to the following individuals and organizations:

Jeffrey Weiss
Dan Green
Susan Victor
Deborah Bracken
Ron Contarsy
Cloverdale Press
Judith Phillips, Stress Management Consultants
Della Smith
The New York Heart Association
The American Heart Association
Metropolitan Life Insurance Company
Russell Fleischmann and Maureen Sullivan, International Paper Company's Health Fitness Center
Susan Dresner
Argonne National Laboratory

A special thank you to Jane Hughes Paulson for research and assistance.

Contents

Introduction

Fitness and health are two of the primary concerns of today's executive woman. Working women are becoming increasingly aware that without their good health, personal and professional goals cannot be accomplished. The Executive Body: A Working Woman's Guide to Life Style and Total Fitness was written to be a resource for today's woman. It is a guide for professionals and aspiring executives who want information and direction on making health their number one priority.

As a fitness professional I have designed exercise, stress management, and nutrition programs for thousands of working women. I recognize that it is not easy to find the time for exercise in schedules that are already jam-packed with myriad responsibilities. But learning how to incorporate fitness into a hectic life style can be the key to long-lasting energy, stamina, and health.

The Executive Body will provide you with the tools and resources to integrate exercise, stress management, and nutrition into your daily life, at the same time suggesting ways to make your life run more smoothly. The programs for getting in shape, coping with stress, and eating right are all designed to help you make the best use of the time you spend getting fit and staying fit. Even women with the busiest of schedules will find that they can make fitness "fit in."

As the director of Employee Fitness Enterprises, a consulting firm for corporate fitness programs, I personally experience the pressures and time constraints of today's profes-

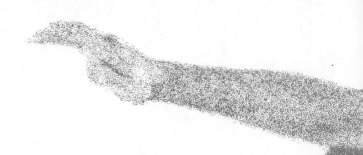

sional woman. I have found that the answer to coping with career and personal demands is to make certain that my health comes first. I believe the programs and techniques for achieving physical and mental well-being that work for me will be as helpful for you.

How to exercise? When to exercise? Where to exercise? These are the questions that The Executive Body will answer to help you make fitness a part of your life.

Exercise

More than ever, fitness is a concern of today's working woman. Frequently the concern centers on the lack of time available to exercise, the impact of exercise on weight control, or the problem of discipline. Attitudes toward fitness for women have changed dramatically in the last decade. Yet the problem of how to stay committed to a regimen and the importance of foresight in planning a program often are not even addressed. By not exercising, women—whose work styles (and life styles) place enormous limits on their time and energy—may find they are neglecting one of the most crucial elements in their climb to success.

You can learn how to coordinate fitness into your daily routine. When exercise becomes a natural part of your life, your body won't let you slack off, because not exercising means lethargy of the body and mind. Integrating fitness into your life style is one of the best ways of maintaining good health. Physical activity actually increases energy, and daily exercise can help ensure a body and spirit that are strong and resilient. When you have your health, your potential is unlimited!

Morning Fitness— From Bed to Bath to Getting Dressed

Getting up in the morning. It's the bane of much of the work force because there never seems to be enough time for everything that needs to be done—including sleep. The alarm goes off, there's the jump out of bed to silence the incessant ringing and the guilty feeling when you get back under the sheets for just a few more minutes of precious sleep. Finally, you push your tired body from the bed and move to the shower to banish the morning drowsiness. From that point on, it's business as usual. There's breakfast to make, dressing for work, perhaps family responsibilities, then the dash to beat the rush hour traffic. Wouldn't it be nice if you could ease yourself into the hectic morning routine by starting the day relaxed and energized?

There is a way to beat this A.M. shock. If you think you can't find the extra time to exercise before leaving for work, rest assured that this is not an ordinary exercise regimen. It does not require an exercise mat or equipment. It is not even necessary to change your clothes. It is a program of specially designed movements that are integrated into your early morning activity. This program is not time-consuming, nor does it require any special degree of ability.

The exercises ease your muscles into alertness with movements that increase circulation by bringing blood to the body's extremities. The movements loosen tight areas and help relieve stiffness in the neck, back, and shoulders. Many of the exercises are designed to be done in bed, so you can use those few minutes after the alarm goes off to wake up drowsy muscles and energize yourself.

It's important to understand that how you feel when you wake up correlates with the quality of your sleep. If you've had a fitful, restless night, then getting up in the morning will seem like punishment. You can help assure a good night's sleep by taking into consideration a number of factors before going to bed.

Regular Schedule

Try to establish a standard time for sleeping and waking. The body's internal clock is thrown off schedule when regular sleeping patterns are changed by more than about an hour.

Nighttime Exercise

Do not exercise vigorously before going to bed. Any dynamic exercise that increases the heart rate will energize the body and keep you awake long after you want to fall asleep.

Attitude

Going to bed feeling tense and perhaps guilty because you have left things undone will affect your ability to fall asleep. Consider sleep as a positive and normal part of life. Try to relax before bed with relaxation exercises, a warm bath, or some soothing music.

Food Consumption

Avoid eating late at night or your digestive system will be working while it and you should be at rest. You should also limit fluid intake before going to bed; otherwise you may be awakened by the need to urinate.

Temperature Control

Extreme temperatures will affect the quality of your sleep. If the room temperature is too warm or too cool you will sleep fitfully. Most people sleep better when the temperature is slightly on the cool side, around 65–68 degrees Fahrenheit.

Sound and Light

If you are sensitive to sounds (street noise, neighbors, air conditioners, etc.) or require complete darkness to sleep, then you need to make your room environment conducive to rest. Dark window shades can help cut out light, and thick draperies can muffle outside noise. Additionally, ear plugs and an eye mask will further shut out intrusive sounds and light.

Your Mattress

A good mattress is crucial to restful sleep. Ideally it should offer firm support with some resiliency. Sleeping on a bed that is too hard or too soft puts a strain on the muscles and can create back or neck problems.

Sleeping Position

The arrangement of your body while you sleep strongly influences how your muscles feel the next morning. Back problems are aggravated and new ones develop if the spine is arched during rest. The best position is on your side with hips and knees slightly bent. If you prefer sleeping on your back, place a pillow under the knees to prevent swayback. While sleeping on the stomach is not recommended, a pillow under the stomach will take some of the strain off the back.

MORNING FITNESS EXERCISES

The following exercises done daily will help you wake up from head to toe. They start in bed and keep you in motion as you head for the kitchen or bathroom. While beds do not really provide enough support for exercise, these movements overcome the problem. They are not calisthenics but slow, controlled motions that prepare the body for movement. They are also a good warm-up before any intensive exercise in the morning.

NOTE: Osteoarthritis, a degenerative joint disease, afflicts nearly everyone as part of the aging process. As a precautionary action to preserve mobility, the Arthritis Foundation recommends that joints should be exercised through their full range of motion daily. The morning fitness exercises focus considerably on joint mobility, and the series is a valuable preventive measure.

When you first wake up there's nothing better than a head-to-toe stretch to ease muscle stiffness. This initial stretch will also begin to increase blood circulation.

1. Lying on your back with knees bent, place arms over head (remove pillow for an unobstructed area) with elbows bent so there is no tension. The torso should be pressed slightly into the bed so there is no arch in the back. Exhale.
2. Inhale and stretch the body to its fullest length in 5 counts. The fingers and toes should be extended and reaching to their maximum. You may experience a tingling feeling in the hands and feet as circulation increases.
3. Relax muscles and return to initial position.

Repeat 4 times.

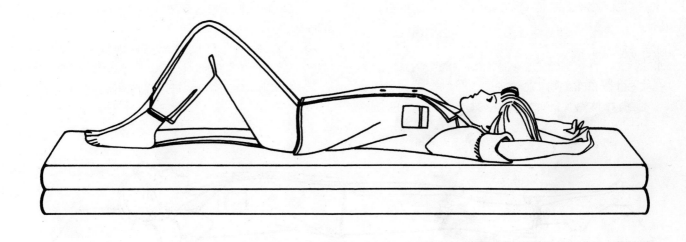

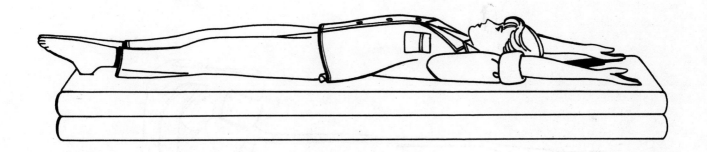

2. Neck and Shoulder Stretch

This gentle loosener for the neck and shoulders will release the tightness from these areas. It feels particularly good if you wake up with neck tension due to an awkward sleeping position.

1. Lying on your back, extend legs straight on bed but don't hold them stiffly. Place hands behind head with elbows open to the sides.

2. Bring elbows together, then lift the head and roll chin to the chest. The head should be lifted gently, not jerked, to prevent any strain on the neck. Hold position for count of 4.

3. Return head to bed by gently rolling back. Open elbows. Repeat several times until neck and shoulder muscles feel loose.

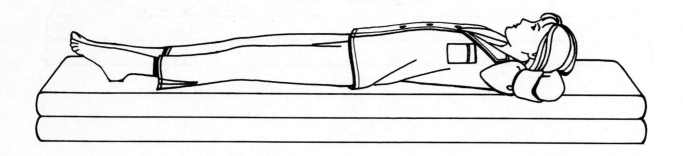

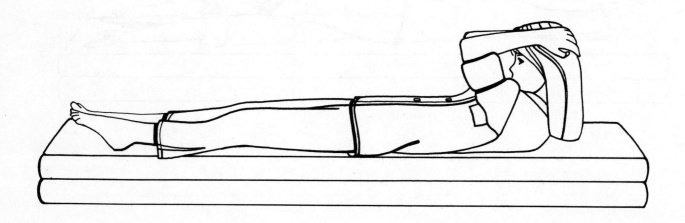

3. Spine Stretcher

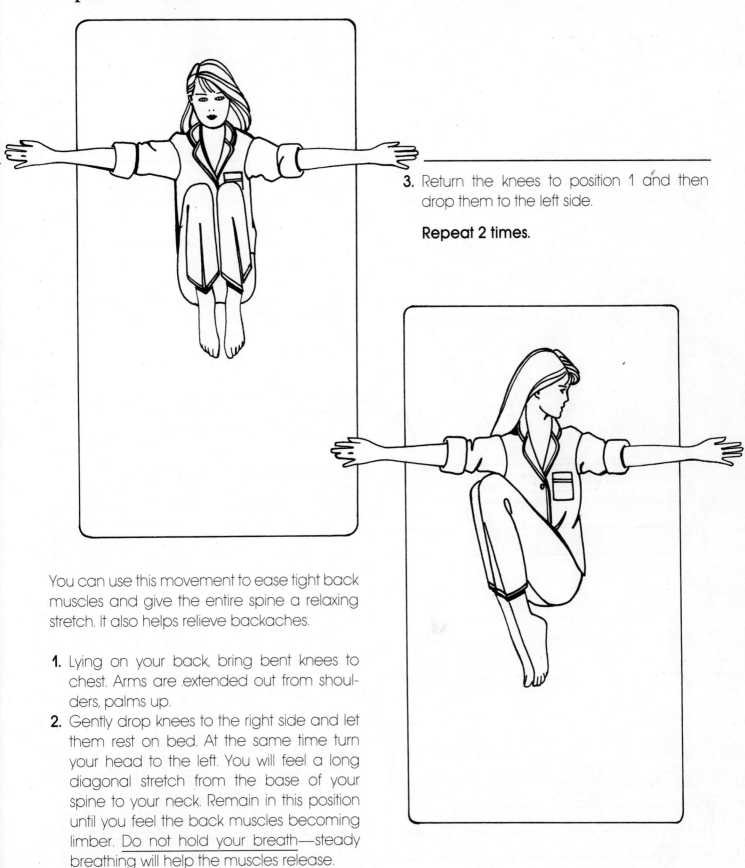

3. Return the knees to position 1 and then drop them to the left side.

Repeat 2 times.

You can use this movement to ease tight back muscles and give the entire spine a relaxing stretch. It also helps relieve backaches.

1. Lying on your back, bring bent knees to chest. Arms are extended out from shoulders, palms up.
2. Gently drop knees to the right side and let them rest on bed. At the same time turn your head to the left. You will feel a long diagonal stretch from the base of your spine to your neck. Remain in this position until you feel the back muscles becoming limber. Do not hold your breath—steady breathing will help the muscles release.

4. Hip Joint and Lower Back Warm-Up

This exercise increases mobility in the hip joints as it gently lengthens the lower back muscles.

1. Lying on your back, bend knees and place feet about 6 inches from buttocks.
2. Clasp right knee with both hands and bring it to your chest. Hold for a count of 8.
3. Slide the left leg out so it is extended straight on the bed and continue to hold the right knee for another count of 8.
4. Release the right knee and place the right foot on the bed. Slide the left foot toward you and bring the left knee to the chest. Repeat the exercise with the left leg.

Repeat 2 times.

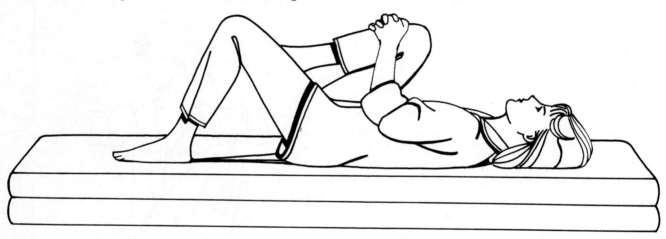

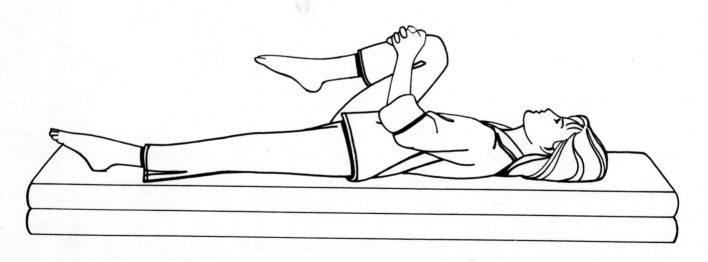

5. Spine Curl-Up and Body Stretcher

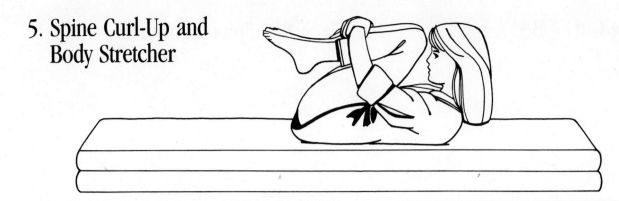

This multipurpose movement provides benefits to the back, arms, and legs, and it also strengthens the abdominal muscles.

1. Lying on your back with arms at sides, use the stomach muscles to bring bent knees up to chest.
2. Wrap arms around knees, drop chin to the chest, and curl head toward the knees. If you are very flexible, your forehead may be able to touch your knees.
3. Return your head to the bed and extend arms and legs to the ceiling. With up-stretched limbs, rotate the ankles and hands inward and outward.
4. Return to position 2.
5. Relax body by extending legs on the bed and placing arms at sides.

Repeat 3 times.

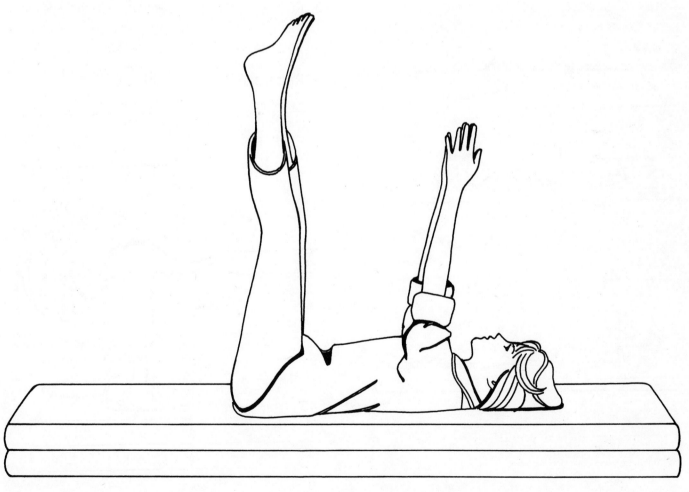

6. Getting Out of Bed

7. Seated Spine Loosener

There are many ways of rising from a bed, but most of them put a great deal of strain on the back. When you use the lower back and neck to sit up, enormous pressure is placed on those areas. You can avoid back problems and easily get up with these three movements.

1. With knees bent slightly, face the edge of the bed.
2. Place the hand of your top arm in front of you on the bed and use it to push yourself up to a seated position. The other hand can also give you support to help raise the torso.
3. Swing your legs over the bed and you're seated and ready to go!

You can stretch the muscles around the vertebrae from the base of the head to the tailbone with this exercise.

1. Sitting on the edge of the bed, place hands behind head with elbows open to the sides.
2. Bring elbows together, drop chin to chest, and roll down the spine (articulating each vertebra until you reach the tailbone). Let head rest on knees. Hold for count of 6.
3. Reverse and roll up, starting at the base of the spine. The chin stays on the chest until you are completely uncurled.

Repeat 3 times.

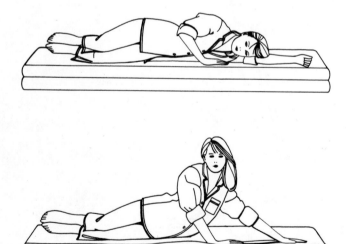

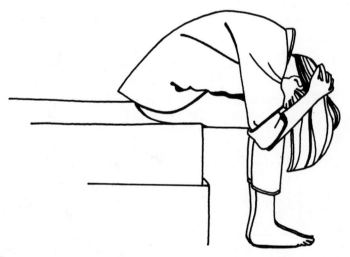

8. Standing Torso Stretch

You can head for the bathroom or kitchen and still keep your body working to get out any leftover kinks or tension.

1. Standing, wrap arms around chest as if you are grabbing the material of a T-shirt.
2. Pretend you are taking off the T-shirt. Arms are wrapped around the body and they lift

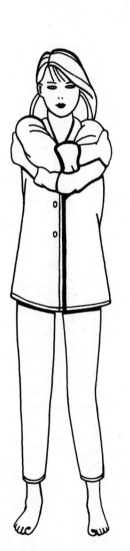
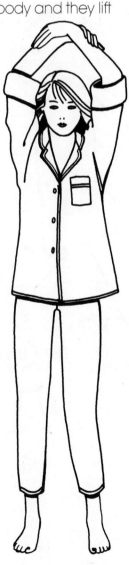
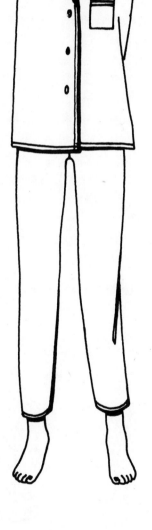

above the shoulders and head. Stretch the arms above the head.
3. Lower arms to your sides.

Repeat 4 times.

9. Calf Muscle Toner

Making double use of your time is the beauty of this toning exercise. As you brush your teeth at the bathroom sink, you can lean your weight against the sink rim to stretch tight calf muscles.

1. With toothbrush in one hand, place the other hand on the sink rim. Legs are in an open lunge position. The left knee is bent and the right leg is extended back with the heel slightly lifted. Toes are pointing forward.
2. Pressing into the hand, let your torso move slightly forward as you stretch the calf muscle by lowering the right heel to the floor. Hold for 6 seconds.
3. Reverse and extend left leg back.

Repeat 3 to 6 times until muscles feel limber.

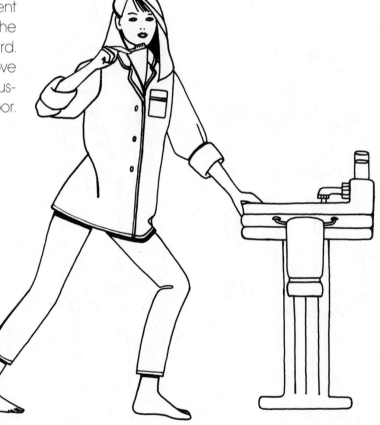

CHAPTER TWO

Intensive Conditioning for At-Home Workouts

This is your guide to a thorough program of exercise that can get the most sedentary body back into shape. It is a no-nonsense plan that focuses on toning specific body areas and improving cardiovascular functioning. You can select portions of the program that are most pertinent to your problems or perform the entire exercise series for total conditioning. This is a program specially designed for the working woman with a focus on counteracting the physical effects of sedentary work styles and incorporating an understanding of busy schedules and time constraints.

The exercise plan is divided into nine sections—five specific body areas/muscle groups plus a warm-up, flexibility exercises, cardiovascular conditioning, and a cool-down. Any exercise session should be preceded by a warm-up to prepare the muscles for movement. After that you can define the extent of your workout according to the time you have available.

The program is streamlined in its approach to achieving strong and supple muscles through efficient muscle action. Each of the muscle group sections contains six specialized exercises to shape up that particular body area. The first four exercises in each section are progressively more challenging. This prevents undue strain on the muscles and gives you graduated control over more difficult exercises. Two advanced exercises are also included in each section. These movements can be included in your workout as you become more accomplished in executing the initial exercises, have additional time for a more comprehensive session, or require more concentrated work on a particular area.

Women who have not exercised regularly throughout their lives may think they are too old to begin or not in "good enough" shape to even consider dressing in workout clothes. Exercise knows no boundaries in terms of age or body shape. Each woman owes it to herself to be the best she can be, and that "best" includes physical conditioning. It is never too late to start a program of exercise. In fact, the determination with which you approach fitness also translates into your attitudes toward achieving career and personal goals.

If you have not exercised in weeks, months, even years, be patient and exercise moderately at first. Muscles, bones, and joints need to be eased into movement. Be prepared to start slowly and restrain yourself from overdoing initially. Women over fifty who have not exercised actively throughout their lives are particularly encouraged to initiate an exercise program to help counteract the bone-thinning condition known as osteoporosis, common in postmenopausal women. Studies have indicated that exercise and nutritional supplements can prevent this condition.

Exercising at home is more convenient for most working women since it eliminates the problems of adjusting personal schedules to exercise class schedules and transportation. You have the option of exercising before work, after work, in the evening, or whatever time suits you.

If you hesitate about exercising because you feel too tired after work or think that too much physical activity in the morning will be exhausting, remember, exercise does not rob you of vitality or make you lethargic. The interesting thing about exercise is that the more energy you expend, the better you feel and the more energy you have. Not only does it improve your muscle tone and body shape, but in addition it changes your state of mind.

For example, if you tend to refrain from exercise after work because you are too tired, you may be mistaking mental fatigue for physical fatigue. Eight to ten hours filled with pressure and deadlines takes a toll on anyone. Do not confuse the strain you feel in your mind with your physical state. Exercise can "clear your mind" by focusing your attention on another activity. Through exercise your powers of mental concentration are used to facilitate muscle action and coordination. You simply cannot think about work when you are trying to execute a demanding exercise routine.

In terms of exercise routines, how do you know how much is enough? "If twenty sit-ups are good, then two hundred must be even better" is fallacious, and possibly dangerous, reasoning. Continued repetitions of an exercise can actually cause injury after a certain point; the muscles can become strained if a particular motion is repeated over and over. With most calisthenic exercises a maximum of twenty-five to fifty repetitions is recommended. Beyond these maximums most people become bored, which leads to inattention, which can also lead to injury.

Any exercise should be done carefully, paying attention to proper execution. This is especially true of calisthenics. It's more prudent to move slowly to make certain you are activating the appropriate muscle groups and working correctly to prevent injury. While calisthenics may be done at a fast pace, the question of speed applies more significantly to aerobic activities that require a rapid and sustained pace for maximum benefits.

What Is Fitness?

Physical fitness is defined as the ability to live life fully and vigorously with muscular, skeletal, and cardiovascular reserves that provide resiliency, strength, and stamina. The sedentary work style of today's executive woman does not promote and in fact diminishes physical resources. Physical activity and specialized exercise can offset the effects of a desk job and give you energy, endurance, and a strong, toned body.

The criteria for general fitness are muscular strength, joint and muscle flexibility, cardiovascular stamina, and proper body alignment. All elements are necessary for total fitness. This means that even though some individuals may be naturally gifted with one factor, flexibility for example, they are not totally fit unless muscle strength, endurance, and alignment are developed. Every person has different strengths and weaknesses, and the purpose of a total fitness program is to balance all the elements.

While many of us know when our bodies are out of shape (a full-length mirror tells no lies), we often learn more about our physical weaknesses when we are unable to do a particular physical task. If you cannot lift an average-size suitcase, race for the bus without getting out of breath, or participate in sports activities without straining muscles, then your body is telling you that it is less than totally fit.

The Executive Body's Intensive Conditioning Program will not only help you attain and maintain a satisfying fitness level, it will also enhance your self-image as you work toward a toned and trimmed body.

Getting Ready for the Shape-Up

Motivation and discipline are the keys to success in both fitness and the workplace. You can ensure results when you work out regularly with enthusiasm and intent. Here are some guidelines to help make your program the most rewarding, enjoyable, and energizing.

1. Consult with your physician before participating in this program or any new exercise regimen.
2. At-home exercising does offer lots of scheduling flexibility, but it is helpful to plan a definite time when you will work out. A specific time provides a structure and psychological readiness. This is not to say that you cannot stray from the scheduled time,

but initially it is a motivational tool and an aid to commitment. Also, select an area for exercising that is well ventilated, light, and pleasant.

3. Before exercising, always wait at least one and a half hours after eating. Too much food or liquid in the digestive tract can make you feel uncomfortable or nauseated, or can cause cramping. It's best to exercise before a meal if you are on a weight-reducing plan because the activity will reduce your appetite. (During exercise the stomach's blood supply is reduced, which makes you lose the desire for food.)

4. Use a mat or rug to cushion the body for exercises done on the floor, particularly those performed on the back. If you feel any discomfort fold a small hand towel and place it under sensitive areas.

5. Dress comfortably in nonrestrictive clothing that permits freedom of movement. Jewelry and eyeglasses should be removed.

6. Add music while you exercise, because a steady rhythm can help your body move with greater ease. A slow musical selection will provide a soothing, relaxing state of mind that is particularly conducive for flexibility stretches and cool-downs.

7. Muscle stiffness is likely to occur if you have not exercised recently, but don't let this deter your resolve to continue the program. A warm bath will ease muscle aches, and additional flexibility movements will help decrease stiffness. Muscle soreness is an indication that you are activating muscles that have not been used. This is a positive sign that your exercise efforts will increase flexibility and strength.

8. As you do the exercises, concentrate on the instructions to ensure proper body alignment. You want to execute the movements without creating tension in other body areas. Remember to breathe deeply and evenly. Holding your breath causes muscular tension, decreasing efficiency of motion and inhibiting flexibility.

9. Be patient with yourself. Flaccid muscles don't become firm overnight and marathon endurance is not developed instantly. Progressive challenges and steady progress are the best route to increasing your general fitness.

10. If you feel pain during the course of any exercise, stop immediately. Reread the instructions to make sure you are doing the exercise correctly and proceed slowly and carefully. If the discomfort persists, discontinue the movement for the present time.

WARMING UP

Warming up is a necessary part of any exercise session because it prepares the body for movement and reduces the possibility of injury to muscles and joints. A good warm-up readies you for exercise by increasing your circulation, which literally "warms" the muscles and raises body temperature slightly. Warm muscles are more pliable and respond to stretching and strengthening exercises more easily than "cold" muscles, which resist movement. A warm-up also increases joint flexibility and mobility by moving limbs and other body parts through a range of motion. This is important to help prevent ligament strains and joint inflammation.

The warm-up conditions the body so you can move freely and adapt to the movements of particular exercises without strain. Take a tip from professional athletes and dancers, who make warming up the foundation of their training. They always prepare the body for motion with a series of exercises that gradually prepare the muscles for more demanding movement.

The following warm-ups can be done in approximately five minutes. If your muscles are feeling particularly tight, you may want to spend more time by increasing the suggested repetitions. Don't be tempted to skip the few minutes it takes to warm up or you could find yourself sidelined with needless aches and pains. In addition, the warm-up alone is a great reviver if you are feeling tired and need an energy booster.

1. Two-Minute Jog

An easy run (keep it stationary if space is limited) for 1½ to 2 minutes is the most efficient way to increase circulation throughout the body. The jogging makes your heart work harder, and more blood and oxygen are circulated to the body's extremities. Make sure you bend your elbows and pump them back and forth while running.

2. Body Tension Releasers

Shake each arm and leg vigorously for 5 seconds. This helps tight muscles to "let go" and loosens stiff joints. You can also shake the head and torso while bending over from the waist.

3. Neck Relaxer

You should feel the neck muscles releasing and lengthening with this exercise.

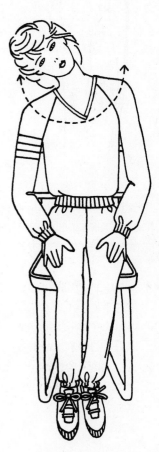

1. Make a half-circle with the head by first tilting it to the right as though you are listening to your shoulder with your ear.
2. Roll the head to the left, dropping the chin to the chest, then completing the half-circle.
3. Return the head to an upright position.

Repeat 4 times. Then reverse, starting to the left side.

4. Shoulder and Arm Rotations

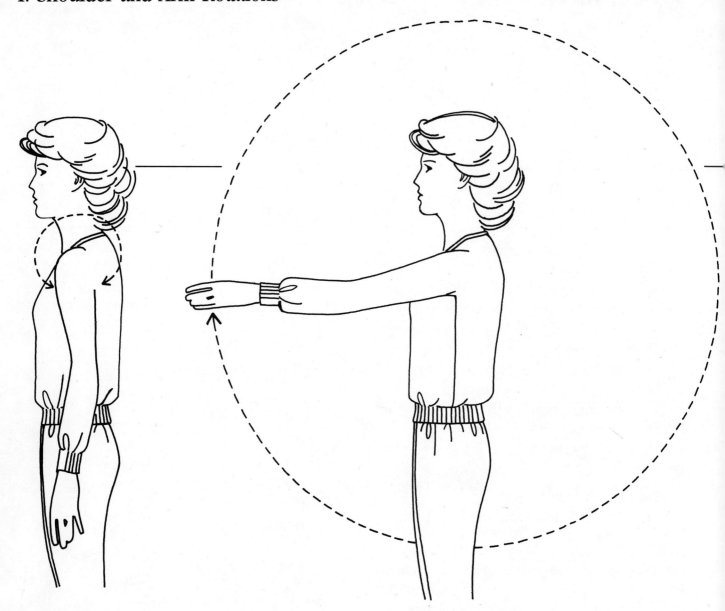

The following motions will increase mobility in the shoulder socket and warm up the muscles surrounding the joint.

1. Standing, with arms hanging at sides, imagine that you are drawing a circle with your right shoulder. Push the shoulder forward, lift it up, and pull it back. Repeat 4 times.
2. Reverse the circle by pushing the shoulder back first, then lifting it and finally bringing it forward to complete the rotation. Make 4 rotations.

3. Using the entire arm, imagine this time that you are drawing a circle in space. Stretch the arm forward, lift it to the ceiling, then extend it behind you and complete the circle. Repeat 4 times.
4. Reverse the circle by extending the arm behind you, up to the ceiling, and forward. Make 4 rotations.

Repeat on the left side.

5. Torso and Back Stretch

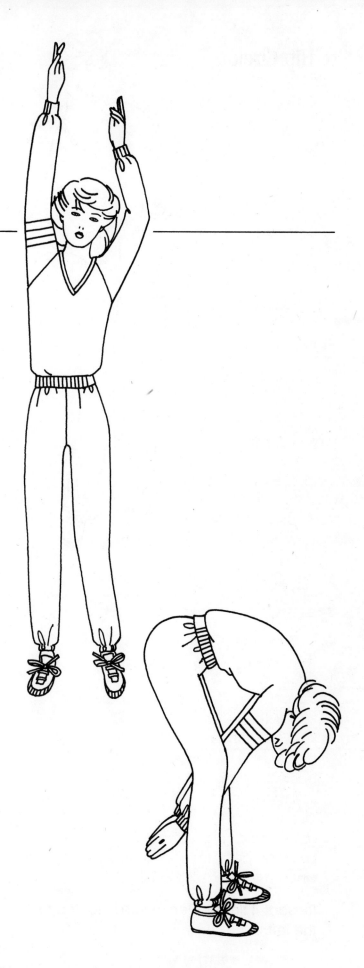

You can warm up the midsection of the body and relieve tight back muscles with these two movements.

1. Standing with legs about shoulder-width apart, stretch arms above the head.

2. As though you are climbing a ladder, reach the right arm for a ladder rung and then the left arm for a higher rung. Stretch arms 8 times. With each reach you should feel a lengthening in the torso.

3. Bend the knees slightly, drop the torso over the legs, and gently reach the arms through the legs, holding this position for a count of 8.

Start the exercise again with the reaches and repeat 4 times.

6. Hip Circle

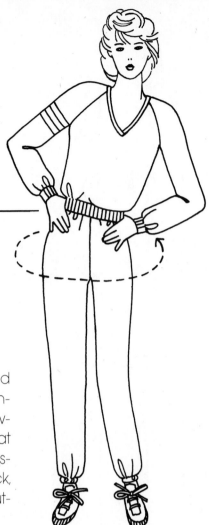

ABDOMINAL MUSCLES

The waist, pelvis, and hip joints are involved in the following movements that loosen tense muscles in the back, stomach, and buttocks.

1. Standing with legs about hip-width apart, bend the knees slightly and place hands on waist.
2. Keeping the stomach lifted, begin to make a circle by pushing the right hip to the right side.
3. Continuing the circle, push the pelvis slightly forward.
4. Push the left hip to the left side and finish the circle by letting the hips release to the back. This causes a slight arch in the back, so it is important to keep the stomach muscles working to prevent any strain. (If you have a back problem, don't finish the circle by going back. Instead move the hips side, forward, side; side, forward, side.)

Repeat 4 times. Then reverse, starting to the left.

The stomach area is a point of vanity for many women, and if only for appearance's sake there is great motivation for toning the abdominal muscles. Beyond the visual results, strong stomach muscles are crucial for a healthy back. Weak abdominals and their effect on posture are a factor in lower back pain. A regular program of exercise that focuses on strengthening the stomach muscles is an important measure in preventing back problems.

Abdominal muscles that are flaccid and weak cause the stomach to protrude, resulting in what is commonly referred to as a "pot belly." The extended belly offers no support for the back, causing it to hyperextend, which places enormous strain on the lower spine. When the posture is improved by strengthening the abdominals and lengthening the shortened back muscles, there is almost instantaneous relief for the back. The support provided by the stronger stomach muscles also helps to counteract the effects of sitting at a desk for hours each day.

In the quest for an attractive figure, women have been influenced by fashion magazines that present a lithe, flat-stomached model as the ideal. Most women are not built like models, and the completely flat abdomen is not only an impossible pursuit for many but an undesirable one as well. A slight roundness to the stomach is natural because of the reproductive organs that are located in the abdominal area. Exercise can improve your appearance, tone the muscles, and make your stomach flatter to a degree, but it's important to recognize that a feminine curve is normal and does not mean that you are not exercising rigorously enough.

Abdominal exercises must be done correctly or muscle bulk develops. You can gain strength and tone without bulk if you do the exercises slowly and methodically, not simply rushing through them in an effort to get it over with as quickly as possible. For the best results you want to concentrate on using gradual muscle contraction instead of momentum to work the body. Remembering to breathe steadily is especially important.

The following series of exercises provides a thorough conditioning of the abdominal muscles. In addition to strengthening the rectus abdominis (the long vertical muscle that is activated in the familiar sit-up), there are movements that involve the internal obliques and external obliques (cross diagonal muscles) and the transversus abdominus (horizontal muscle fibers). These form a natural girdle for the body. All four muscle groups must be used for a complete conditioning.

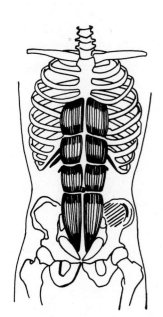

Rectus Abdominis

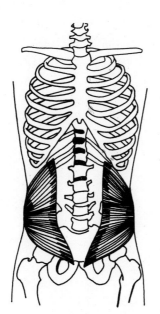

Internal Oblique

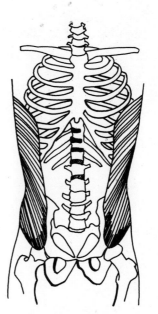

External Oblique

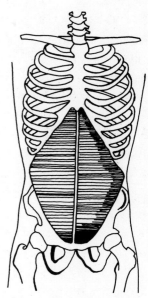

Transversus Abdominis

Pelvic Tilt

NOTE: Pregnant women frequently experience lower back pain resulting from the pressure on the lower spine created by the increasing weight of the fetus. Developing the strength of the abdominal muscles can significantly ease the back discomfort of a pregnancy weight gain. These exercises can be performed by the expectant mother, but she should get her physician's approval before starting any fitness program during pregnancy.

As you do the abdominal exercises, include a movement between the exercises to stretch the spine and relax the abdominals. The pelvic tilt releases and lengthens the muscles of the stomach and is excellent for the back. Alternate one or two repetitions of the pelvic tilt after you do each of the abdominal exercises that follow.

1. Lying on your back with arms at sides, bend knees and place feet about 12 inches from buttocks. Knees and feet should be hip-width apart.

2. Exhale and tilt the pelvis up. Roll up the spine by first lifting the lower back, then the middle back, and finally the upper back. The shoulders remain on the floor.

3. Roll down the spine and articulate each vertebra by first lowering the upper back, then the middle back, and finally the lower back. Let the pelvis release and relax on the floor.

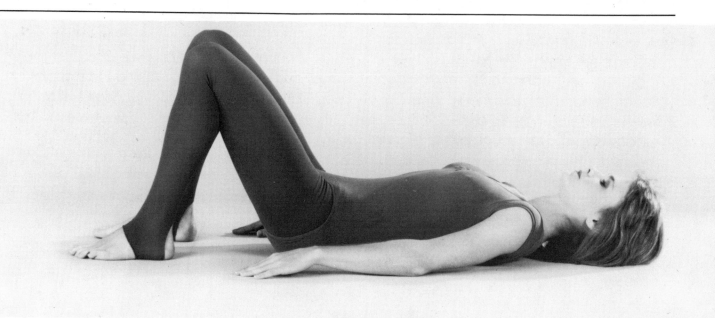

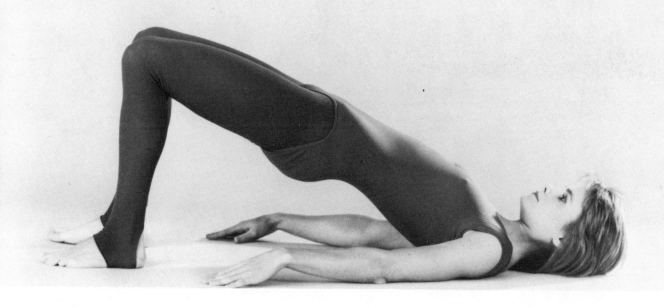

ABDOMINALS

1. Abdominal Toner

Repetitions: 3, working up to 6

1. Lying on your back with arms at sides and knees bent, bring chin to chest, and lift shoulders and upper back off the floor. Reach hands alongside knees.
2. With arms straight and hands fisted, beat first downward 20 times. The pressure of the "beats" forces you to use the abdominal muscles to hold the body steady. Slowly inhale and exhale twice during the beating motions (inhale on 5 beats, exhale on 5 beats, etc.)
3. Relax the arms and return the body to the floor.

Once you bring the chin to the chest, concentrate on activating the stomach muscles immediately by pulling the muscles in toward the spine. Try to imagine that the muscles are creating a flow of energy that is directed lengthwise up through the rib cage and into the chest. This will help prevent you from gripping the muscles and causing them to build bulk.

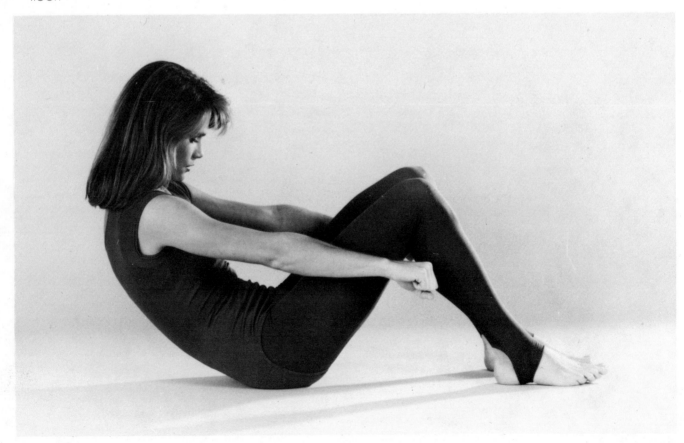

2. Diagonal Stomach Strengthener

Repetitions: 4 to each side, working up to
10 to each side

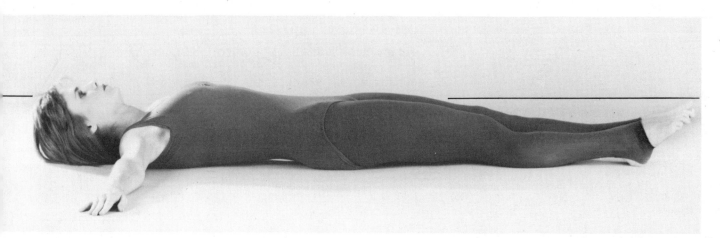

1. Lying on your back, stretch legs and extend arms out from shoulders. Inhale.
2. Exhaling, bend right knee (slide foot on floor) and lift torso. As you lift the torso, the left arm crosses your chest and reaches for your right knee.
3. Inhale and return torso and arm to floor.

4. Repeat to opposite side by bending left knee and reaching with the right arm.

Concentrate on exhaling as you raise the torso. The exhalation helps you to "scoop out" and flatten the entire abdominal area.

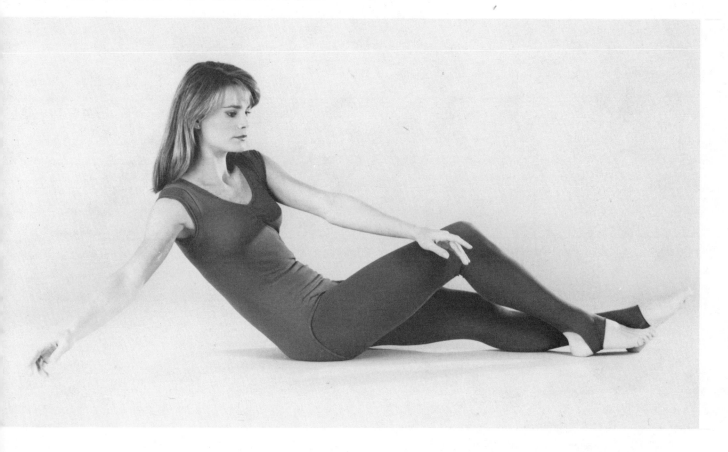

3. Roll-Down

Repetitions: 3, working up to 8

1. Sitting, bend knees and place feet flat on the floor. Spine should be straight.
2. Drop chin to chest and roll halfway down to the floor, curving the spine. Shoulders should be curved forward, completing a "C" shape formed by the torso. Lift arms toward knees. Hold position for 10 seconds.
3. Return to initial position by using the stomach muscles to initiate your movement. The roll-up starts at the base of the spine and works its way up through the back until the spine is perpendicular to the floor.

As you roll down, it will feel as though you are pulling the abdominal muscles into the spine. This reversed sit-up isolates the abdominal muscles and prevents you from using the hip flexors that do most of the work in a regular sit-up.

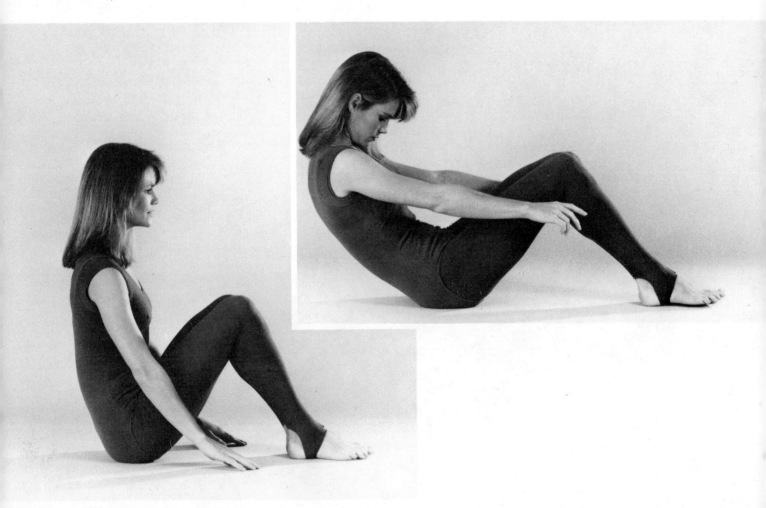

4. The Bicycle

Repetitions: 10 on each side, working up to 20

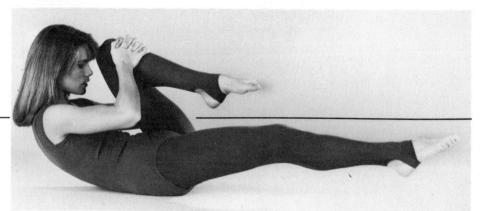

1. Lying on your back with legs extended, lift right leg about 4 inches off floor. Raise shoulders, clasp hands around left knee, and bring forehead toward knee.
2. Change legs (they move simultaneously) by bringing right knee to chest as left leg extends straight. The extended leg does not touch the floor at any time during the exercise.

   Be sure that the forehead, not the chin, is trying to touch the bent knee. If the chin is thrust forward instead of resting on the chest, tension develops in the back of the neck.

   If you need a physical reminder to hold the stomach in, place hands on abdomen instead of clasping knees.

   After completing the repetitions, continue the exercise with a variation that involves the external and internal obliques.

3. Lying on your back with legs extended, lift right leg about 4 inches off floor. Place hands behind head and raise shoulders. Bend left knee into chest and twist the body slightly to touch right elbow to left knee.
4. Change legs (right knee bends into chest as left leg extends straight) and touch left elbow to right knee.

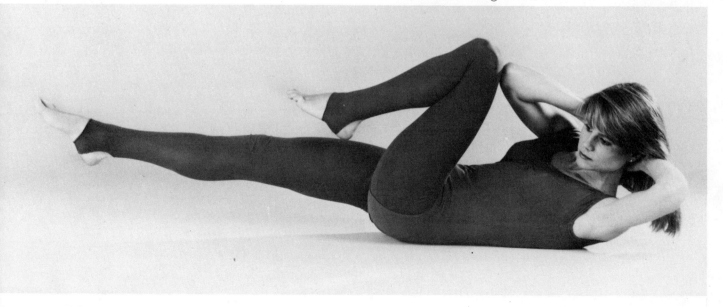

ADVANCED ABDOMINALS
5. The "Reacher"

Repetitions: 3, working up to 6

1. Lying on your back, bend knees to chest.
2. Extend legs to ceiling.
3. Open legs to a V-shape, then raise torso, and reach arms through legs.
4. As though you are pulling on a rope, reach with the left arm and then the right arm for 8 pulls.
5. Bring legs together, bend knees, and hug them to your chest.
6. Place feet on floor, then lower torso and head to floor. Relax.

Keep abdominals activated throughout the exercise, particularly when the arms are reaching through the legs.

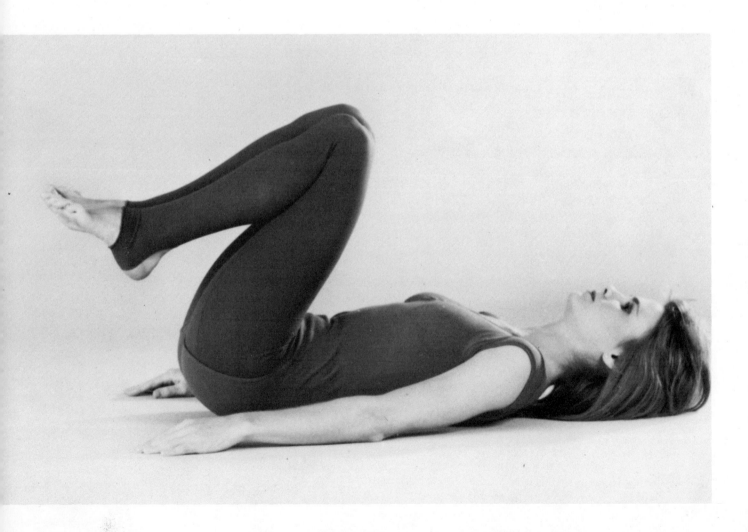

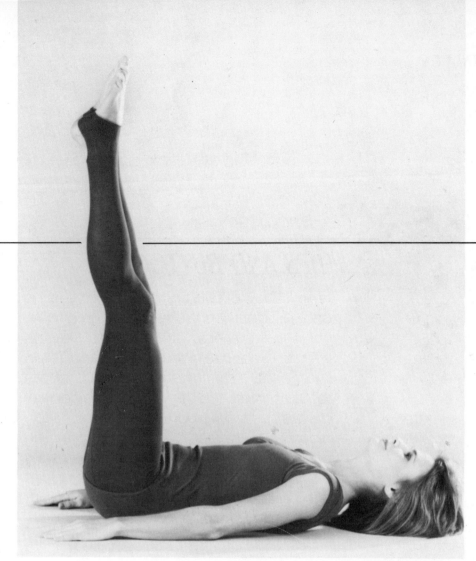

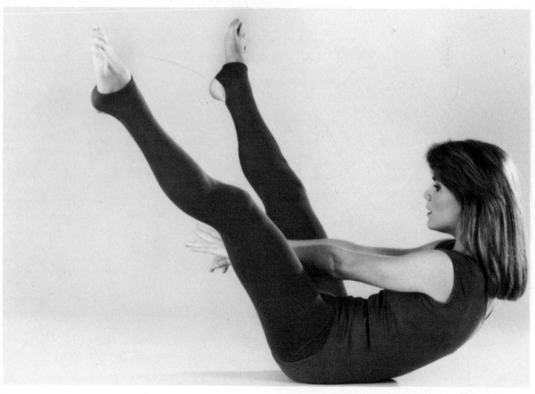

6. Raised Leg Sit-Up

Repetitions: 5 to each side, working up to 10

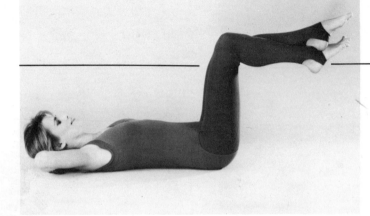

1. Lying on your back, bend knees, lift calves parallel to the floor, and cross ankles. Place hands behind head. Inhale.
2. Exhaling, raise the torso and touch the left elbow to right knee.
3. Return torso to floor.
4. Continue exercise by alternating sides.

HIPS AND BUTTOCKS

Sitting all day takes its toll. Most women see the tangible effects of a sedentary job in a figure that is bottom-heavy. The hips and buttocks seem to expand relentlessly, and panic sets in when once loose-fitting skirts and pants become uncomfortably tight across the derriere. The desk-bound woman does not have to forfeit figure or career, because exercise can tone and firm the hip and buttock muscles and provide a sleeker, trimmer appearance.

The gluteus maximus is the large, fleshy muscle that forms much of the buttocks. When the gluteus maximus and the muscles that lie un-

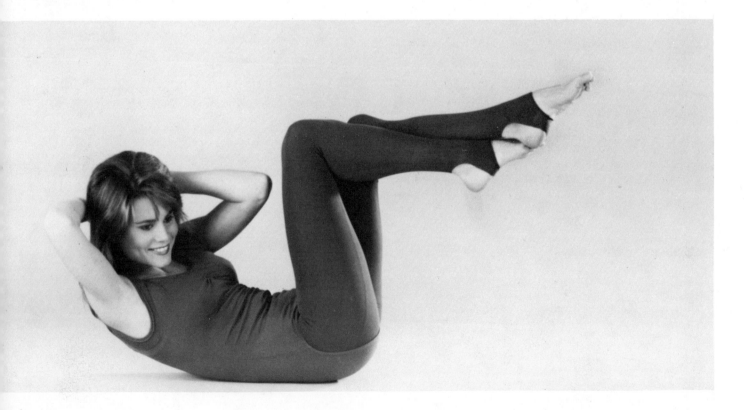

derneath it (the gluteus medius and gluteus minimus) are not used regularly they become flaccid, creating the "fanny spread" experienced by many inactive women. The key to counteracting the loss of tone in the gluteals is through movement. The exercises in this section specifically engage muscle groups that shape the hips and buttocks and will give you a smoother, firmer appearance.

In addition to the exercises there are two preventive measures you can include in your daily routine: (1) walk as much as possible, and (2) sit correctly. Walking activates the hip and buttock muscles and tones them naturally. It is important to get out of your chair and move around every hour or so. The activity lifts the buttock muscles and improves circulation, as well as generally making you feel better physically and mentally.

Just as important as walking is knowing how to sit correctly. All too often there is a tendency to slump slightly, causing body weight to compress the muscles surrounding the lower spine and the gluteals. This not only contributes to fanny spread but will exacerbate any back problems.

When you sit, the weight of your torso should be evenly distributed on the ischia, the bones that form the base of the pelvis. To find the ischia, sit and place your hands underneath the buttocks. You will feel a protuberance under each buttock. If you are sitting properly, the ischia are perpendicular to your chair and prevent the gluteals from taking the strain of the trunk's weight.

1. Lying on your back with arms at sides, bend knees and place feet about 8 inches from buttocks. Feet and knees are hip-width apart.
2. Exhaling, proceed to do a pelvic tilt (see p. 32) by lifting the lower back, middle back, and upper back.
3. Remaining in the tilted position, tighten the buttocks and lift and lower the heels 8 times. Keep the toes relaxed and on the floor.
4. Roll down the spine and relax.

The torso should be held stationary as you lift and lower the heels. Do not let it bob up and down.

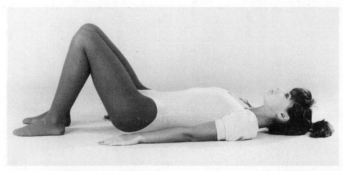

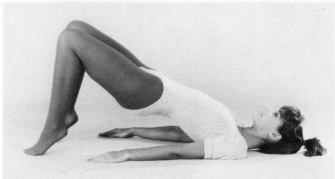

2. Hip Trimmer

Repetitions: 8 to each side, working up to 15

1. Lying on your back, bring knees to chest and extend arms out from shoulders.
2. Keeping the knees together, lower them to the right side.
3. Extend the legs straight, parallel to right arm.
4. Bend knees to position 2.
5. Return the knees to the chest and repeat to left side.

As you drop the knees from side to side and extend them, try to keep the shoulders stationary. Do not let one shoulder lift off the floor as the knees lower to the opposite side.

This exercise is also good for the waist and stomach. Make sure you pull the stomach in and activate the abdominals as you return the knees to the chest (position 5).

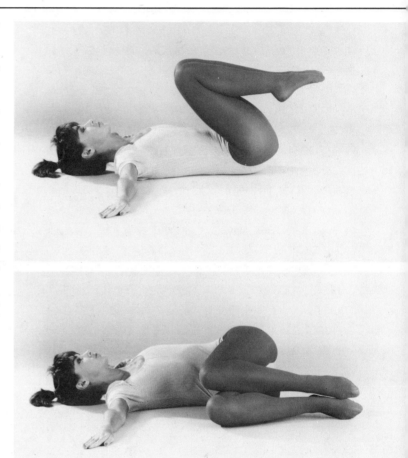

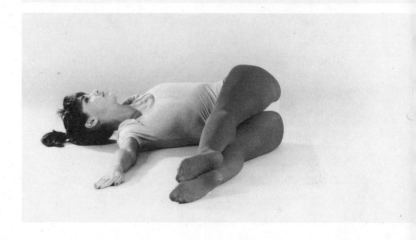

3. The Triangle

Repetitions: 4 sets on each leg, working up to 8

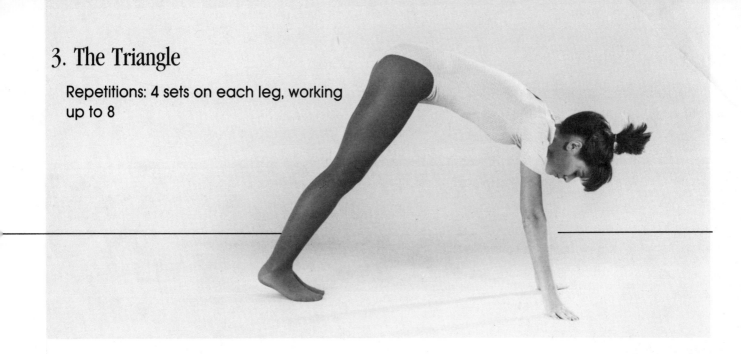

1. Make a triangle with the body by placing the hands and feet on the floor and lifting the hips.

2. Extend the right leg in the air (the leg is slightly rotated outward) and flex the foot. Tighten the right buttock and gently pulse the leg up 8 times.

3. Lower the leg and repeat exercise on the left.

While lifting either leg, keep the head and neck relaxed by directing your focus toward the floor.

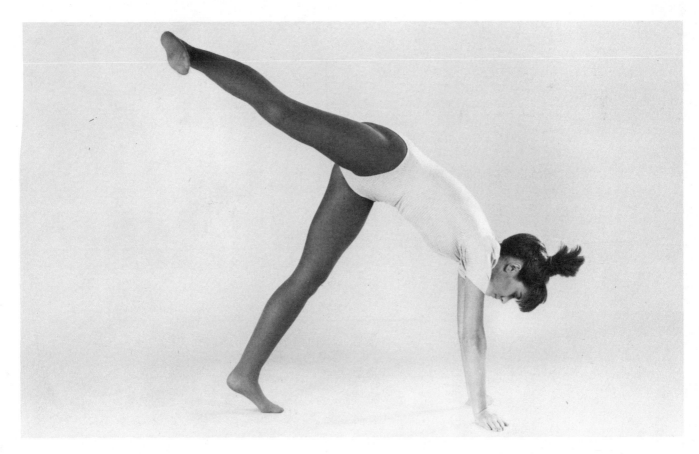

4. Fanny Firmer

Repetitions: 3 on each side, working up to 6

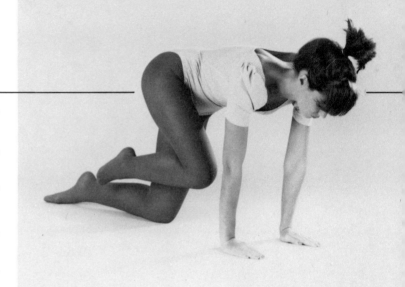

1. On hands and knees, bring right knee to chest.
2. Extend the right leg to the side, parallel to the floor.
3. Make 6 small circles forward with the right leg, initiating the movement from the hip.
4. Reverse the circles and make 6 rotations backward.
5. Bend the right knee to the chest and place knee on floor. Repeat exercise on left leg.

Form and body alignment are important in executing this exercise correctly. When one leg is extended to the side do not let the body weight sink into the opposite hip. The stomach should be lifted to support the back, and the spine should be one long line from the tailbone to the head, as in photo 2.

Between repetitions you can stretch the hip and buttock muscles by sitting back on the heels and extending the arms forward.

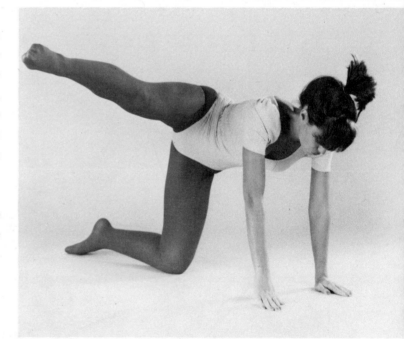

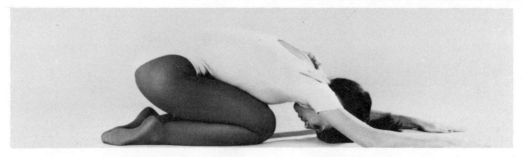

ADVANCED HIPS AND BUTTOCKS

5. Leg Extension

Repetitions: 5 to each side, working up to 10

1. Sitting, bring the soles of feet together to form a diamond shape with the legs. Hands are placed on the floor for support.
2. Keeping your hands on the floor, fold the right knee over to touch the left knee.
3. Extend the right leg straight to the side about 3 inches from floor. Hold for count of 4.
4. Bend right knee to touch left knee.
5. Open right knee to right side to original diamond position. Repeat to left side with left leg.

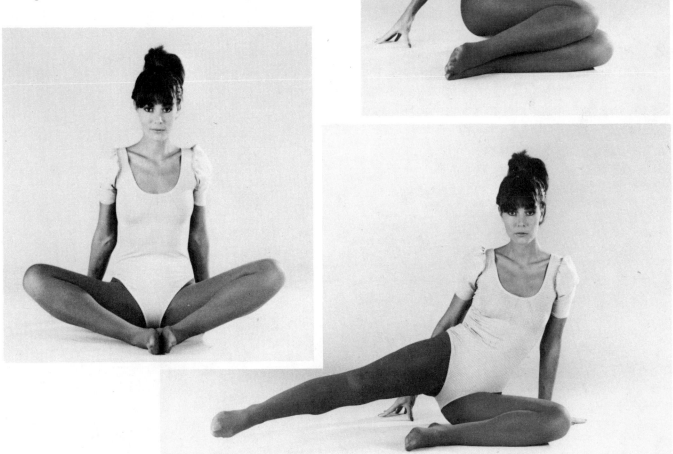

6. The Shaper

Repetitions: 5 sets on each side, working up to 10

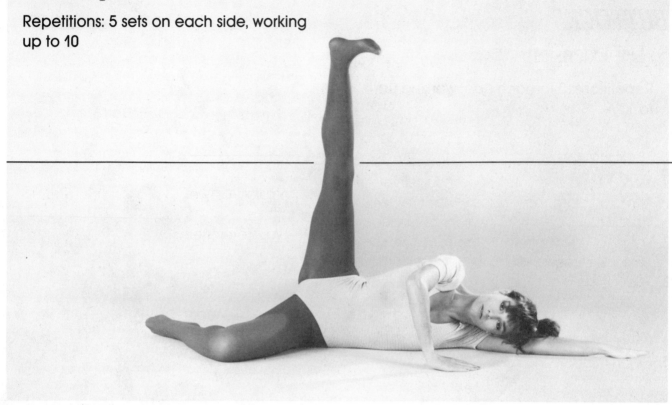

1. Lying on your side, bend bottom leg. Extend top leg straight up and flex the foot.
2. Lower top leg in front of bent leg and gently pulse top leg downward 6 times. The toes of the flexed foot should be pointed toward the floor for maximum results.
3. Lift top leg to original position.
4. Bend top leg to relax the muscles. Repeat exercise, then change sides.

As you lie on your side do not let your body weight sink into the supporting elbow and shoulder. Lift the chest and rib cage and keep the stomach muscles working throughout the exercise for control.

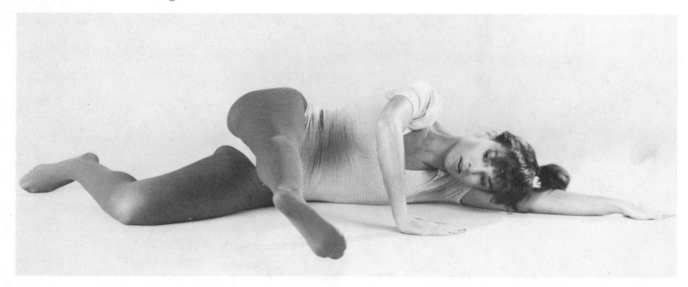

WAIST

How often do you bend, twist, or stretch during the course of a day? If infrequently, then chances are your waist is not as trim as it could be. But don't despair. Of all the body areas, the waist responds to movement most quickly. Specific exercises for the midsection can zoom in on a thick waist and tighten slack muscles.

Like the stomach, the appearance of the waist is strongly affected by posture. Slouching creates the look of thickness in the torso and can make even the most fit body appear unshapely. As you stand, it is important to lift the rib cage out of the waist. Do not mistake raising the shoulders for improving posture. The support starts with the abdominals and continues with the rib cage lifted high and the shoulders resting squarely and comfortably without tension on top of the trunk. This elongates the torso, making your waist appear trimmer immediately as well as giving you a confident, commanding stature.

Waist exercises primarily involve stretching and twisting movements that tone flaccid muscles and prevent sagging midriffs. In addition to the exercises that follow, it also helps to make a concentrated effort to include stretching and bending movements during the workday. A little extra twist when you reach for materials on your desk or stretching the arm a bit higher after replacing books on a shelf will complement your at-home conditioning program.

As you do the exercises, be patient if your torso feels tight. The motions should be done slowly to give the muscles time to stretch. If you feel any discomfort or strain, make the movement smaller. You can increase the range of motion as your muscles become stronger and more flexible.

1. Waist Stretch

Repetitions: 8 to each side, working up to 15

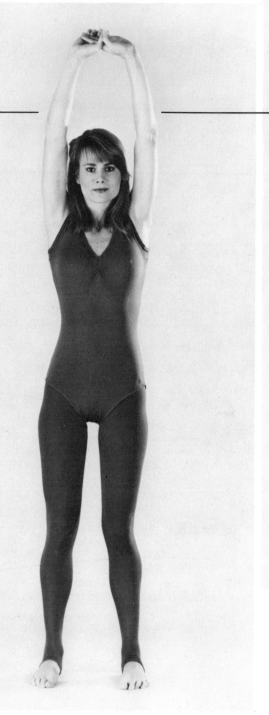

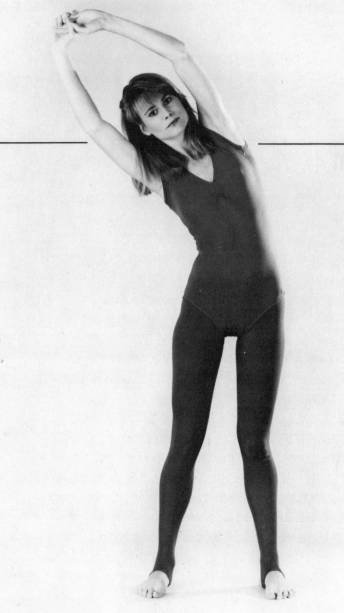

3. Reach the arms up and over to the right side, making an arc with the body. Hold for 5 seconds.
4. Return arms to center and relax by letting elbows bend (position 1). Then repeat to left side.

Remember to keep the stomach lifted to support the back. If you feel any strain in the lower back, move the arms slightly forward when you stretch to either side.

1. Standing with legs hip-width apart, clasp hands above head. Elbows are relaxed and slightly bent.
2. Lifting rib cage out of the waist, stretch arms high.

2. Knee Drop

Repetitions: 20 to each side, working up to 35

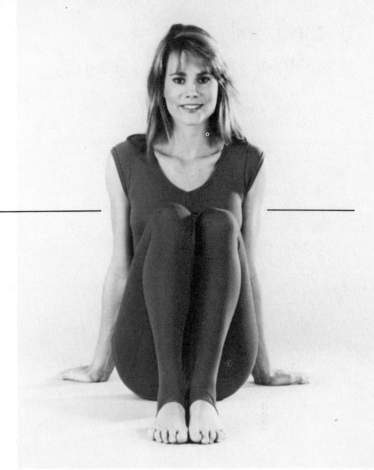

1. Sitting, bend knees and place feet flat on floor. Hands are next to the buttocks helping to support the body.
2. Drop knees to right side, looking to your left to accentuate the twist in the torso.
3. Return knees and head to center.
4. Alternate sides and continue exercise by dropping knees to the left and turning head to the right.

If you feel no discomfort, a brisk tempo is recommended for the knee drops. Each movement gets one count, so the rhythm is <u>drop, center, drop, center</u> to the count 1, 2, 3, 4, etc.

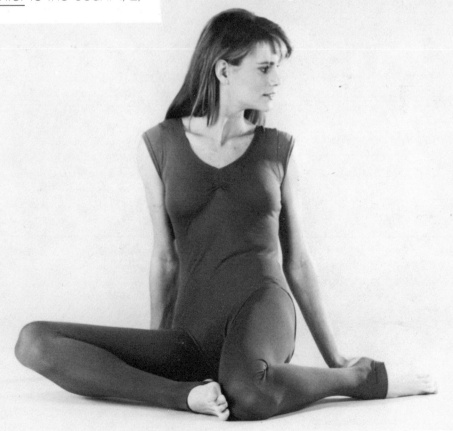

3. Torso Circle

Repetitions: 6 to each side, working up to 12

1. Sitting cross-legged, stretch right arm up and over head to the left side. The left hand is placed on the floor to support the body.
2. Circling the right arm forward, bring it in front of the body as you drop the head and torso toward the floor. The left arm now extends forward as well.
3. Continuing the circle, the torso arcs to the right as the left arm reaches to the right side and stretches over the head. The right hand rests on the floor.
4. Complete the repetitions and then reverse the circles by stretching the left arm over the head to the right side.

The abdominals are working throughout the exercise, especially when the torso drops forward (position 2).

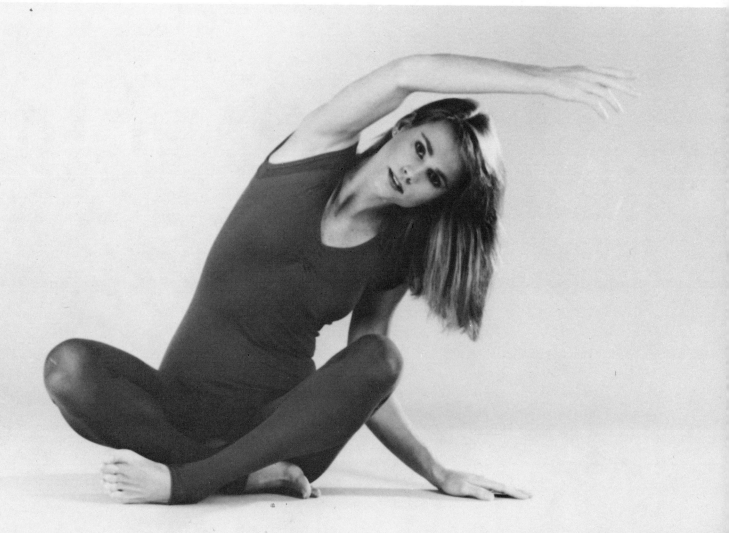

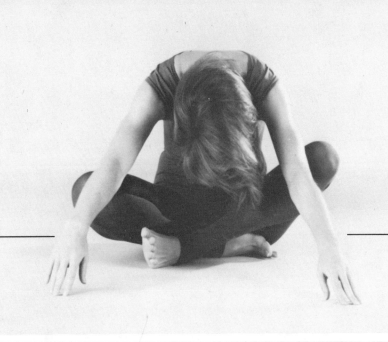

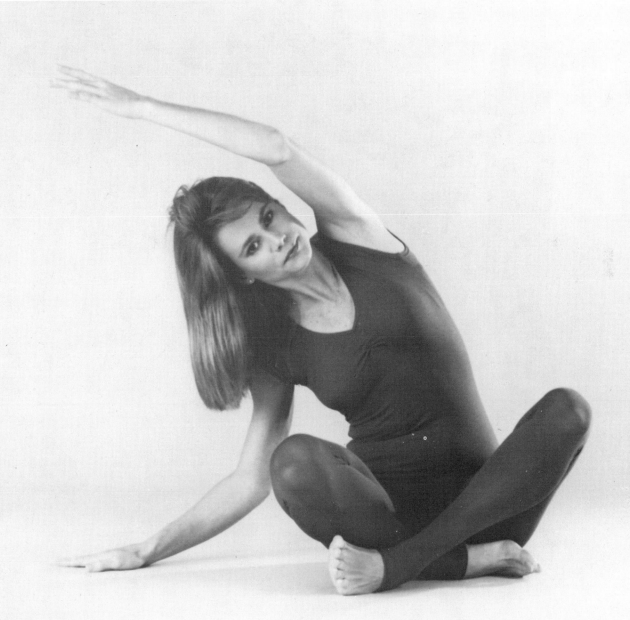

4. The Windmill

Repetitions: 20 to each side, working up to 35

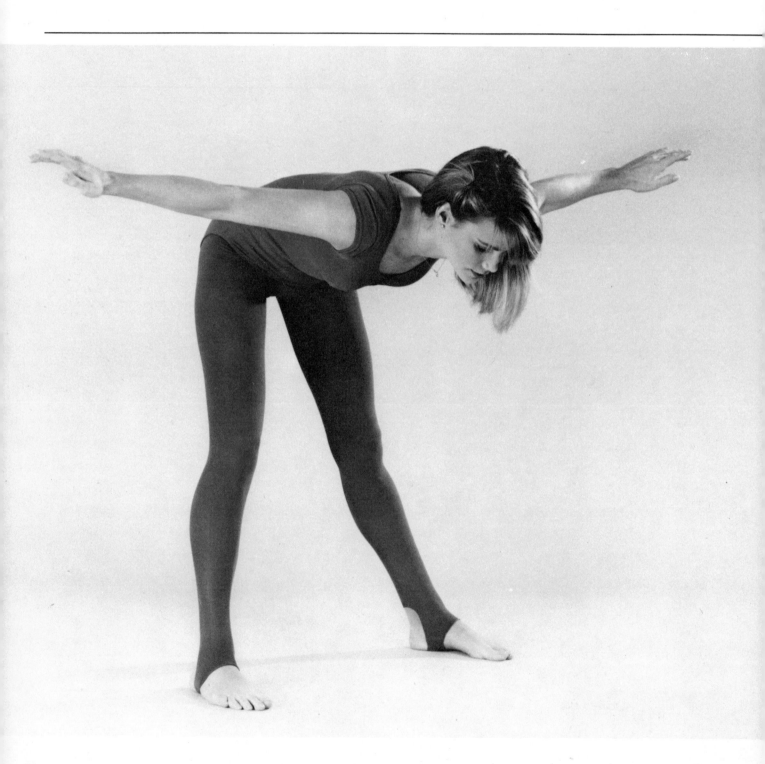

1. Standing with legs shoulder-width apart, bend the torso forward so it is parallel to the floor. Arms are stretched out straight from the shoulders. Bend the knees slightly to prevent strain on the back.
2. Twist to the right and touch right foot with left hand.
3. Twist to the left and touch left foot with right hand.

When the knees are bent it is important that each knee is centered over each foot. Do not let the knees roll in.

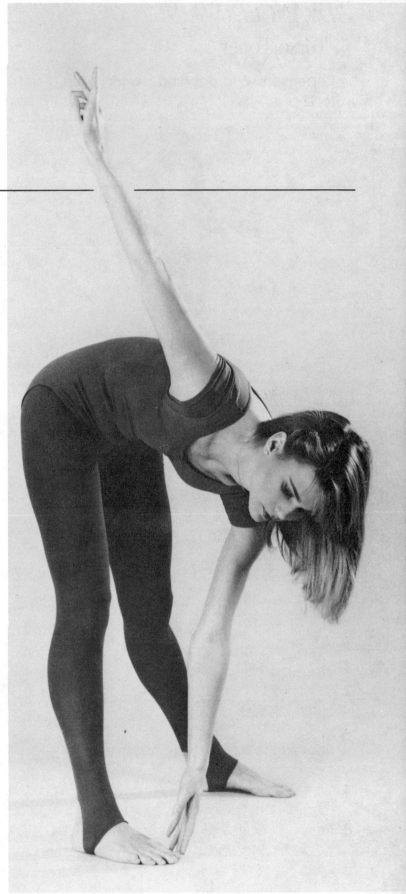

ADVANCED WAIST
5. Torso Toner

Repetitions: 6 to each side, working up
to 12

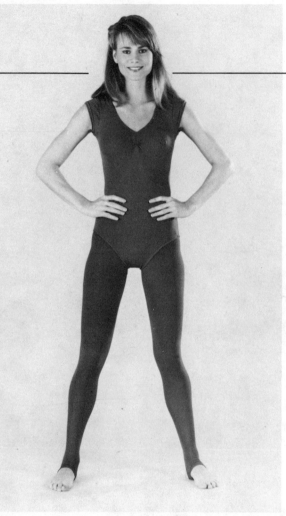

To achieve the maximum torso stretch to the side and front diagonal, imagine that your fingertips are being pulled by an invisible force to help extend the body farther into space.

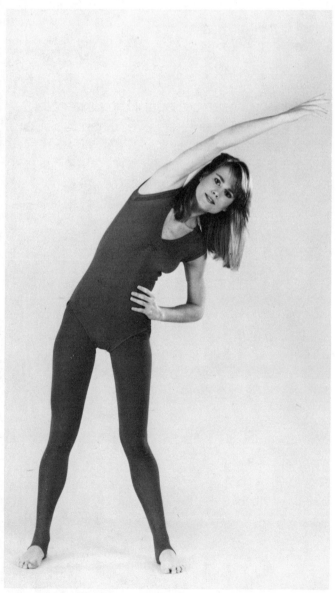

1. Stand with legs shoulder-width apart and place hands at waist.
2. Stretch right arm up over head and bend to the left side.
3. Bend the torso forward and reach with the right arm to the left diagonal, flattening the back parallel to the floor,
4. Lift the torso up, return to position 2, and then stretch the right arm a bit farther.
5. Return to position 1 and continue exercise by alternating sides.

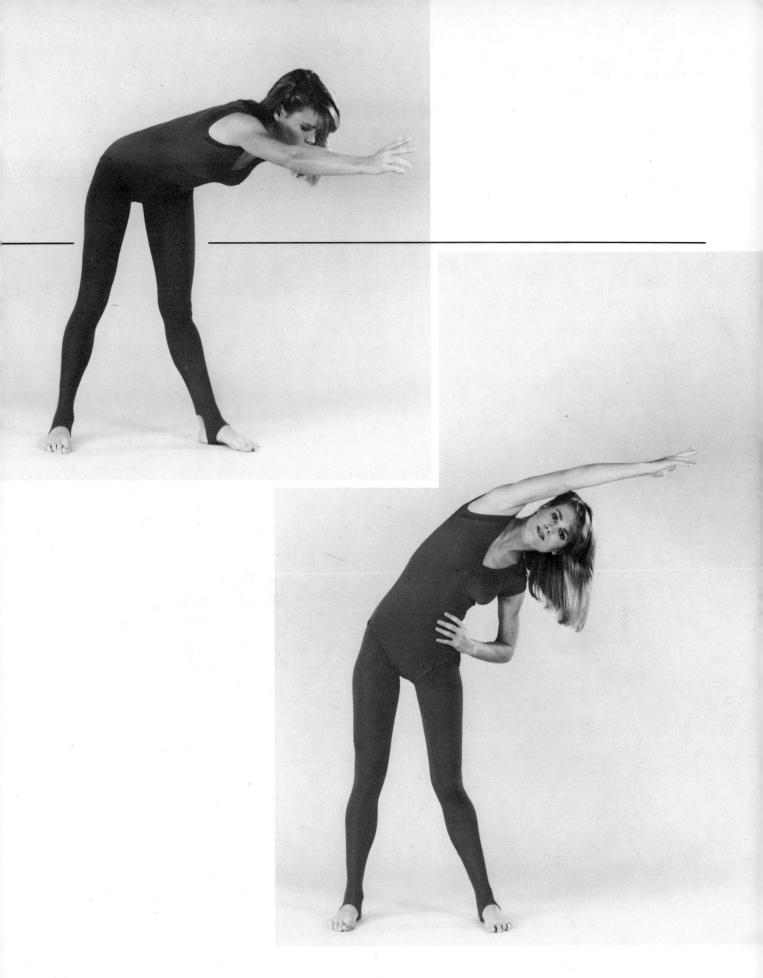

6. Waist Cross

Repetitions: 6 to each side, working up to 12

1. Lying on your back, stretch legs and extend arms from shoulders.
2. Bend right knee to chest, then extend right leg straight up.
3. Cross right leg over torso toward left hand as you turn head to the right.
4. Raise leg again as in position 2 and return head to center. Bend right knee and extend leg on floor to starting position.

5. Alternate sides and continue exercise with left leg.

As the leg crosses over the body, keep both shoulders on the floor to get maximum twist in the waist.

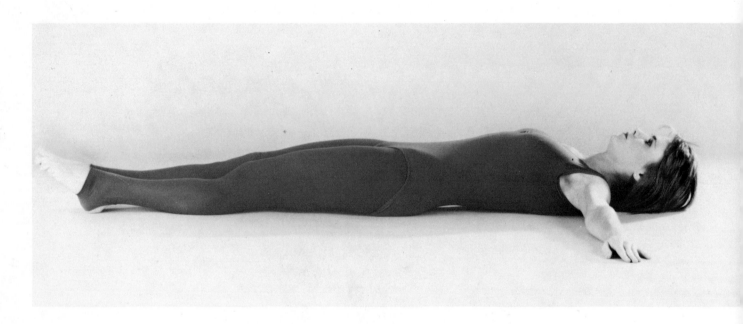

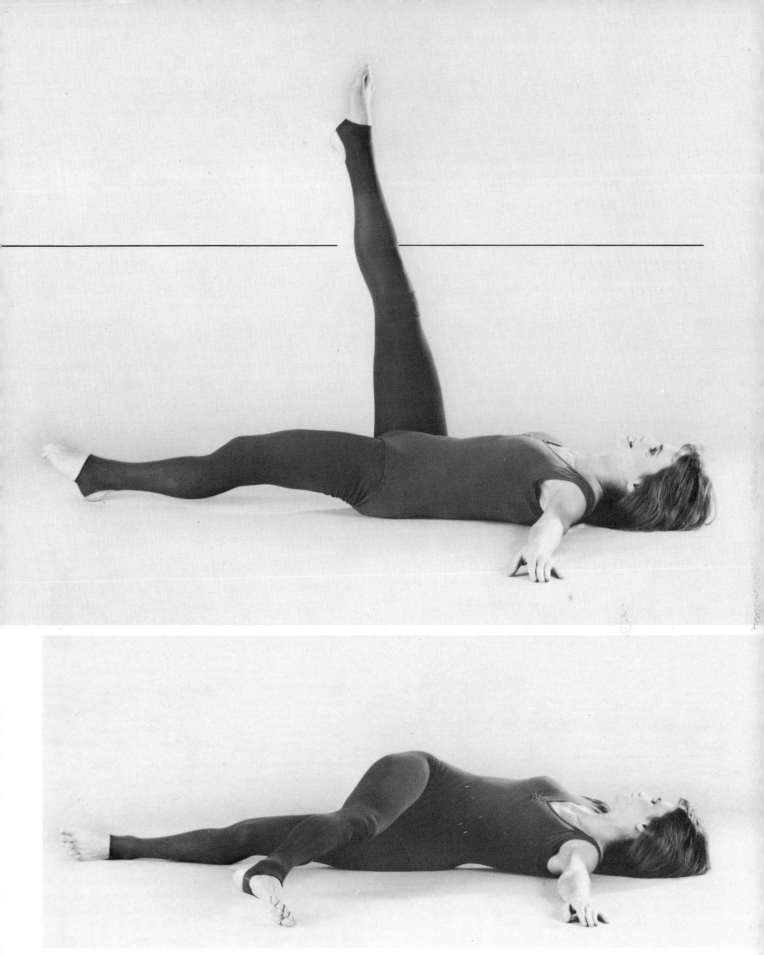

UPPER ARMS

Flabby upper arms are a problem experienced by many women who are inactive, and it's a disconcerting figure flaw for several reasons: (1) it usually reflects a lack of strength in the upper body, (2) it affects the appearance of the bust, and (3) it is a sign of aging. Exercise and body weight are two major factors affecting a woman's physical appearance. But while total body shape is influenced by one's weight, weight loss is not the only answer for improving the upper arms. In fact, exercise is critical for the biceps and triceps. A substantial weight loss without exercise will leave the upper arms with sagging tissues and unattractive loose skin. The exercises in this section will strengthen and tone the upper arms. In addition to developing the biceps and triceps, movements for the deltoids (shoulder muscles) and pectorals are included to increase overall strength for the upper torso. Exercising these muscle groups will result in more shapely upper arms and defined shoulders, and in improved support for the breasts.

To progress with the program, weights should be used for specific exercises. Added weight provides resistance to challenge the muscles and makes them work harder. While many of the myths surrounding the use of weights by women have been dispelled, it is important to reiterate that a woman will not develop the bulk associated with male body builders. Testosterone, the hormone responsible for creating muscle bulk, is predominant in the male body, and females lack adequate amounts of the hormone to create such dramatic physical changes in their bodies. Essentially, weights help tone and firm a woman's muscles and create smooth definitions of the muscle groups.

Three- to five-pound free weights (also called dumbbells) and/or weighted wrist cuffs are the only equipment needed for the following exercises. These can be purchased inexpensively from most athletic supply stores. You can also create your own weights from ordinary household items such as soup cans. Just make sure that you are using equal poundage in each hand to prevent any muscle imbalance.

NOTE: Exercises with weights should be done every other day. This enables the body to rebuild muscle tissue that breaks down as part of the training, which is a natural part of the strengthening process.

1. Shoulder Warm-Up

Repetitions: 3 sets of 6

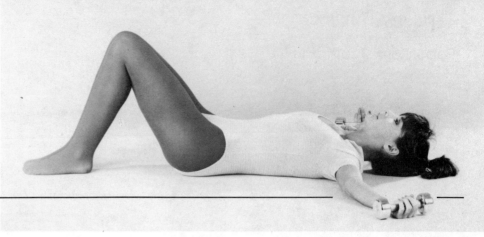

1. Lying on your back, bend knees and stretch arms straight out from shoulders. Hands are fisted or holding weights with palms facing ceiling.
2. Raise arms slowly until they are perpendicular to floor and parallel to each other.
3. Lower arms to floor slowly and with control.

4. Bend arms at elbows and bring fists toward chest.
5. Open elbows and return arms to floor.

Each repetition should be done slowly, remembering to exhale at points of exertion (positions 2 and 4).

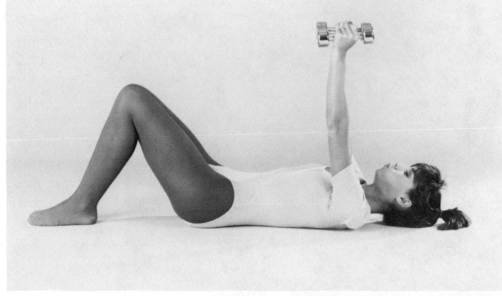

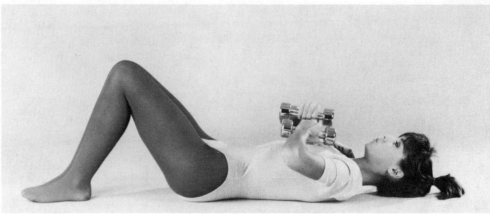

2. Triceps Toner

Repetitions: 3 sets of 10

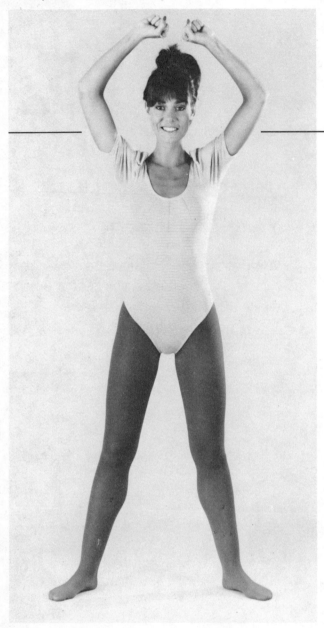

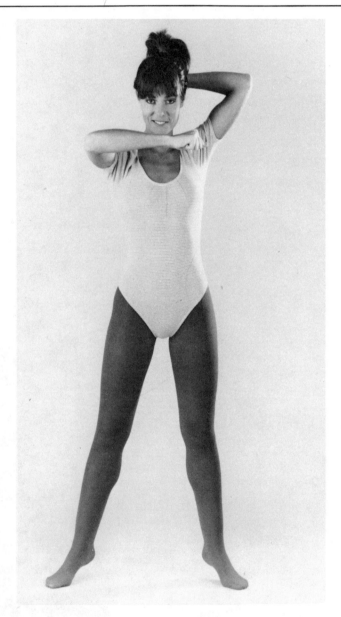

1. Standing with feet shoulder-width apart, bend elbows above head to form a diamond shape. Fist hands.

2. Bring right forearm in front of face as left forearm lowers behind head.

3. Continue by raising arms to starting position and then bring left forearm in front as right forearm lowers behind head. You have just completed one repetition.

Free weights or wrist cuffs can be used to provide greater muscle resistance. When using weights, this exercise is done at a slow, controlled pace. Without weights the movements can be done more briskly.

3. Pectoral Strengthener

Repetitions: 3 sets of 10

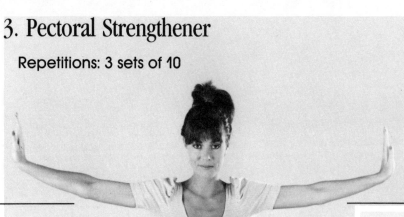

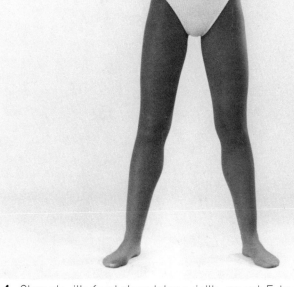

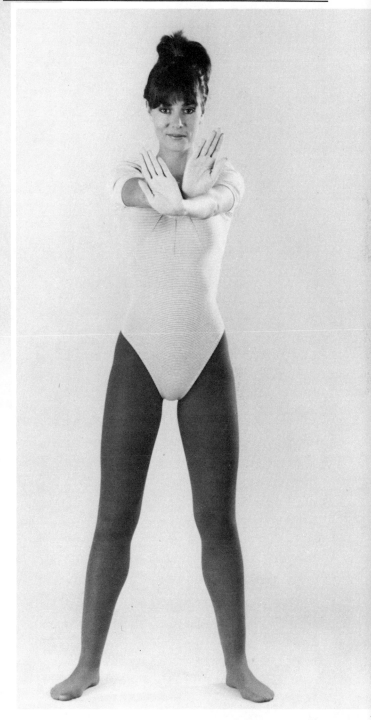

1. Stand with feet shoulder-width apart. Extend arms straight out to the sides at shoulder level and flex hands.

2. Keeping hands flexed, bring arms in front of chest and cross right wrist over left wrist.

3. Cross left wrist over right wrist.

4. Open arms to position 1. You have just completed one repetition.

If you are not holding weights, this exercise can be done at a brisk tempo to a rhythm that is counted <u>one</u> (cross wrists) <u>and</u> (cross wrists) <u>two</u> (open arms). Take it a bit slower and with more control if you are using weights.

4. Biceps Builder

Repetitions: 3 sets of 8

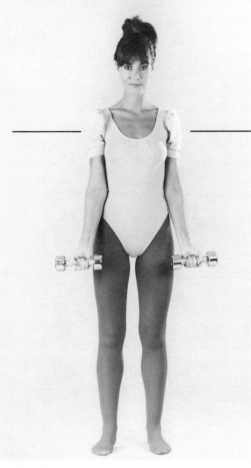

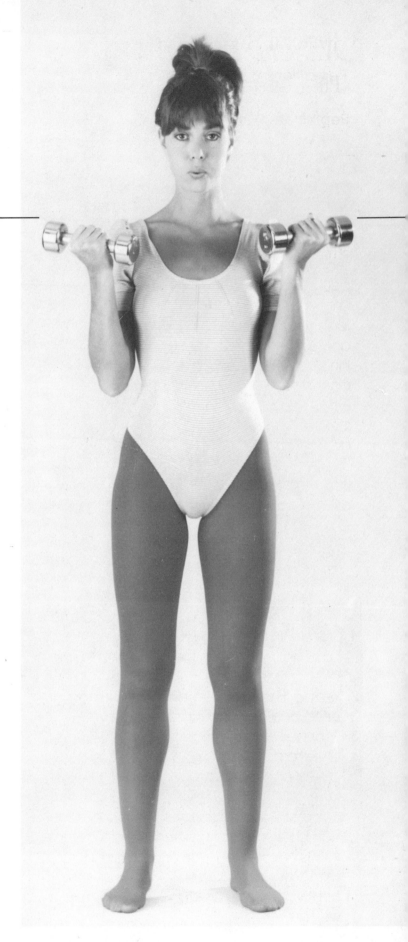

1. Grasp a dumbbell in each hand, stand with feet apart and arms extended downward in front of your body. Inhale.
2. Exhaling, bend elbows and curl hands to shoulders.
3. As you inhale, slowly extend arms down to starting position.

Do 2 sets moving both arms together and 1 set alternating arms.

Keep back straight and elbows against sides of body as you bend and extend arms.

This exercise is best done with free weights. Use dumbbells or soup cans.

ADVANCED UPPER ARMS
5. Push-Up

Repetitions: 6, working up to 15

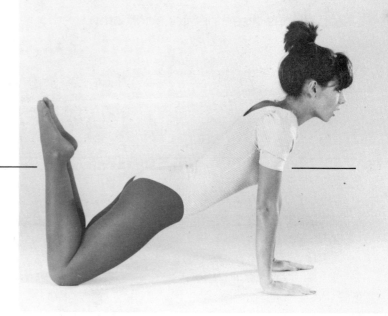

1. Lying face down, place hands on floor at shoulders and bend knees. Exhaling, press palms into the floor and push yourself up until arms are straight. Your head, neck, torso, and hips should form a 45-degree angle to the floor.
2. Inhaling, bend elbows and slowly lower the body until the chest touches the floor.
3. Exhale and press into the palms, pushing the body up to the 45-degree position again.

Body alignment is particularly important in push-ups to guarantee that the chest and arm muscles are being used properly. The common mistake of lifting the buttocks first should be avoided. If possible, do the exercise in front of a mirror and watch to make sure the upper body creates one long line.

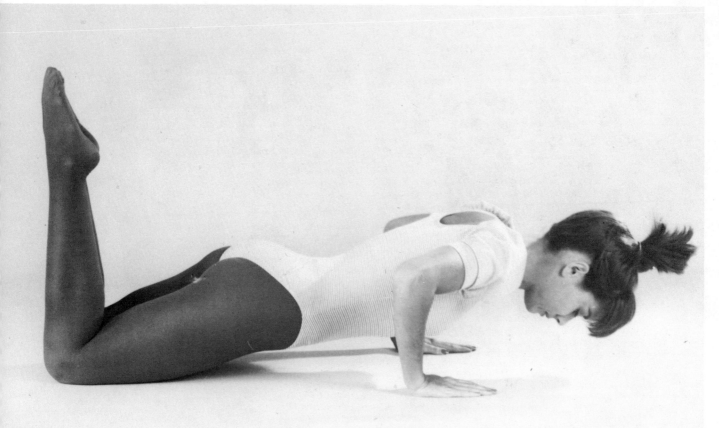

6. Triceps Extension

Repetitions: 3 sets of 8 for each arm

---

1. Bending over from the hips, extend back so it is parallel to floor. Place right hand on a low table or other flat surface for support. Left upper arm is touching the side of the body with the elbow bent and hand in front of the shoulder. Inhale.
2. Exhale and extend left arm back and up.

The upper arm should not lose contact with the left side.
3. Inhale and return arm to starting position. Complete sets and repeat with right arm.

This exercise should be done with weights for best results.

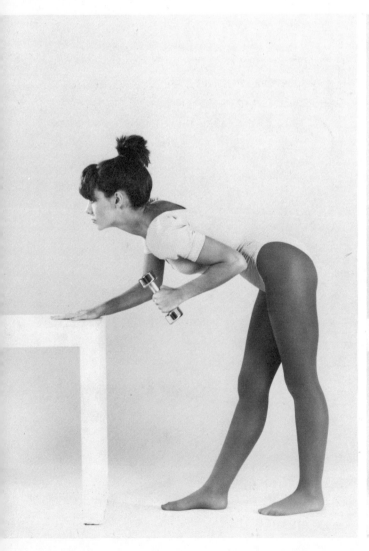
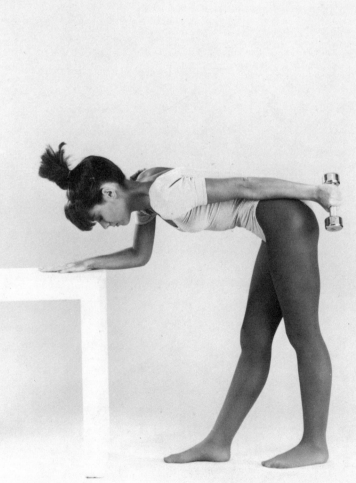

FLEXIBILITY EXERCISES

Flexibility exercises should be included as a regular part of any conditioning program. Not only do stretches limber and loosen the muscles of the body, they also increase joint mobility and improve circulation. In fact, the tense, harried executive would do well to stretch every day to relax muscles that grip in response to stress. Tight muscles have to release to achieve flexibility, and by using breath, imagery, and gravity you can achieve a more supple body while easing out tension.

The key to a successful flexibility program is patience. Muscle elasticity develops gradually and should not be rushed. It is a mistake to imitate the extreme stretches of conditioned athletes because you risk muscle strain and serious injury. Use the photographs in this section as a guide to positioning the body, but limit your range of motion at first if you have not exercised or stretched recently. With continued practice your muscles will become more flexible and enable you to stretch farther.

You can gain maximum results from the following stretches if you set aside enough time so that you don't feel rushed. The effectiveness of the exercises is achieved by holding the position for a specified count while focusing on your breathing. You may feel as though you are not working hard enough, but think of it as a different kind of work. Learning how to release muscles and stretch without tension takes just as much concentration as a rapid series of leg lifts.

Frequently there is a temptation to bounce while stretching because it seems as though flexibility will increase. It is critical that any inclination to do this be suppressed. Bouncing is counterproductive because it causes the muscles to contract at the same time you are trying to lengthen them. And the resistance created by the bouncing motion increases the likelihood of injury.

Those new to exercising sometimes have difficulty distinguishing "good" versus "bad" pain. As you stretch you will probably feel a mild discomfort initially as the muscles lengthen. This is a "safe" sensation and indicates that you are gently easing muscles into an elongated state. If you feel pain, though, stop immediately. Pain is an indication that you are pushing yourself too far and forcing a position. Always remember to let your body adjust to a new position slowly and gradually.

1. Spine Stretch

Repetitions: 2 to each side

1. Lying on your back, bend knees and cross left leg over right leg. Arms are extended straight at shoulder level.
2. Gently drop knees to right side as you look toward the left hand. This creates a diagonal twist in the torso and lengthens the muscles along the spine from the tailbone to the neck. Hold position for 30 seconds.
3. Slowly return knees to center.

4. Repeat to the other side by crossing right leg over left leg and dropping knees to the left.

Take deep breaths throughout the exercise; A deep inhalation and controlled exhalation will supply oxygen to the muscles and help tight areas release.

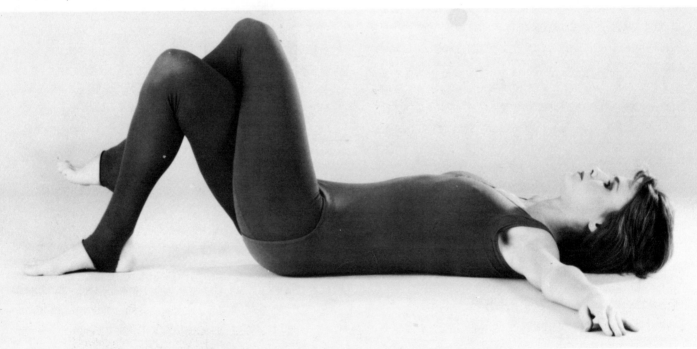

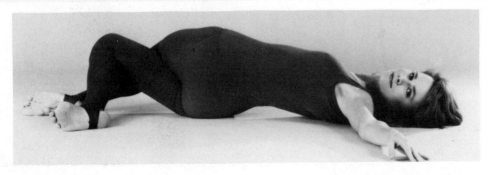

2. Forward Bending Stretch

Repetitions: 2 for each leg

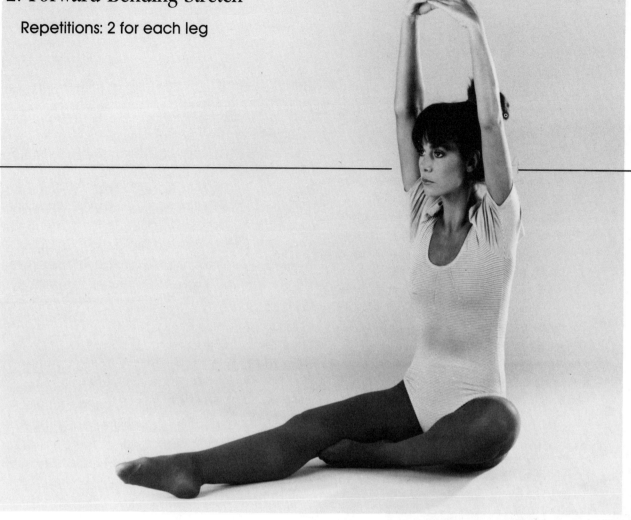

1. Sitting with the right leg extended forward, bend left leg and place the sole of the foot against the right thigh. The left knee points to the left side. Clasp hands above head and stretch arms straight up. Inhale.
2. Exhaling, fold the body slowly over the right leg and grasp the knee, calf, ankle, or toes, depending on your flexibility. Hold position for 20 to 30 seconds. Breathe continually.
3. Return to starting position by stretching the arms out and raising the torso up. Repeat.
4. Change sides and repeat on the left leg.

The head, neck, and shoulders should be relaxed when the torso is folded over the leg. The chin is dropped and resting on the chest.

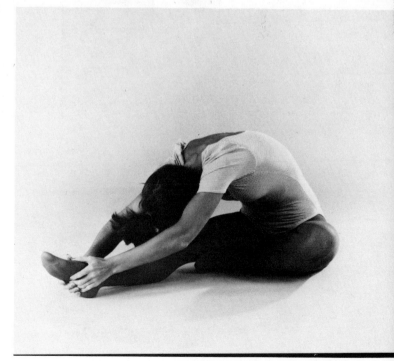

3. Torso Arc

Repetitions: 2 to each side

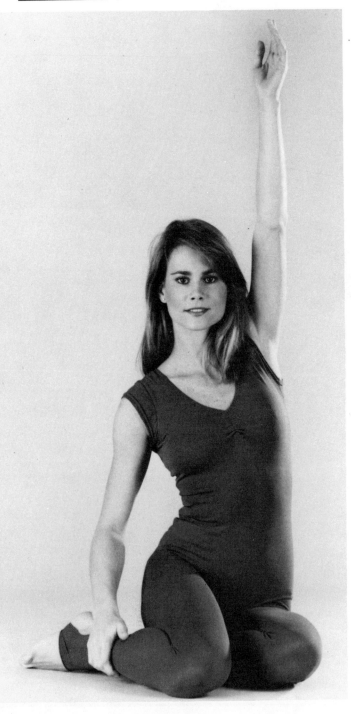

1. Sitting on the left hip, bend knees and fold them to your right side. Left arm is raised to the ceiling. Inhale.
2. As you exhale, stretch left arm up and over the head to the right. Right hand is placed on the floor to provide support for the body. Hold for 20 seconds and continue breathing.
3. Inhale and lift arm to starting position. Repeat. Change sides.

When you stretch the arm, concentrate on lifting the rib cage out of the waist. This will increase the length of the torso as you bend to the side and provide a longer stretch. The stomach muscles are also working to support the trunk.

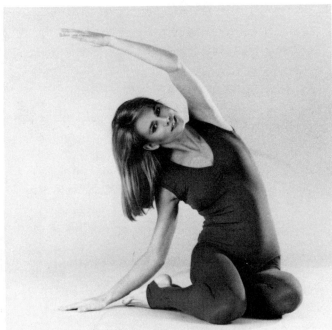

4. Chest, Shoulder, and Arm Stretch

Repetitions: 6 to each side

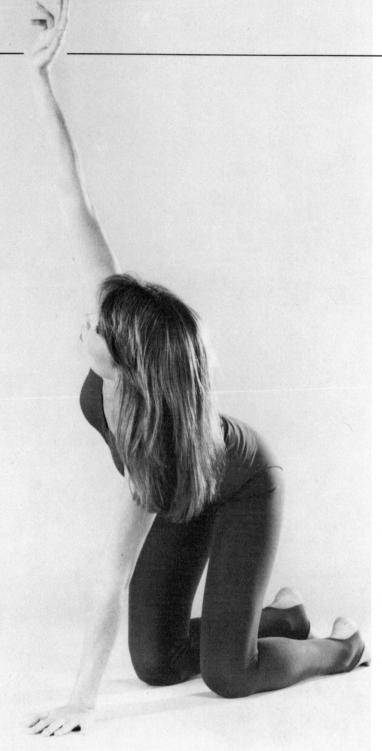

1. On hands and knees, slowly raise right arm to the side and up to the ceiling as you inhale. Turn head to look at right hand as you turn the chest to the side.
2. Exhaling, slowly lower the arm and curve it under the chest and the left arm. Complete repetitions on right side and change sides.

This exercise is particularly beneficial after sitting at a desk all day. Contracted shoulder and chest muscles are lengthened by the opening and curving motions of this stretch.

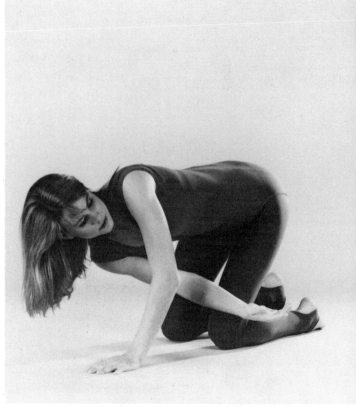

ADVANCED FLEXIBILITY EXERCISES

5. Back and Thigh Stretch

This two-part exercise elongates the muscles along the spine and stretches the quadriceps (the muscles in the front of the thighs).

PART I: SPINE STRETCH

Repetitions: 3

1. Lying on the stomach with the forehead on the floor, place hands under shoulders.
2. Stretching the chin out on the floor, slowly raise the head, neck, shoulders, and chest off the floor by pressing into the palms. Keep the pelvis on the floor and concentrate on the arch made by the upper spine. Hold for 10 seconds. Keep the breath smooth and controlled.
3. Slowly return the torso to the floor by first lowering the chest, then the shoulders, and finally the neck and head.

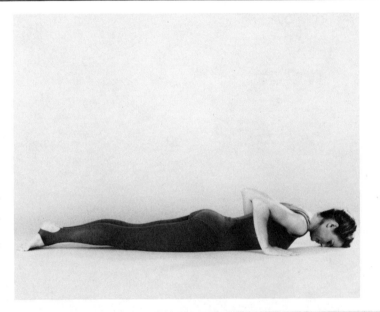

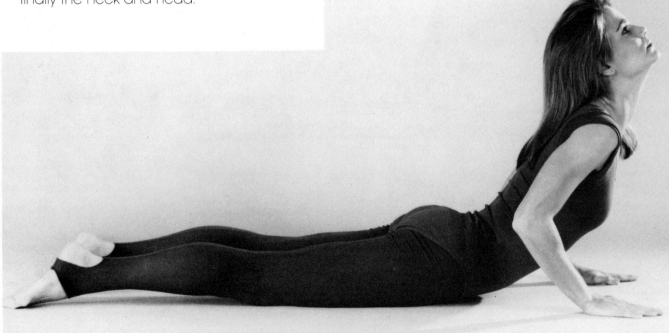

PART II: SPINE AND THIGH STRETCH

Repetitions: 3

1. Lying on the stomach with the forehead on the floor, bend the knees (keep thighs on the floor) and grasp the ankles.
2. Slowly lift the head and chest and then raise the thighs. The arms should be kept straight. Hold for 10 seconds and breathe steadily.
3. Lower the body to the floor and release the legs.

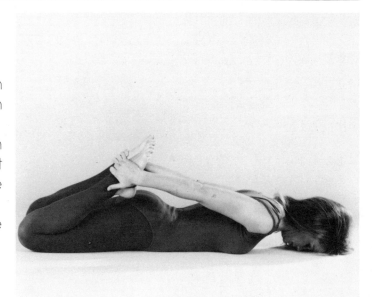

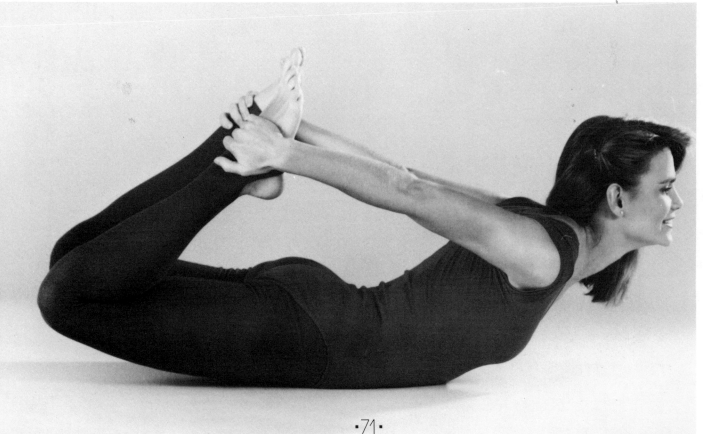

6. Hamstring Stretch

Repetitions: 3

1. Lying on your back, lift legs and bend them to form a diamond shape, touching feet together and opening knees to the sides.
2. Straighten legs to form a V-shape and place hands on the inside of the knees, calves, or ankles, depending on your flexibility. Hold position for 10 seconds and focus on using the breath. Breathing steadily helps you to release and lengthen the muscles.
3. Return legs to starting position. Bring knees together and hug them to chest.

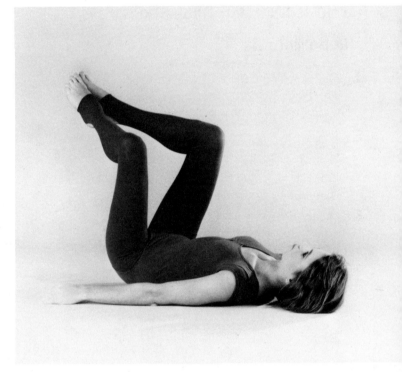

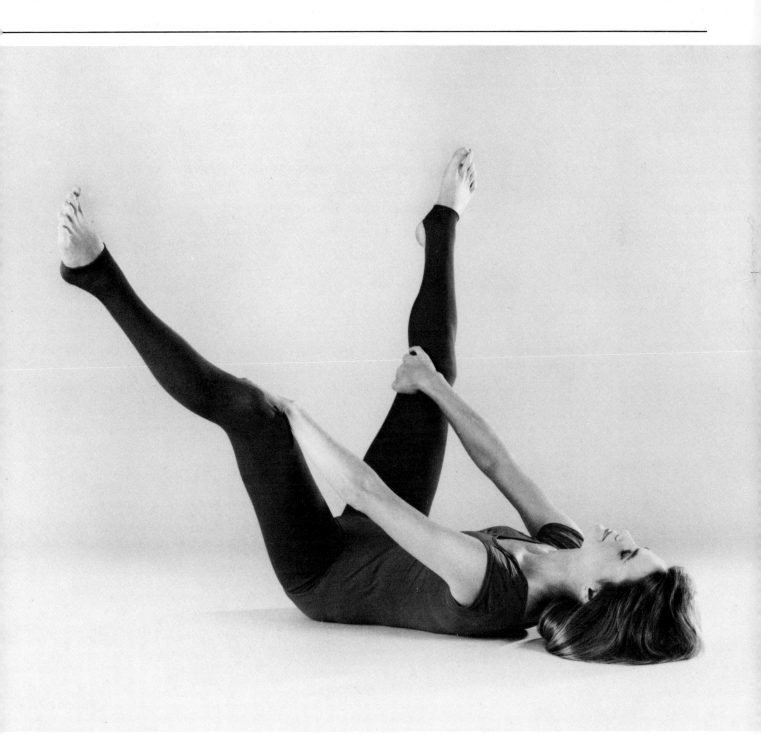

LEGS

Thighs. Calves. Ankles. Most women feel that at least one part of their legs could use some improvement. A sedentary life not only affects the muscle tone and appearance of the legs, it is also a prime contributor to the circulatory problems experienced by many women. Sitting for hours daily not only makes muscles flaccid and unshapely, it also decreases blood flow to the extremities. Exercising regularly will help counteract the physical effects of a desk job in addition to helping prevent problems such as varicose veins and swollen ankles.

The best all-round exercise for the legs is walking, because the physical motion loosens stiff joints and provides overall tone. Walk as much as you can and opt for stairs instead of elevators whenever possible. Do be aware that your choice of footwear plays an important part in the way you look and feel. It is essential to limit the wearing of very high-heeled shoes because they shorten the calf muscles and create an imbalance in muscles and body alignment. High heels are not rec-ommended for walking any significant distance because they are the number one cause of twisted and wrenched ankles. While running shoes are not the designer choice to accompany a business suit, it is generally acceptable to wear sneakers on the way to work and change to more fashionable footwear after arriving at the office.

If your legs need additional conditioning to supplement that provided by walking, then specific exercises for the thighs, calves, and ankles will help you shape up any problem spots. By focusing on movements that stretch, tone, and strengthen particular muscle groups, you can create better-looking legs. Exercise can slim down heavy thighs and calves as well as making skinny legs more attractive.

As with any exercise, it is imperative to warm up before starting the following movements. The hamstrings (the long muscles that run down the back of the legs) can be particularly vulnerable to strain or injury if they are "cold." Two minutes of jogging in place will increase circulation, bring a greater blood supply to the legs, and prepare the hamstrings for more intensive work.

1. Total Toner

Repetitions: 10, working up to 20

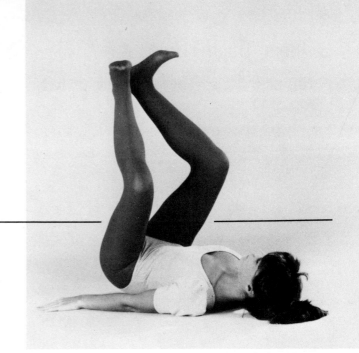

1. Lying on your back, lift legs and bend knees to form a diamond shape. Feet are flexed and pointed to sides with soles parallel to ceiling and heels touching. Inhale.
2. Imagine that an invisible weight is placed on the soles. Exhale and slowly push this

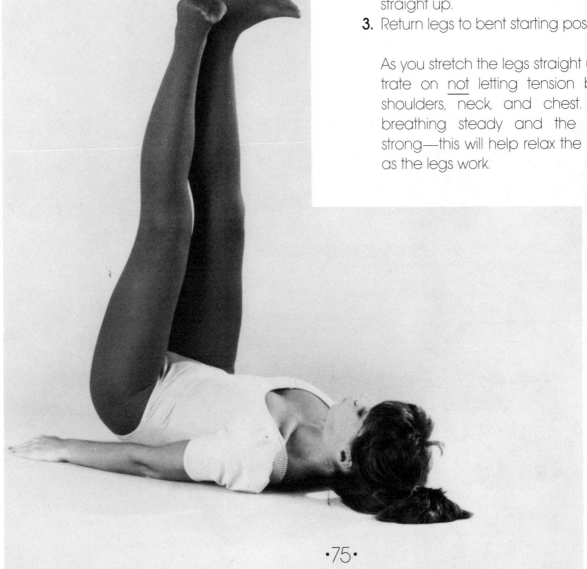

imaginary weight until legs are stretched straight up.
3. Return legs to bent starting position.

As you stretch the legs straight up, concentrate on <u>not</u> letting tension build in the shoulders, neck, and chest. Keep your breathing steady and the abdominals strong—this will help relax the upper body as the legs work.

2. Inner Thigh Trimmer

Repetitions: 3 sets of 10, working up to 6 sets of 10

1. Lying on your back, bend knees and place feet flat on floor about hip-width apart. Tilt the pelvis and roll up the spine until you are supported by your shoulder blades. (This is the Pelvic Tilt, described in detail on p. 32.)

2. Keeping the torso stationary (do not let it bob up and down), bring the knees together to touch and then open them.

3. Repeat the close-and-open motion 10 times and then roll down the spine to the initial position.

In addition to firming the thighs, this exercise is a good toner for the buttocks.

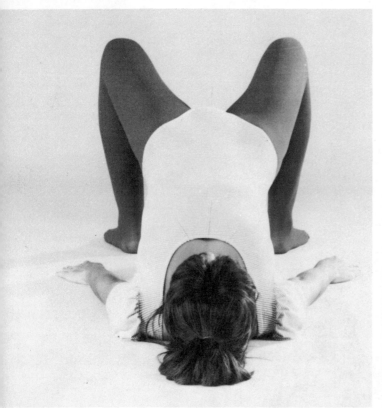 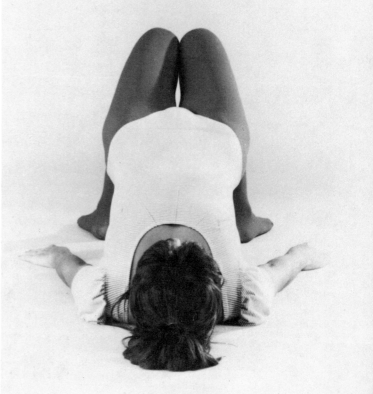

3. Side Lift

Repetitions: 4 sets (each set includes 8 lifts), working up to 8 sets

1. Lying on your side, with arm extended and head resting on arm, stretch legs long. Tighten buttocks and lift top leg about 6 inches.
2. Lower and lift leg 8 times.
3. Lift top leg and slowly bend knee, bringing heel toward buttocks.
4. Straighten leg.

You have just completed one set. Continue repetitions, then change sides and repeat with other leg.

Do not skip the knee bend between sets. This bend stretches the front of the thigh and prevents the leg muscles from gripping and cramping.

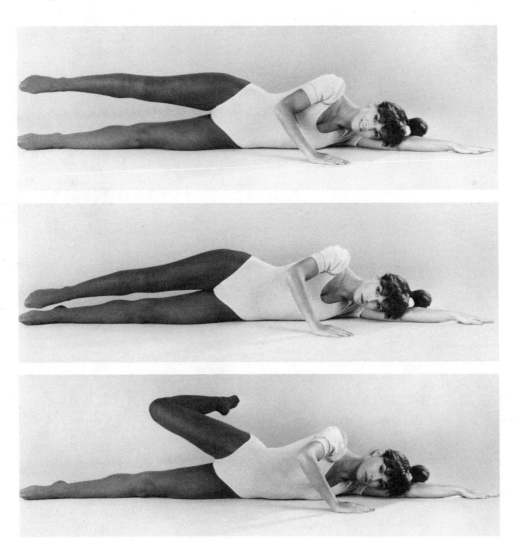

4. Stretch and Flex Leg Toner

Repetitions: 15 on each leg, working up to 25

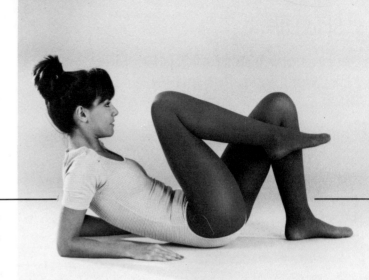

1. Leaning back on elbows, bend knees and place feet flat on the floor. Bring right knee to chest.
2. Stretch right leg straight up.
3. Flex foot and slowly lower leg to floor. Complete repetitions on right leg and repeat exercise with left leg.

For maximum benefits, it is important to control the leg as it lowers to the floor. Instead of letting the leg drop rapidly, use a count of 4 to complete the motion.

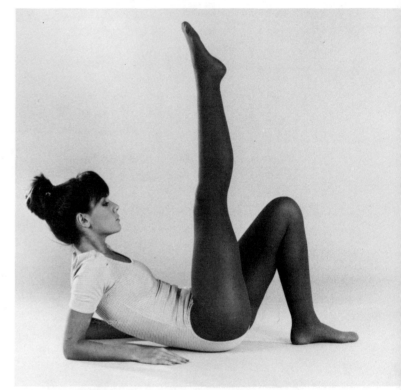

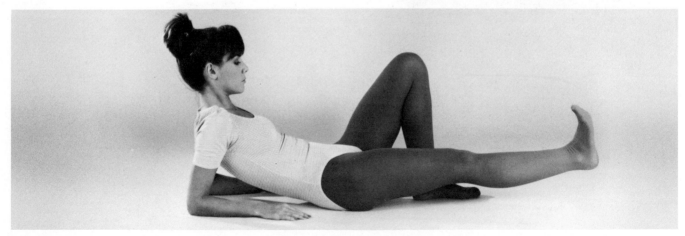

ADVANCED LEGS

5. "V" Lift

Repetitions: 10 on each side, working up
to 20

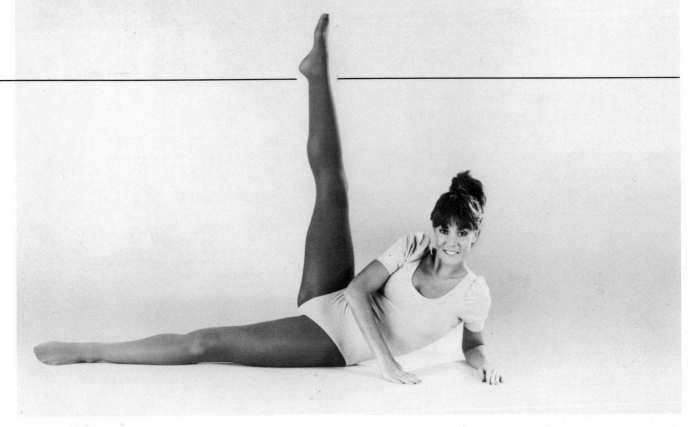

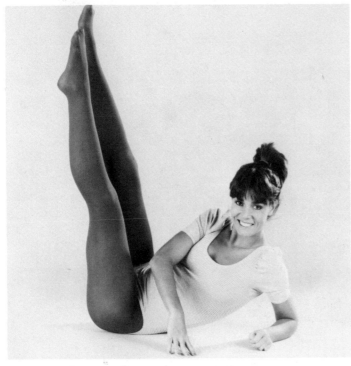

1. Lying on left side and supporting yourself
   on one elbow, stretch left leg straight on
   floor and extend right leg toward ceiling.
2. Lift left leg up to touch right leg. (As you lift
   the left leg, the right hip will drop slightly to
   help balance the body.)
3. Return left leg to floor.
4. Lower right leg to touch left leg. You have
   completed one repetition.

Finish the suggested repetitions on left side
and repeat on the right side. The abdominal muscles should be working throughout
the exercise.

6. Thigh Firmer

Repetitions: 6 on each side, working up to 12

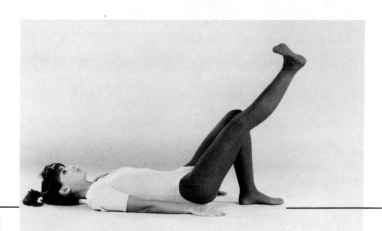

1. Lying on back, bend left knee and extend right leg straight, parallel to the left thigh. Rotate the right leg outward so that the inside of the right knee touches the side of the left knee. Flex the right foot.
2. Lower the right leg about 3 inches from the floor.
3. Point the right foot and raise the leg to the starting position. Complete the repetitions and repeat with left leg.

The rotation of the leg in this exercise helps to shape the thigh. Concentrate on initiating the rotation from the top of the leg at the hip joint.

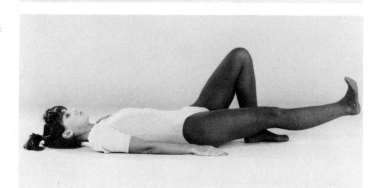

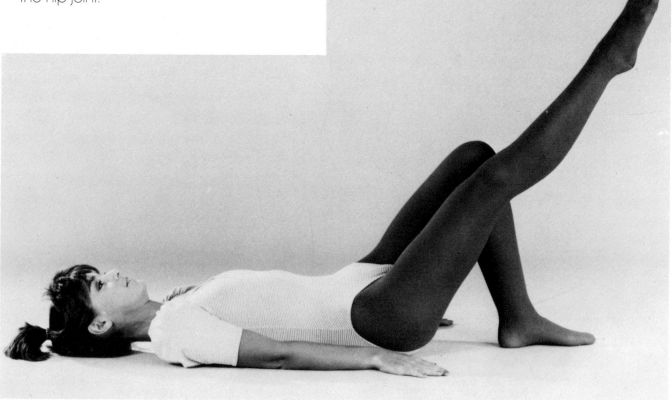

AEROBICS

Aerobic exercise spans a variety of activities, including swimming, bicycling, jogging, skiing, rope skipping, squash and racquetball, skating, and even brisk walking, to mention a few. Simply put, the activity must cause your body to demand more oxygen over a specific period of time.

Aerobic is defined as "living, active or occurring only in the presence of oxygen," and in relation to exercise, it promotes the supply and use of oxygen. The value of aerobic exercise is widespread in its impact on an individual's health. Not only does aerobic exercise contribute to a more efficient heart and improved cardiovascular system, it is also one of the best methods of weight control and tension release in addition to providing an energy boost.

Many women think that "aerobics" is synonymous with dancing. While enthusiasm for aerobic dancing has heightened awareness that aerobic training is an essential component of a personal fitness program, some people have become confused by the term. Aerobic dancing is only one method of fitness training but not the only form of cardiovascular conditioning. To those women who are not devotees of dance, this may come as a relief.

To gain an aerobic training effect from your exercise program, it is necessary to sustain your heart rate within a specified target zone for a minimum of twenty minutes, three times a week. This means that while five or ten minutes of active exercise may make you feel better (and energized), it does not qualify as aerobic training.

You can calculate your heart rate target zone with the following formula based on age:

220 minus age equals age estimated maximum heart rate (beats per minute)

For example, the calculation for a thirty-five-year-old woman is:

220 − 35 = 185 (beats per minute)

The target zone is between 70 percent and 85 percent of the age estimated maximum heart rate. For the thirty-five-year-old woman the range is 130 to 157:

185 × .70 = 130   185 × .85 = 157
Target zone   Target zone
low end   upper end

It is important to monitor your heart rate by checking your pulse throughout the aerobic activity to ensure you are within the boundaries of your target zone. You can take your pulse in one of several ways: by placing two or three fingers on the inside of your wrist, in line with your index finger, by placing two fingers on one of the carotid arteries (which can be felt on either side of the neck under the jaw), or by placing the fingers on your temples. Count the beats for ten seconds and multiply by six. This gives you the number of heartbeats per minute.

If your heartbeat registers above the 85 percent target zone, then reduce the intensity of your activity so it falls within the appropriate boundaries. If it falls below 70 percent, then increase your exertion to bring the heart rate into the training zone.

Women who have not exercised vigorously recently should ease into an aerobics program and progressively increase their exertion. Initially it is wise to start at a 60 percent level or even less to gradually condition the body. As your body gets stronger and stamina increases, you will safely be able to exercise in the recommended target zone of 70 to 85 percent.

Aerobic activity is a key factor in weight control. Women who have battled weight problems throughout their lives will find that a regular program of aerobic activity can help them lose pounds and keep them off successfully. Essentially, weight problems are the effect of lack of activity. Increasing exercise time can be the solution for many women who have found restrictive diets to be unsuccessful, unpleasant, and boring. Aerobic exercise will increase your metabolism—the rate at which your body burns calories. In fact, in addition to the higher metabolic rate that occurs during exercise, there are also benefits afterward. For example, when you exercise vigorously, the body continues to burn more calories following the activity than it would during normal resting. For as long as six to eight hours after a continuous forty-five-minute aerobic workout, you can expect to burn about twice as many calories resting as you would if you had remained inactive.

Additionally, appetite is better regulated in people who participate in a regular program of aerobic exercise. Excess pounds often develop because people eat when they are not hungry and food becomes a source of gratification to offset emotional needs. This may sound familiar if you find yourself heading for the refrigerator whenever you are depressed, tense, or anxious. Aerobic activity can help you channel emotions that normally might lead you to the kitchen. After exercising vigorously there is little desire for food (the digestive system is less active then because the blood supply has been decreased in the stomach). The activity is an aid in regulating appetite and identifying "bona fide" hunger.

You may ask how it is possible to fit three twenty-minute sessions of aerobic activity into a full schedule each week when just squeezing in body-conditioning exercises is a feat. The answer is, aerobic activities can become a part of your everyday life. It's important to mention once again that walking is one of the best forms of exercise. It takes less planning to accomplish a daily quota of brisk walking than to arrange your schedule to make sure you can go swimming several times a week. Walking does not necessitate a change of clothing other than switching to a pair of sturdy shoes, and it can be done anytime, anywhere.

Combining priorities such as fitness and family is a way to take the full advantage of limited time. For example, bicycling outdoors is a great way for a working mother to be with her children and exercise too. An added fitness benefit is that a child's energy can be an inspiration and motivation.

Stationary bikes are also appealing to busy women because they offer the ability to accomplish two tasks at once. Watch the television news as you pedal and you can catch up on world events while you keep your heart beating within its target zone. One note of caution, though: a leisurely pedal will not sufficiently raise the heart rate. You have to pump your legs vigorously to gain the aerobic benefits of bicycling.

Boredom is the primary threat to most fitness regimens, and therefore it is essential to make every effort to create a program for yourself that is enjoyable and invigorating. For example, if you consider running "cruel and unusual punishment," then it is unlikely you will be a runner for long. Select several activities that you like or have always wanted to try. By providing some options for diversity there is a greater chance you will achieve a successful ongoing regimen.

As you determine the types of aerobic activities you want to pursue, also consider your preference for individual or group activities. Some women need the support and enthusiasm of a class situation—for example, aerobic dance courses—to stay with a program. The motivation provided by an instructor may also be a critical element for progress. But some women prefer solitary activities because they offer more scheduling flexibility. Additionally, while competition can be stimulating in group activities, some women would rather

leave the competitive drive at the office and opt to compete only against themselves in distance running, swimming, or walking.

In selecting an activity, think about what is most appropriate for your body and consider its strengths and weaknesses. Women who have been plagued by back, knee, or foot problems would do best to try activities other than running or rope skipping. Both place enormous strain on the joints of the body and are particularly stressful for weak knees and ankles. A non-weight-bearing sport such as swimming is ideal because the body is supported by water, thereby preventing joint irritation. Bicycling is also "safe" for most individuals, as the joints are not acting as shock absorbers against the jolts that occur with running.

Aerobic dancing is enjoyed by millions, but be discriminating in choosing a class and the facility where it is taught. Instructor qualifications vary depending on the organization. Ideally an instructor should hold a degree in movement education, dance, or exercise physiology, and have current CPR (cardiopulmonary resuscitation) certification.

Most organizations will permit you to observe a class before making a financial commitment for a series. This observation visit provides the opportunity to assess the instructor's teaching style and personality.

The facility for an aerobics dance class can pass or fail on the basis of the floor on which you dance. Never participate in a class where you will be jumping on a concrete floor. Aerobic dancing on a stone-hard surface can create severe leg problems ranging from ligament and cartilage damage to shin splints. A wood floor is the recomended surface because wood provides "give" and helps to cushion jumping movements.

Finally, whether you choose to jog, participate in racquet sports, or join aerobic dance classes, remember that your feet must be protected. Investing in the proper footwear can help prevent discomfort or injury. In addition to running shoes that provide essential cushioning, manufacturers have now developed specific styles for aerobic dancing and racquet sports. These styles are lighter-weight than running shoes and are more flexible to adapt to the lateral movements.

As with the body-conditioning program, it is essential to warm up before starting an aerobic workout. Use the warm-up exercises in Chapter 1 to raise the body's temperature and prepare it for more demanding movement.

Finish your aerobic session by gradually lowering the intensity of your activity. It is important not to stop suddenly but rather to keep moving at a decreased pace. This prevents the pooling of blood in the extremities. Within five to ten minutes your heart rate should be below 100 beats per minute. You can also include some of the following cool-down movements to stretch tight muscles and help lower the heart rate.

If you have been running, dancing, skipping rope, or walking briskly, complete your aerobic session with movements that will lengthen muscles that have shortened during the activity. These exercises should be done slowly for maximum results.

1. Calf Stretch

Hold for 1 minute on each leg.

1. Standing in a lunge position, with both feet pointing forward, bend right knee and extend left leg back. The heel of the left foot can be raised slightly.
2. Slowly lower the left heel to the floor. As the heel presses to the floor you will feel a stretch in the calf muscle. Hold position.
3. Repeat with right leg extended back.

As you lower the heel to the floor, do not bounce it up and down. Flexibility is achieved by sustaining the lowered heel position.

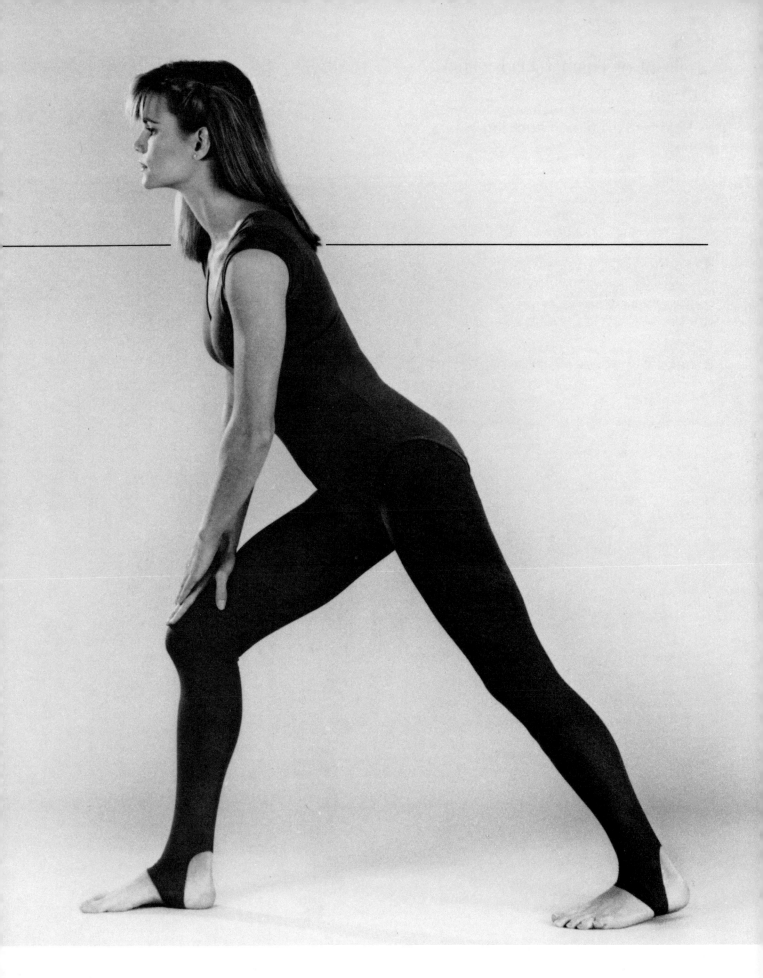

2. Front of Thigh (Quadriceps) Stretch

Hold for 1 minute on each leg.

1. Standing on the left leg, bend right leg behind you and clasp instep with right hand.
2. Gently press instep into hand to increase the stretch in the front of the thigh. Hold position.
3. Repeat with opposite leg in bent position.

Keep stomach muscles activated throughout this stretch to prevent arching the spine.

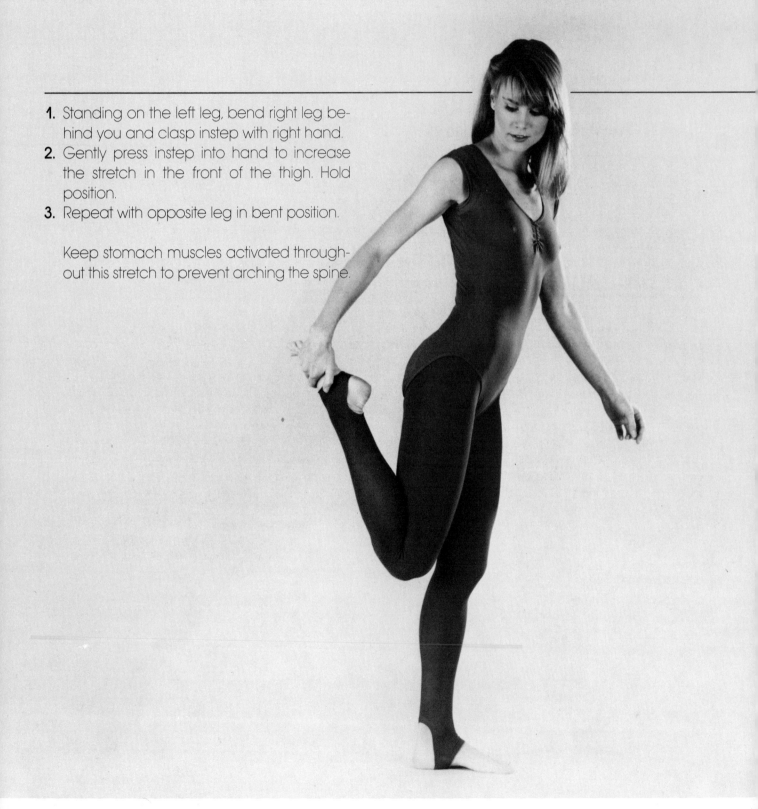

3. Back Stretch

Hold for 30 seconds; repeat twice.

4. Back of Thigh (Hamstring) Stretch

Hold for 30 seconds; repeat twice.

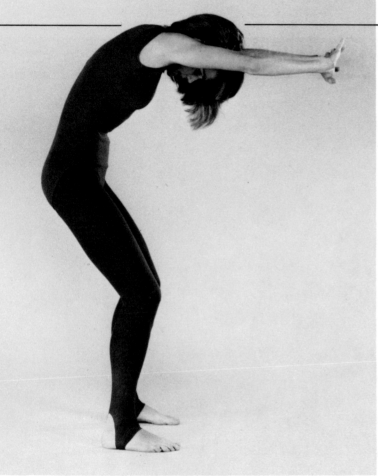

1. Standing with legs hip-width apart and feet pointing forward, bend knees and drop torso over legs. Clasp hands around ankles and rest chest on top of thighs. Head and neck are relaxed and hanging toward the floor. Gently press chest into thighs and hold position. Release position and repeat.

This hamstring stretch prevents strain on the knee joints and lower spine.

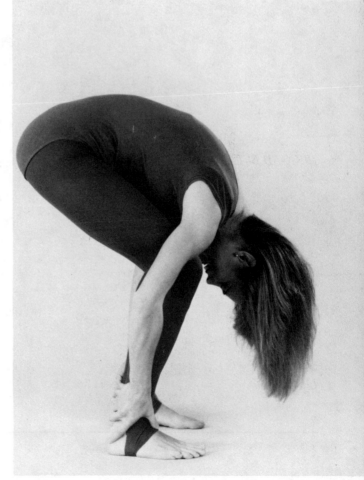

1. Standing with legs about hip-width apart and feet pointing forward, bend knees slightly and make a "C" curve with upper body. Clasp hands and push arms forward. Relax head and neck by letting chin rest on chest. Hold position. Release position and repeat.

This stretch lengthens back muscles that tighten when the back is arched. The "C" curve is particularly helpful in relieving backaches.

INTENSIVE CONDITIONING FOR AT-HOME WORKOUTS
EXERCISE REFERENCE CHART

	Exercise	Repetitions	Goal
WARM-UP	Two-Minute Jog	1½–2 minutes	
	Body Tension Releasers	30 seconds	
	Neck Relaxer	4	
	Shoulder and Arm Rotations	4	
	Torso and Back Stretch	4	
	Hip Circle	4	
ABDOMINALS	Abdominal Toner	3	6
	Diagonal Stomach Strengthener	4	10
	Roll-Down	3	8
	The Bicycle	10	20
	(and Variation)	10	20
	* The "Reacher"	3	6
	* Raised Leg Sit-Up	5	10
	Pelvic Tilt	2 after each abdominal exercise	
HIPS AND BUTTOCKS	Buttocks Toner	4	10
	Hip Trimmer	8	15
	The Triangle	4	8
	Fanny Firmer	3	6
	* Leg Extension	5	10
	* The Shaper	5	10
WAIST	Waist Stretch	8	15
	Knee Drop	20	35
	Torso Circle	6	12
	The Windmill	20	35
	* Torso Toner	6	12
	* Waist Cross	6	12
UPPER ARMS	Shoulder Warm-Up	3 sets of 6	
	Triceps Toner	3 sets of 10	

* Advanced exercises

	Exercise	Repetitions	Goal
UPPER ARMS cont.	Pectoral Strengthener	3 sets of 10	
	Biceps Builder	3 sets of 8	
	*Push-Up	6	15
	*Triceps Extension	3 sets of 8	
FLEXIBILITY	Spine Stretch	2, hold for 30 seconds each	
	Forward Bending Stretch	2, hold for 20–30 seconds each	
	Torso Arc	2, hold for 20 seconds each	
	Chest, Shoulder, and Arm Stretch	6	
	*Back and Thigh Stretch (Parts I and II)	3 of each, hold for 10 seconds each	
	*Hamstring Stretch	3, hold for 10 seconds each	
LEGS	Total Toner	10	20
	Inner Thigh Trimmer	3 sets of 10	6 sets of 10
	Side Lift	4 sets of 8	8 sets of 8
	Stretch and Flex Leg Tone	15	25
	*"V" Lift	10	20
	*Thigh Firmer	6	12
AEROBIC ACTIVITY		20 minutes, 3 times weekly	
COOL-DOWN	Calf Stretch	1, hold for 1 minute for each leg	
	Front of Thigh Stretch	1, hold for 1 minute for each leg	
	Back Stretch	2, hold for 30 seconds	
	Back of Thigh Stretch	2, hold for 30 seconds	

*Advanced exercises

When you want to squeeze a fast workout into a busy schedule, the following exercise regimens can be your guide to a quick fitness session. Each workout offers exercise options that can help you stay fit in minimum time.

The number of exercises that are suggested for each workout is an estimate. If you need to work more slowly to guarantee proper body alignment, you may do fewer exercises in the allotted time. It is more important to concentrate on executing the movements correctly than to rush.

10 Minute Workout

While ten minutes is not long enough for a total body conditioning program, you can make the most of the limited time by focusing on a single body area or muscle group. On days that are very busy, ten minutes of activity can provide an energy boost and a chance to exercise a particular problem area.

Suggested Exercise Plan

Warm-up (approximately 5 minutes) + three exercises from one of the body area/muscle group listings in the Exercise Reference Chart. To prevent muscle strain, the advanced exercises should not be done in the 10 Minute Workout.

Example:
Warm-up + Abdominal Exercises (Abdominal Toner, Diagonal Stomach Strengthener, and Roll-Down)
or
Warm-up + Waist Exercises (Waist Stretch, Knee Drop, and Torso Circle)

20 Minute Workout

Twenty minutes offers the time to include exercises for additional body areas as well as more intensive work. In this time period it is possible to complete all the exercises (regular and advanced) for two body areas/muscle groups. If you feel that you are not ready to execute the advanced movements, concentrate on doing the first three or four exercises of several of the body area listings in the reference chart. As with the 10 Minute Workout, it is important to start the exercise session with a warm-up.

Suggested Exercise Plans

PLAN A

Warm-up + six exercises from two of the body area/muscle group listings in the Exercise Reference Chart.

Example:

Warm-up + Hips and Buttocks Exercises
(Buttocks Toner, Hip Trimmer, The Triangle, Fanny Firmer, Leg Extension, and The Shaper)
and
Flexibility Exercises (Spine Stretch, Forward Bending Stretch, Torso Arc, Chest, Shoulder, and Arm Stretch, Back and Thigh Stretch, and Hamstring Stretch)

PLAN B

Warm-up + four exercises from three body area/muscle group listings.

Example:

Warm-up + Abdominal Exercises
(Abdominal Toner, Diagonal Stomach Strengthener, Roll-Down, and The Bicycle)
and
Upper Arms (Shoulder Warm-Up, Triceps Toner, Pectoral Strengthener, and Biceps Builder)
and
Leg Exercises (Total Toner, Inner Thigh Trimmer, Side Lift, and Stretch and Flex Leg Toner)

30 Minute Workout

A thirty-minute exercise session provides the opportunity for more extensive body conditioning work or a twenty-minute aerobic activity with a warm-up and cool-down period. The 30 Minute Workout enables you to do three or four exercises for nearly every body area/muscle group or to execute the complete exercise program for three body areas.

If it is possible to include a half-hour workout several times a week, ideally you want to alternate body-conditioning work with aerobic exercise. This provides a balanced program of cardiovascular activity with strengthening, toning, and flexibility work.

Suggested Exercise Plans

PLAN A

Warm-up + aerobic activity + cool-down

Example: Warm-up + bicycle riding + cool-down

PLAN B

Warm-up + three or four exercises from five body area/muscle group listings in the Exercise Reference Chart.

Example:

Warm-up + Abdominal Exercises (Abdominal Toner, Diagonal Stomach Strengthener, Roll-Down, and The Bicycle)
and
Hips and Buttocks Exercises (Buttocks Toner, Hip Trimmer, The Triangle, and Fanny Firmer)
and
Waist Exercises (Waist Stretch, Knee Drop, Torso Circle, and The Windmill)
and
Flexibility Exercises (Spine Stretch, Forward Bending Stretch, Torso Arc, and Chest, Shoulder, and Arm Stretch)
and
Leg Exercises (Total Toner, Inner Thigh Trimmer, Side Lift, and Stretch and Flex Leg Toner)

PLAN C

Warm-up + six exercises from three of the body area/muscle group listings.

Example:

Warm-up + Upper Arm Exercises (Shoulder Warm-Up, Triceps Toner, Pectoral Strengthener, Biceps Builder, Push-Up, and Triceps Extension)

and

Waist Exercises (Waist Stretch, Knee Drop, Torso Circle, The Windmill, Torso Toner, and Waist Cross)

and

Hips and Buttocks Exercises (Buttocks Toner, Hip Trimmer, The Triangle, Fanny Firmer, Leg Extension, and The Shaper)

Fitness During the Workday— Noontime Alternatives

The alternatives explored in this chapter are not suggested to upset your workday schedule or make you feel guilty about failing to exercise. They are suggestions that can offer new possibilities of integrating physical activity into a workday that may already seem completely booked. While the ideal fitness regimen of four thirty-minute sessions weekly may appeal to you, perhaps it's just not possible for you to schedule more than two. You don't have to be Wonder Woman, nor are you training for the Olympics. Your concern is health and making your body function as well as possible within the limits established by your professional/personal life.

How many times have you worked straight through lunch, sat at your desk for hours, and felt exhausted by three-thirty P.M.? Fitness during the workday means taking care of yourself. You will be more productive and will feel better physically and emotionally. Taking time to eat right is essential. Equally important is physical activity, which requires conscious action on your part.

All too often a sedentary work style becomes habitual. Executives may feel that it just takes too much time and effort to go out of the office for lunch. The standard rationalization usually goes something like this: "Eating at my desk means more time for work, and not taking a break enhances my concentration." Actually the opposite effect occurs. After several hours without movement or change of environment, the body becomes physically and mentally fatigued. Pushing yourself to continue working without a break is generally fruitless because the body becomes restless and the attention span is diminished.

Ideally, movement should be integrated into your workday. Walking to the water fountain or up a flight of stairs can provide the muscle action that will shake you out of your physical lethargy. Just a change of environment provided by a brief visit to another part of the office can affect mental outlook and concentration. Some physical movement and visual diversion can help ensure job productivity throughout the day.

The lunch hour is the built-in break that can be used to greatest advantage. While many lunches may be of a business nature for you, if they get you out of the office, then at least an environmental change is provided. But if you are on your own during noontime, you can use that hour or so to relax and reenergize your body through exercise. There is nothing like activity to release the tension of morning pressures and stress.

Not every situation works for every woman, nor do all activities appeal to all women. You may say that changing your clothes to work out at noon is just too much trouble when you need to look your best for an afternoon meeting. There will be times when you may forgo all physical activity because there are emergency deadlines. Or perhaps you won't go to the gym because the weather is inclement and you do not want to become disheveled before an important appointment. These are all reasonable statements.

Fitness Center Programs

Before exploring exercise programs outside the office, first check the opportunities that may be available at your company. Corporations of all sizes, from Fortune 500 firms to small, privately owned companies, have begun instituting their own fitness programs for employees. The extent of the programs, the facilities, and the availability of trained professional staff vary from company to company. Some corporations have built fitness centers with equipment and services rivaling those of the most elaborate health clubs. Other companies provide more modest programs, but these can be just as effective in promoting physical fitness and health monitoring.

Many firms offer their fitness facilities only to upper-level management as an executive perk. Others establish eligibility on the basis of age, while some offer membership to all staff and include spouses. In most instances the centers require that employees make at least two visits per week to ensure commitment and to achieve the benefits of an ongoing program.

The corporate fitness centers provide a wide range of exercise activities. Most of them are equipped with stationary devices to maximize the use of limited space and include treadmills, rowing machines, Universal or Nautilus equipment, free weights, and exercycles. More expansive facilities include rooms for group classes such as aerobics, yoga, or calisthenics and provide special sessions on lower back problems or flexibility exercises.

If your company has an in-house fitness center, becoming a participant offers many advantages. The convenience of the facility cannot be matched. Most centers are open from 7 A.M. to 7 P.M., and in some cases executives have the option of taking time during the workday to exercise rather than at lunchtime or before or after work. (These midmorning or afternoon sessions are valuable energy revivers and tension releasers.) Most of the centers have exercise physiologists who help you develop a program personally geared to your strengths and weaknesses in addition to providing instruction, guidance, and motivation.

These on-the-premises fitness centers have locker rooms and showers, so you can leave a workout really feeling comfortable about going back to your job. Some even have saunas and steam rooms and provide shorts, T-shirts, towels, and hair dryers.

In the United States and Canada hundreds of companies now have fitness programs for employees. For further information on fitness centers in corporations, contact Association for Fitness in Business, 1312 Washington Boulevard, Stamford, Connecticut, 06902.

Companies that have neither the space, budget, nor personnel to establish an in-house program frequently offer top management the option of membership in an executive health center convenient to the office. Many major metropolitan areas have this type of fitness center, with programs specially geared to the executive. They guarantee participants a complete workout that can be accomplished in less than an hour (including changing clothes and showering). The centers provide exercise gear so executives need not tote workout clothing, and they are normally open from early morning till early evening. The programs usually concentrate on cardiovascular fitness, muscular strength, and flexibility and are directed by medical personnel, exercise physiologists, and exercise specialists. Many of these centers highlight the one-to-one contact between trainer and client and provide a continual monitoring of members' progress.

Health Clubs

If none of these programs is available, you may want to consider joining a health club. Some corporations will underwrite the cost of the membership, and there are health clubs that offer reduced fees to corporate groups.

Health clubs offer a wide range of services, equipment, and specialized instructors, but these fitness centers can vary dramatically in the quality of management, facilities, and personnel. Before investing your money or your firm's resources in a membership, it is prudent to establish a checklist of standards that a club should fulfill to ensure maximum satisfaction for you.

1. Location
   If you plan to use the club during the workday it is essential that it be convenient to

your office. A location that is more than a ten-minute drive or walk from your job is a deterrent from the start. Convenience is critical when you want to squeeze in an exercise session during lunch hour.

2. Operating Hours

Does the club's schedule match yours? If it opens after you start work, closes early, and you would frequently miss the noontime sessions due to work obligations, then this club will not serve your needs. It's best to look for a club that offers the greatest flexibility in terms of early morning and evening hours, weekend availability, and lots of lunch hour classes.

3. Instructors

One of the most important criteria of a reputable club is the standard it sets for hiring instructors. Find out if the staff is required to hold degrees or certification in movement education, exercise physiology, or athletic training. A knowledge of anatomy, body chemistry, and first aid is essential. There are too many "exercise experts" who have limited understanding of how the body works and these instructors can be hazardous to your health.

You should also watch the staff in action to observe their style in interacting with members. Is individual attention given to clients, or do the instructors spend more time chatting with one another and working out themselves?

4. Size of Membership

Many clubs place no limit on membership size and plan on attrition to keep the facilities from becoming overcrowded. Visit the club during the hours you are most likely to use it to see if there is adequate space. Ask yourself if there is enough area to exercise, swim (if the facility has a pool), shower, and get dressed without feeling crowded.

5. Activities

Before joining a club, identify the kinds of activities you want. If you are only interested in calisthenics and aerobics classes, then don't join a club where your membership fee covers equipment and activities you will never use.

6. Classes

In your visit to a prospective club, be sure to observe the classes that you would want to join. Take note of the following points:

- Is class size limited? Classes with more than twenty-five participants offer little opportunity for individual instruction or correction. It's important that a teacher see your body in action to watch for proper execution of exercises. Without input from an instructor you can unknowingly injure yourself.

- Does the same instructor teach an ongoing class or do instructors rotate? If there is a different teacher each time you take the class, there is no opportunity for an instructor to monitor your progress or for regular evaluation of your physical strengths and weaknesses. Again, this limits the input you receive about your body.

Ideally you want the same instructor to lead the class at all times.

- What kind of atmosphere is created by the instructor? A good teacher provides motivation and challenge to a class. The pace of the class should be geared to the level of the participants, and the instructor should be personable and approachable.

7 Club Environment and Upkeep
Cleanliness and well-maintained equipment and facilities are important for your personal well-being and physical health. The locker room and showers should be spotlessly clean and the exercise areas well lit and pleasant.

Private Instruction

Some executive women find that while they want and need active exercise, their erratic schedules make it difficult for them to attend a health club or fitness class regularly. Additionally, a group class may not serve their purposes because with limited time to exercise they want to make the most of a session by focusing on their particular needs. The solution in these cases is to consider a private class with an instructor who can create a program tailored to your needs. There are personal trainers who will come to your office or home and design a program of specialized exercise for you.

For example, if you want a session at work that will tone, strengthen, and relax your body without working up a sweat, your instructor may create a class based on yoga-type exercises. On the other hand, the woman who wants to lose weight may want a trainer to develop a program that focuses on aerobics. Your instructor is your consultant and is there to lead you in the exercises, supply motivation and reinforcement, and provide feedback about your performance and progress.

These one-to-one sessions don't require a lot of space, and you may find that your office is a suitable area. (If your office is too small, perhaps you can use a conference room or another private space that is not regularly scheduled for meetings.) An in-office class is a valuable time-saver and the ultimate in privacy and convenience. Your instructor arrives (this is the ultimate motivation!), you change your clothes, close the door to your office, and start exercising. In only thirty minutes a good personal trainer should be able to provide you with a thorough workout that covers all the major muscle groups.

The best way to find a private instructor is through a personal recommendation. If no referrals are available, contact exercise salons, dance studios, or health clubs and inquire whether any of the instructors provide private classes and make office or home visits. Interview potential teachers, request references, and make your selection based on personal compatibility as well as professional credentials. The cost is more than you would pay for a group class, but it is a personal service.

Other Options

While exercise sessions are a great diversion mentally and offer enormous physical benefits, you can integrate fitness into the workday in other ways as well. Again, walking is one of the best all-round forms of exercise—it increases the heart rate and works the cardiovascular system, involves all the major muscle groups in movement, and requires no special equipment. If possible, get out of the office during lunch and walk to a nearby park for some fresh air and new scenery. Take a book, have a picnic, or just let your mind wander. Even in the winter, a brisk walk in the cold, crisp air can do wonders. When you get back to work you'll feel refreshed, relaxed, and able to concentrate clearly in the afternoon.

When you absolutely cannot get away from the office, don't let that be an excuse for letting tension and pressure take over. Lunchtime is a good opportunity to use relaxation techniques. Take full advantage of less office activity, noise, and people to slow down and center yourself. The following relaxation countdown will release tension quickly and help you focus on the tasks at hand.

RELAXATION COUNTDOWN

1. Roll your eyes up (this helps you keep them closed).
2. Close your eyelids.
3. Breathe deeply three times.
4. Count backward from 10. After saying each number to yourself, tell yourself that you are becoming more relaxed.
5. When you reach number 1, just sit and enjoy the silence in the mind and the body for several moments.
6. Think about opening your eyes.
7. Roll your eyes down.
8. Open your eyelids and stretch your body slowly.

CHAPTER
FOUR

Traveling and Staying in Shape

Traveling takes a particular toll on the working woman. Out-of-town trips usually mean days of continual meetings and evenings spent with business associates over dinner. It can be a grueling schedule and one that leaves little time (or energy!) for fitness and taking care of yourself. It is easy to understand how a regular exercise regimen can be neglected during business trips simply because there does not seem to be time for anything other than work. While it is possible to rationalize why traveling can be a legitimate excuse for easing up on exercise, the reasons for continuing with a fitness program "on the road" are more compelling.

Business trips can be draining, physically and mentally. Instead of experiencing exhaustion during and after travel, it is possible to retain stamina and energy. This chapter offers guidelines and suggestions to help ensure that you keep fit when you are on the road. How to fight jet lag, how to feel most comfortable during air travel, how to continue your exercise routine while away, and the best places to stay are discussed to provide the executive woman with the resources for healthful traveling.

Fighting Jet Lag

Traveling across time zones presents the problem of jet lag, which is the bane of many frequent fliers. Jet lag is the disorder that arises when your biological rhythms regulating the body's functions are disrupted. Sleep/wake

·100·

patterns, digestion, body temperature, and even hormonal secretions are influenced. Jet lag symptoms include drowsiness, insomnia, headache, loss of appetite, indigestion, constipation or diarrhea, and irritability.

Studies conducted by Charles F. Ehret, Ph.D., a scientist at the Argonne National Laboratory, revealed that humans do not have to be the passive victims of disrupted body clocks. Jet lag can be avoided by implementing changes in sleep and diet patterns prior to flying. The following tips can help you prepare for new time zones without jet lag.

Sleep

It takes about one day per time zone crossed for our bodies to adapt to new destinations. Most business travelers do not have the luxury of arriving three to five days in advance of a transcontinental or transoceanic meeting. However, it is possible to adjust your body clock to the new destination before you leave by trying to adapt to the sleep/wake cycle of the city to be visited. This means going to bed and getting up according to the time it would be in your destination city. While it may not be practical to totally conform to your destination's time zone, any alteration of your patterns will help you adjust more quickly when you arrive.

When you are in-flight, synchronize your body to the sleep/wake hours of your destination. Set your watch ahead or behind and adjust your behavior to that of your destination.

For example, if you fly during your day, but their night, you should try to sleep inflight. You will then be synchronized with the new time zone when you arrive during their day. This way you are coordinating your body's rhythms to the light/dark cycle of the new time zone. If possible, schedule your arrival during daylight. It is easier for the body to adjust. Once you arrive, try to go to bed and wake up according to the local time.

Diet

Dr. Ehret has developed an eating plan to relieve jet lag that is based on high-protein and high-carbohydrate meals and on alternating feast and fast days. High-protein meals provide you with extended energy for up to five hours because they stimulate the adrenaline system. High-carbohydrate meals supply a burst of energy for about an hour but then induce sleepiness. When you alternate eating heavily (feasting) with eating lightly (fasting), this respectively replenishes and diminishes energy reserves, helping your body adjust to a new time zone more quickly. The anti-jet-lag diet also includes caffeinated beverages that contain the energy-inducing chemicals methylated xanthines, which can help to reset body clocks.

If you are flying within the United States the following anti-jet-lag diet plan should be started two days before departure. Travelers flying to overseas destinations should initiate the eating plan four days before the flight.

You can send for a free wallet-sized copy of the "Countdown" chart by mailing a self-addressed stamped envelope to: Office of Public Affairs, Argonne National Laboratory, 9700 South Cass Avenue, Argonne, Ill. 60439.

The chart illustrates that four days prior to an overseas flight you should eat extra portions of high-protein foods for breakfast and lunch (day 1). Dinner should be a high-carbohydrate meal.

Day 2 is a fast day. Calories are kept to a minimum to help deplete the liver's store of carbohydrates and prepare the body's clock for resetting. All meals should be light, restricted to foods such as salads, soups, fruits, and juices. Continue the program for the next two days.

It is recommended that you avoid caffeinated beverages on all days but the flight day. (If you need a caffeine boost on any day before your flight, you can indulge only from 3 P.M. to 5 P.M.) On flight day, if you are traveling from the East Coast to the West Coast, drink coffee, tea, or cola only in the morning. Eastbound travelers should have caffeinated drinks only between 6 P.M. and 11 P.M.

Once in-flight, begin to adjust to your destination's local time by resetting your wristwatch. Skip meals until breakfast of your new time zone, then eat a high-protein "feast" breakfast. This should be followed later in the day with a "feast" high-protein lunch and a high-carbohydrate dinner.

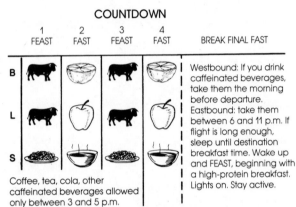

THE ARGONNE ANTI-JET-LAG DIET

COUNTDOWN

	1 FEAST	2 FAST	3 FEAST	4 FAST	BREAK FINAL FAST

Westbound: If you drink caffeinated beverages, take them the morning before departure. Eastbound: take them between 6 and 11 p.m. If flight is long enough, sleep until destination breakfast time. Wake up and FEAST, beginning with a high-protein breakfast. Lights on. Stay active.

Coffee, tea, cola, other caffeinated beverages allowed only between 3 and 5 p.m.

FEAST on high-protein breakfasts and lunches to stimulate the body's active cycle. Suitable meals include steak, eggs, hamburgers, high-protein cereals, green beans.

FEAST on high-carbohydrate suppers to stimulate sleep. They include spaghetti and other pastas (but no meatballs), crepes (but no meat filling), potatoes, other starchy vegetables, and sweet desserts.

FAST days help deplete the liver's store of carbohydrates and prepare the body's clock for resetting. Suitable foods include fruit, light soups, broths, skimpy salads, unbuttered toast, half pieces of bread. Keep calories and carbohydrates to a minimum.

Source: U.S. Government Printing Office: 1982–654-824. Reprinted by permission of Argonne National Laboratory.

In-Flight Comfort

Sitting too long anywhere can make you feel tired, but hours aboard a pressurized airplane can leave you lethargic, stiff, and weary. If the first stop after arriving at your destination is a business meeting, then it makes sense to take certain precautions that will ensure your top performance. Air travel can be made easier and more comfortable when you use foresight.

What you wear can influence how you feel during your flight and once you deplane. While a fitted suit may be most appropriate for your meeting, opt for less restrictive clothing during travel time. Most women experience some bloating and water retention on a plane. Tight-fitting clothes can be very uncomfortable. A knit dress with a jacket is an excellent choice for traveling and business. The knit fabric has some "give" and the jacket creates a professional look and can be removed during flight.

Low-heeled shoes are a necessity when flying. This is not the time to "break in" a new pair of pumps. Many travelers experience swollen feet during air travel because they are confined to a seat and circulation suffers. The pull of gravity causes blood to pool in the body's extremities, creating puffiness in the feet and ankles. Ideally, you should bring along an extra pair of shoes that are slightly larger to accommodate any swelling.

Airplane cabins are very dry, and it is easy to become dehydrated during the flight. Drink plenty of fluids on board—water and fruit juices are best.

Avoid alcoholic beverages. They are the worst drink for any traveler. Alcohol contributes to dehydration and affects your body clock, hindering your ability to adjust to new time zones.

The low humidity of airplane cabins tends to dry out the skin and make the eyes feel irritated. Counteract these drying effects by bringing some travel-size skin care aids on board with you. A small mineral-water mister can restore lost moisture to the face, and a cream or lotion moisturizer will help lock in the water. A lubricating eyewash can make you feel revived when you deplane. You might also want to bring a purse-sized cologne along to give you an extra lift.

The importance of exercise during air travel cannot be stressed too highly. You can make a long flight more comfortable and arrive at your destination in top form physically and mentally if you do some movements on board. This will stimulate circulation and loosen muscles and joints that tense up when motion is restricted by confining seats. Getting out of your seat and simply walking up and down the aisle will give your body a chance to stretch and make you feel less lethargic. In addition to walking, there are a number of movements you can do in your seat that will improve circulation and provide relief for stiff body areas. The following exercises are designed to be done while sitting. In addition to these movements, many of the On-the-Job Tension-Releasing Exercises (see Chapter 12) are ideal during a flight because they too are done while seated.

1. Neck Stretch

Hold each position for 5 seconds and repeat 4 times.

1. Sitting with your back straight, drop your chin and try to let it touch your chest.
2. Lift chin toward ceiling and let your head bend back. You should feel a long stretch down the front of the neck.
3. Center the head on the neck and turn the head as far as you can to the right.
4. Return the head to the front and turn it as far as you can to the left.

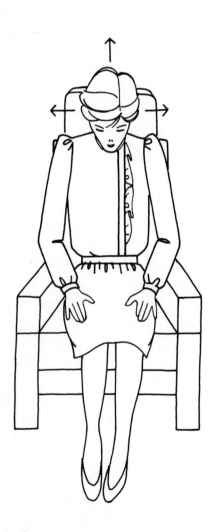

2. Walking in Place

Repeat for 1 minute.

1. Sitting with your back straight and stomach pulled in, lift the right leg up about 4 inches. The motion is initiated in the hip joint and simulates a walking action.
2. Replace foot on floor.
3. Repeat with left leg and alternate legs continuously.

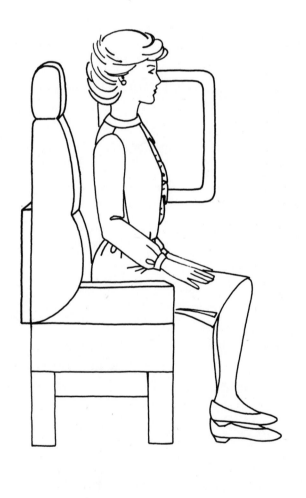

3. Foot Flexor

Repeat 15 times.

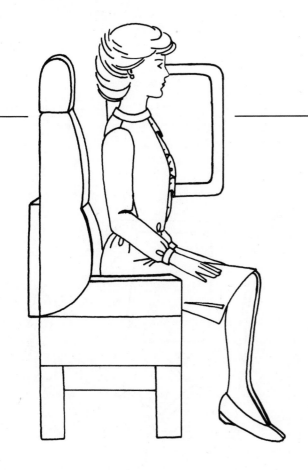

1. Sitting with your back straight, press into the balls of the feet. As you press, the heels lift off the floor.
2. Rock back on the heels and lift the toes off the floor. You will feel a slight pull in the back of the calves as the muscles stretch.

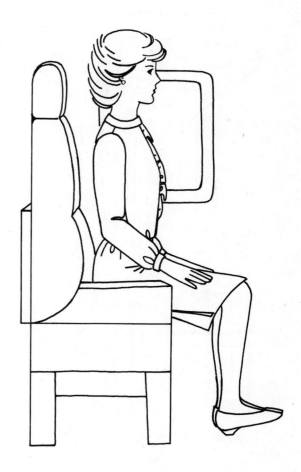

4. Back Twist

Repeat 10 times.

---

1. Sitting with your back straight, clasp hands behind head and open elbows to the side.
2. Bending the torso forward, twist so that the right elbow touches the left knee.
3. Return to initial position and repeat to the opposite side.

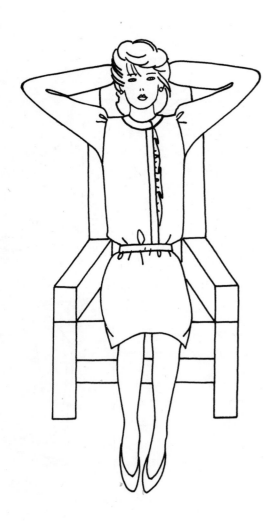

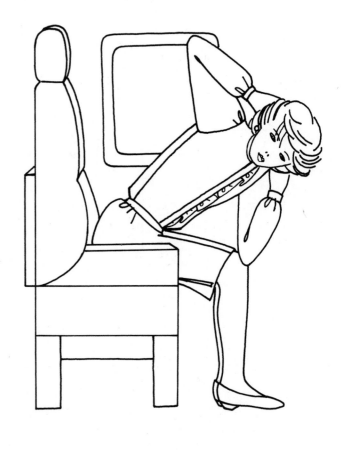

5. Arm and Shoulder Stretch

Repeat 10 times.

1. Sitting with your back straight, interlock fingers in front of chest (palms of hands face chest). Keeping fingers interlocked, turn palms outward and stretch arms above your head.
2. Gently press the arms back (initiating the movement from the shoulders).

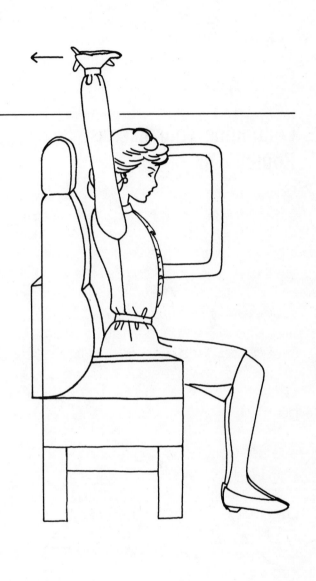

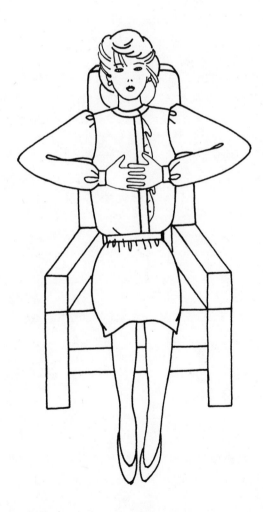

Continuing Your Exercise
Routine Out of Town

Staying in shape on the road takes perseverance. It is easy to fall into a pattern of returning to your hotel room after a long day and collapsing. There are two main reasons for making sure you incorporate fitness activities during your out-of-town stay: (1) keeping up your exercise regimen on business trips gives you extra stamina and energy to concentrate through day-long meetings and conferences, and (2) you won't return home five pounds heavier and feeling guilty about a weight gain.

The when, where, and how of integrating exercise workouts during travel are points that need to be considered before leaving on a business trip. The key to staying with your exercise routine is to plan for it. Take along portable fitness aids that will ensure your working out. These "carry-alongs" are the tools you need for fitness activities—leotard, shoes, tennis racquet, exercise tapes, portable cassette player, swimsuit, etc. If you work out with weights, there are now inflatable free weights designed particularly for travelers that can be filled with water when you arrive at your destination. By guaranteeing that your exercise gear is with you, you are off to a good start to continuing your fitness routine, and you do not have the excuse "I didn't bring a swimsuit so I'll just skip the pool while I'm at the hotel."

Any kind of workout that can be done in your room puts you one step ahead. Out-of-town meetings usually mean a full schedule of business activities that can keep you going from the early morning to late evening. Since active exercise late at night may prevent you from falling asleep, your alternatives are early morning, lunchtime if you have any scheduling leeway, or the after-work period from 5 to 7 P.M. (a pre-dinner workout will help curb inclinations toward overeating at lengthy business dinners).

Many women find that their most valuable traveling exercise aids are instruction tapes and a lightweight, portable cassette player. The exercise tapes provide the discipline of a regular routine to follow, and the workout can be done at your convenience.

A plus in recent years to frequent travelers is the recognition by hundreds of hotels and motels that fitness is a major concern of their guests. For instance, approximately 60 percent of all Marriott hotels throughout the world currently offer guests special in-house fitness facilities, and Sheraton Hotels cater to joggers with a variety of recreational services. Many of their hotels provide printed maps of jogging/running routes in the vicinity and some have running tracks, a number of which are equipped with exercise stations.

The services and equipment at many hotels are extensive and rival the amenities offered by exclusive health clubs. These facilities have been designed to focus on the needs of the traveler who wants to keep in shape year-round. Registered guests usually have complimentary use of all hotel fitness facilities, although some hotels require nominal fees for equipment rental, court time, and golfing. The hotels and motels that offer exercise and recreational activities solve the problem of making fitness "fit in" during business travel. Hotel fitness centers are staffed from early morning to evening, making workouts possible throughout the day.

The list that appears in the back of the book is a guide to hotels and motels throughout the United States and Canada that provide spa/sauna facilities. This can be a helpful aid to ensuring that staying fit while traveling is both possible and enjoyable.

Combining fitness with a few vacation days is a unique way to relax when work takes you abroad. Crossing the Atlantic by ship takes only four and a half days and it is an excellent way to diminish jet lag. In addition, the physical vitality gained on a cruise is always welcome before embarking on a hectic schedule of business meetings.

Fitness programs have been developed by several cruise ship companies, and they offer advantages that surpass the expediency of air travel. One company, the Cunard Line, has created a spa at sea with its "Golden Door" program on the Queen Elizabeth 2. They offer a particularly unique program with individualized prescriptions for total fitness through a variety of exercise classes, personal consultations, and specially prepared high-energy, low-calorie foods. Sitmar's West Coast ship Fairsky is equipped with a well-designed running track and exercise room. The line also offers special meals.

A cruise ship can transport you to your destination feeling healthy, fit, and relaxed. Remaining physically active is possible with the variety of recreational sports and classes that are provided, and you can even lose weight on special fitness cruises.

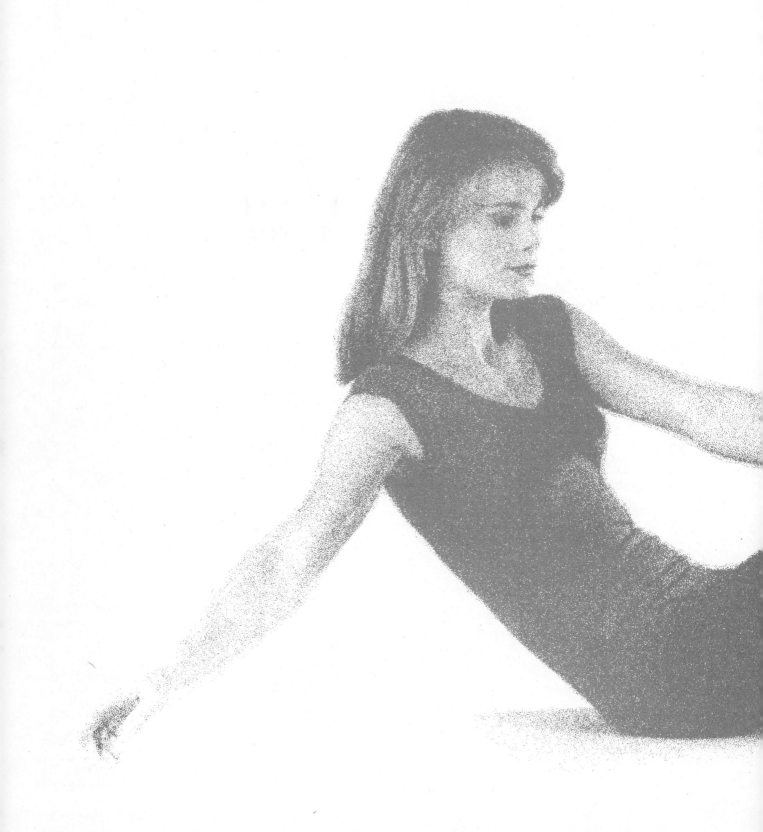

Nutrition

Eating for health. It is a simple statement but one that is often overlooked by many professional women. Hectic schedules can cause meals to be afterthoughts which are grabbed on the run when hunger pangs strike or else frequent highly caloric business lunches and dinners. Neither of these eating patterns contributes to good health or maximum energy. Healthful eating for working women means knowing when to eat and learning what foods provide energy most efficiently. This knowledge will guide you to making the best food choices for your diet.

We have become a nation obsessed with thinness and weight control—particularly for women. However, nutrition is often ignored in the quest to become thin so many women develop eating habits that are harmful to their bodies. It is important to recognize that thinness does not necessarily equal health. Medical studies have revealed that people who weigh 10 to 20 percent under their ideal weight are more apt to have a higher mortality rate than obese individuals.

Actuarial research done by the Metropolitan Life Insurance Company for its Height and

WEIGHTS AT AGES 25–59 BASED ON LOWEST MORTALITY. WEIGHT IN POUNDS ACCORDING TO FRAME (IN INDOOR CLOTHING WEIGHING 3 LBS., SHOES WITH 1" HEELS).

Height Feet	Height Inches	Small Frame	Medium Frame	Large Frame
4	10	102–111	109–121	118–131
4	11	103–113	111–123	120–134
5	0	104–115	113–126	122–137
5	1	106–118	115–129	125–140
5	2	108–121	118–132	128–143
5	3	111–124	121–135	131–147
5	4	114–127	124–138	134–151
5	5	117–130	127–141	137–155
5	6	120–133	130–144	140–159
5	7	123–136	133–147	143–163
5	8	126–139	136–150	146–167
5	9	129–142	139–153	149–170
5	10	132–145	142–156	152–173
5	11	135–148	145–159	155–176
6	0	138–151	148–162	158–179

Source of basic data: 1979 Build Study, Society of Actuaries and Association of Life Insurance Medical Directors of America, 1980.

*1983 Height & Weight Table reprinted with permission of the Metropolitan Insurance Companies.

Weight Table show that today's women can weigh more than their 1959 counterparts and still expect favorable longevity. While the table does not mean that people have a license to gain weight, it does indicate that many women may have fewer pounds to lose.

In establishing eating patterns that will be most beneficial to you, remember some of the information you were told as a child—it still applies. Three meals a day are essential (although some nutritionists recommend eating several smaller meals spread throughout the day). By skipping breakfast, lunch, or dinner you are not only making it difficult for you to sustain energy for demanding mental or physical activity, but you are also depriving yourself of important vitamins and minerals. Additionally, weight control is sabotaged when meals are skipped as a way of reducing calories. Most women find that if they skip breakfast or lunch they are ravenous at the next meal and consume excessive calories. It is important to remember that calories are the energy-producing components of food and if selected prudently throughout the day, they will provide long-lasting stamina without adding weight.

You can calculate the number of calories you need daily with a simple formula that gives your ideal weight. Multiply your height in inches by 3.5 and subtract 108.

Example: 67 inches (5'7") × 3.5 = 234.5 − 108 = 126.5 pounds

Once you have found your ideal weight multiply the total by:

14—if you are not very active
15—if you are moderately active
16—if you are very active

Example: 126.5 × 15 (moderately active) = 1,897 calories daily

If you are trying to lose weight, the safest method is to cut 500 calories per day off your ideal caloric intake. But remember that an increase of physical activity combined with calorie watching is the most effective, long-lasting weight control plan.

Throughout our lives the basic four food groups are presented as the cornerstones of good nutrition. They are the foundation for healthful eating, but some modifications in the daily number of servings and proportions have been made in recent years. Information on the American diet has shown that most people get their largest percentage of calories from refined sugars and fats, a major contributing factor to heart disease and obesity. The recommended dietary goals compared with the standard diet are as follows:

RECOMMENDED	versus	CURRENT
48% complex carbohydrates		22% complex carbohydrates
12% protein		12% protein
30% fat		42% fat
10% refined sugar		24% refined sugar

You can satisfy the requirements of the recommended dietary goals by following these guidelines for daily servings from the four food groups:

1. Vegetable and Fruit Group: 4 servings daily.
   This group provides important sources of fiber and vitamins A and C.
2. Bread and Cereal Group: 4 servings daily.
   Choose whole grain and enriched products for more nutrients and fiber.
3. Milk Group: 2 servings daily.
   Low-fat dairy products can reduce the calories in your meal plan.
4. Meat Group: 2 servings daily.
   Select lean meats and less fatty foods such as fish and poultry. Dry beans and peas can be substituted for animal protein.

By selecting foods from each of these groups you can create a balanced food plan that will supply you with all the necessary vitamins and minerals. Women on weight control programs should emphasize lean meats and low-fat products and try to eliminate refined sugars from their diets. Do note that extended dieting of under 1,200 calories daily is unlikely to provide the U.S. Recommended Dietary Allowance of nutrients. In such cases a daily multivitamin and mineral supplement is advised.

Breakfast— An Essential for Energy and Health

The importance of eating breakfast cannot be stressed too highly. Meals spaced throughout the day are important to balanced nutrition. The body is fueled by sleep, food, and exercise. Take away food and you have lost an essential energy source. Swallowing a vitamin pill in the morning is not the answer to skipping breakfast, because vitamins are best absorbed when there is food in the digestive tract.

Discuss the subject of breakfast with a group of businesswomen and you will find that they place themselves with one of two camps. There is the group that staunchly defends the merits of an early morning meal, and then there are those who do not consider food an issue until noon. The latter cite a variety of reasons for skipping breakfast—everything from avoiding extra calories to a lack of time to boredom with breakfast foods.

There is a myth that skipping breakfast is an aid to losing weight. Americans typically eat little or no breakfast, have a light lunch, and then consume an enormous dinner. Women who are continually fighting extra pounds should know that the calories eaten at the end of the day are less likely to be burned up by activity and more likely to be stored as fat. Since most of our physical activity takes place during the day, breakfast calories are burned early in the day.

A well-balanced breakfast can provide you with lasting energy and a stable blood-sugar level. The problem with starting the day with sugary pastries (besides the obvious non-nutritive calories) is their effect on the body's chemistry. Refined sugar sends the blood sugar level dramatically high, which is followed by a rapid drop a short time later. This significant shift sets a cycle in motion of continuous sugar cravings to bring the blood sugar back to a high level. Indeed, there is a rush of energy that accompanies eating refined sugar, but it is a temporary surge. This "up and down" syndrome is detrimental to prime job performance, besides draining valuable nutrients from your system.

Along with refined sugar it is important to mention the effects of caffeine. While a stimulating cup of coffee or tea can provide a helpful lift and studies have indicated that limited amounts of caffeine can positively affect mental clarity, too much caffeine presents hazards. Women who have high blood pressure, a predilection toward cystic breasts, or digestive problems or who are pregnant should avoid all caffeinated beverages. In addition, excessive amounts of caffeine can cause nervous symptoms.

Women who want to limit the amount of caffeine in their diet can do so by trying one of several alternatives. The obvious options are decaffeinated coffee and herbal teas. Some people find that decaffeinated coffee does not offer the taste satisfaction of regular coffee. You can gradually wean yourself from the caffeine by initially mixing a half-cup of regular coffee with a decaffeinated brand. By progressively increasing the proportion of the decaffeinated you can eventually eliminate

the caffeine without going "cold turkey."

Tea drinkers can substitute a broad variety of caffeine-free herbal teas. The array of herbal teas produced by numerous manufacturers offers many flavor choices. If you drink tea frequently and find that herbal teas are not always available at restaurants or take-out shops, carry a couple of teabags in your purse. You can request a cup of hot water and add your teabag for a caffeine-free drink.

Another alternative to coffee or tea is grain-based beverages such as Pero or Postum. Containing roasted and ground malted barley, barley, chicory, rye, and molasses, these drinks have none of the stimulating substances found in coffee. They are instant products and dissolve in boiling water.

An important consideration in planning breakfast as well as other meals is the inclusion of high-fiber foods in your diet. Fiber is the part of food that is not digestible by the body and it is not limited to bran, which has been the focus of much publicity.

Fiber is present in many foods and can be divided into two categories, soluble and insoluble. Soluble fiber is found in fruits and vegetables, and scientists believe that it helps stabilize blood sugar and lowers fat and cholesterol levels. It is also thought that soluble fiber improves the absorption of water-soluble vitamins. Insoluble fiber, which is contained in whole grains, adds bulk to the diet, thereby countering constipation and making the use of laxatives unnecessary.

Both forms of fiber are useful in weight reduction plans because they are very filling. They give you a satiated feeling, resulting from fiber's property of absorbing water in the digestive tract. This takes up more space in the stomach and makes you feel full.

A recommended daily requirement of fiber has not been established. However, the U.S. Dietary Guidelines and the National Academy of Sciences suggest an increase from 22 percent of caloric intake from complex carbohydrates to 48–55 percent, which automatically insures greater fiber consumption. (This would total approximately 30–40 grams of fiber daily.)

The following charts list the fiber content of fruits and grains typically included in a breakfast meal.

FRUITS

	Serving Size	Total Fiber (grams)
Apple	1 small	3.9
Banana	1 small	1.8
Blackberries	½ cup	3.7
Grapefruit	½ medium	2.6
Orange	1 small	1.8
Peach	1 medium	1.0
Pear	1 medium	2.8
Plums	2 medium	2.3
Strawberries	¾ cup	2.4
Tangerine	1 medium	2.1

GRAINS

	Serving Size	Total Fiber (grams)
CEREALS		
100% Bran Cereal	1 cup	20.0
Corn grits	½ cup cooked	1.9
Grape Nuts	⅓ cup	5.0
Rolled Oats	½ cup cooked	1.6
Shredded Wheat	2 biscuits	6.1
BREAD/CRACKERS		
Graham crackers	2	1.4
Rye bread	1 slice	2.0
Rye crackers	3	2.3
White bread	1 slice	.8
Whole wheat bread	1 slice	2.7

Breakfast at Home

When time is limited but you want to grab a bite to eat before leaving the house, the speediest plan of action for breakfast is a liquid meal. You can sip a nutritious blender drink as you get dressed or organize your briefcase and not lose precious minutes if you are running late. The advantages of a breakfast drink are that you can pack a considerable amount of nutrition into a liquid and preparation time is the absolute minimum (however long it takes you to drop ingredients into your blender and less than 30 seconds to mix them). These two blender recipes are tasty, packed with nutrients, and most important, fast.

▪ FRUIT SMOOTHIE (175 CALORIES) ▪

4 ounces (½ container) low-fat plain yogurt
¼ cup skim milk
½ cup cut-up fruit (strawberries, peaches, or
    blackberries are particularly good)
1 tablespoon wheat germ
2 ice cubes, optional

Spoon yogurt into blender, add skim milk, fruit, wheat germ, and ice cubes. Cover and process on high speed until smooth.

▪ PROTEIN DRINK (200 CALORIES) ▪

1 tablespoon powdered protein (available at
    natural foods stores)
½ banana
1 raw egg
1 cup skim milk
2 ice cubes

Place all ingredients in blender and whip for 30 seconds.

When you are less rushed for time, a sit-down breakfast is a chance to mentally and nutritionally prepare yourself for the upcoming day's activities. Taking time for breakfast at home does not mean lengthy preparation time, and your meal options can include more possibilities than the standard egg fare. A welcome change for breakfast would be to replace eggs with a slice of turkey or chicken or even a piece of fish. There is little difference in calories, and the variety can break the boredom of deciding whether to scramble, fry, or poach eggs.

The number of hot and cold cereals is almost endless. Options range from oatmeal, cracked wheat, and puffed rice, wheat, or corn to wheat germ and a variety of granola-type products (watch the sugar content, though). You might want to try mixing several together to create different textures and tastes.

Be adventurous in your food choices. If you like cottage cheese in the morning, you might want to consider trying farmer cheese, pot cheese, or ricotta cheese in place of your regular brand. Farmer cheese is available in a number of flavors, and it can be an interesting change.

The same principle applies to spreads for bread, toast, and crackers. There are more options than just butter or margarine. If you are watching your weight, a small amount of jam or jelly is a preferable spread to butter—you can save over 80 calories. The variety of fruit jams is extensive and many are now made with less sugar, making them even more appealing to the calorie counter. Nut butters are also a nice change of pace. For example, peanut butter is rich in protein (one tablespoon has 3.9 grams), has fewer calories (1 tablespoon = 86 calories) than butter (102 calories), and contains no cholesterol (versus butter's 35 mg.). You can also purchase no-salt varieties.

The following breakfast menus can be prepared very quickly, and can be used as a guide to creating meals that provide variety. The menus are between 300 and 400 calories, and the combination of foods will provide you with a head start on energy to begin your day.

MENU 1

Calories
60	½ cup unsweetened orange juice
120	¾ cup whole grain cereal
20	1 tablespoon raisins
90	1 cup low-fat or skim milk
70	1 slice whole wheat bread
23	½ teaspoon margarine
383	

MENU 2

85	½ cantaloupe
70	1 egg, scrambled with herbs
70	1 slice whole wheat or rye toast
45	1 teaspoon margarine
90	1 cup low-fat or skim milk
360	

MENU 3

100	½ banana and 1 small orange, sliced
110	2 large graham crackers
120	½ cup cottage cheese sprinkled with cinnamon
330	

MENU 4

55	1 cup strawberries
150	1 whole wheat bagel
150	1½ ounces hard cheese or 1½ tablespoons peanut butter
355	

MENU 5

45	½ grapefruit
70	1 slice whole wheat bread
45	1 teaspoon mayonnaise
120	3 ounces chicken, sliced
90	1 cup low fat or skim milk
370	

"To Go" Breakfasts

Are you the type of person who prefers getting breakfast "to go" from a coffee shop near your office? Healthy eating does not have to be forsaken for convenience, and it is possible to have a breakfast at your desk that is well balanced. Using foresight to make choices—that means thinking about calories, fats, and sugar content—you can select nutrient-rich foods. And contrary to what you might expect, take-out breakfasts do not have to be calorie disasters. By prudently ignoring the display of doughnuts, danish, and coffee cakes, you can order a low-fat, low-calorie meal that will not destroy a weight control program.

If you are used to ordering a buttered roll and black coffee in the morning, it is time to rethink the "to go" breakfast. That selection provides no protein, no fiber, and is a poor source of vitamins and minerals. The best nutritional guideline for choosing a take-out breakfast is to include:

1. Carbohydrates. Select complex carbohydrates such as whole grain breads and cereals and include nutrient-rich fruits.
2. Protein. Select low-fat sources such as cottage cheese, skim milk, and lean meats.
3. Fat. A small amount of fat in the diet is necessary for utilizing fat-soluble vitamins (A, D, E and K).

Use these tips to maximize nutrition for your take-outs:

- Orange or grapefruit juice is easily available at snack shops and is a good source of vitamin C. Try to get an unsweetened juice, though, as canned juices with added sugar provide nothing more than extra calories.

- A piece of fruit has more fiber and fewer calories than juice. Less processing means more useful fiber, and calorie-wise, it takes several pieces of fruit to make one glass of juice.

- Instead of ordering fried or scrambled eggs (coffee shops are notorious for using excessive amounts of butter for cooking eggs), you can save calories and limit saturated fats by asking for a sliced hard-boiled egg sandwich.

- When ordering coffee "light," specify that you want it with milk (most restaurants normally use cream or half-and-half for coffee and tea).

- While bagels and cream cheese are a breakfast favorite, a hefty smear of cream cheese means lots of calories and fat. Order the bagel if you like but ask for a spread of cottage cheese instead.

- Bran and corn muffins generally have less sugar than blueberry muffins. Corn muffins are usually higher in fat but have more vitamin A than the others. Bran muffins are a good source of fiber and will provide more iron and niacin.

- A container of yogurt is an easy desk breakfast but read the label of the brand you select. Fruit yogurts generally have 100 calories more than their unflavored counterparts. Also, the difference between skim-milk and whole-milk yogurt is about 100 calories. A low-fat plain yogurt with a piece of fruit is your best bet nutritionally and calorically.

The following chart lists calorie counts for common foods that you might select for take-out. Use it as a guide to make the best choices for your "to go" breakfast.

		Serving Size	Calories
FRUITS/JUICES	Apple	1 medium	70
	Apple juice	8 ounces	120
	Banana	1 medium	90
	Cantaloupe	½ medium	85
	Grapefruit	½ medium	45
	Grapefruit juice	8 ounces	100
	Orange	1 medium	70
	Orange juice	8 ounces	120
	Prune juice	8 ounces	200
	Tomato juice	8 ounces	45
BREADS	Bagel	1	150
	Muffin, English	1	130
	Muffin, blueberry	1, 3″ diameter	110
	Muffin, bran	1, 3″ diameter	105
	Muffin, corn	1, 3″ diameter	130
	Raisin bread	1 slice	80
	Rye bread	1 slice	61
	White bread	1 slice	76
	Whole wheat bread	1 slice	70
EGGS/DAIRY PRODUCTS	Butter	1 tablespoon	102
	Cheese, American	1 ounce	105
	Cheese, Swiss	1 ounce	105
	Cottage cheese, creamed	½ cup	120
	Cottage, cheese, low-fat	½ cup	80
	Cream cheese	1 tablespoon	55
	Egg	1 medium	70
	Buttermilk	8 ounces	90
	Milk, skim	8 ounces	90
	Milk, whole	8 ounces	160
	Yogurt, low-fat	8 ounces	150

Snacking and Brown-Bagging

Snacking is a way of life for most people, and it can be a useful means of sustaining energy throughout the day. Unfortunately, "snacks" suffer from a bad reputation, associated with sugary items or fried foods that contain lots of fat and calories. Connecting snacks with "junk food" is not surprising. Manufacturers bombard consumers with advertisements for snack foods that lack nutritional value and are full of "empty" calories.

Snacking can be viewed in a different light if you consider it part of your total eating plan —a way to supply your body with essential nutrients. Snacks can provide vitamins, minerals, and fiber to your diet and be a complement to your meals instead of a caloric disaster.

Office snack machines are notorious for containing selections that offer few options for healthful eating. Candy bars, chemical-laden pastries, and salty chips are the usual fare. But machines can also dispense juices, yogurt, fruit, raisins, nuts, and crackers and cheese. If your company currently has the standard fare, it is worth pursuing attempts to bring in another machine or replace some of the poor offerings with a choice of better foods.

The best way to ensure that you have a nutritious snack available when hunger strikes is to supply your own. This broadens the options beyond the vending machines and guarantees that you have control over what you eat. Selecting foods that will both provide and sustain energy is the key to snacking intelligently. Nontraditional snack foods are the secret to between-meal eating that staves off hunger while ensuring good nutrition.

One of the best snacks is a slice of whole grain bread and cheese. The bread provides carbohydrates and protein, while the cheese contributes extra protein and fat. If you have a "sweet tooth," this combination will counter sugar cravings and provide you with a satisfying, filling snack. A slice of whole wheat bread has 70 calories, and one ounce of most cheeses is about 100 calories. Compared to an average candy bar (200 calories), a bread and cheese snack packs more nutrients and complex carbohydrates into fewer calories.

If calories are a real concern, then you could substitute a slice of chicken or other lean meat in place of the cheese (one ounce of chicken without skin is only 40 calories!). Cheese, though, is a good source of calcium (chicken has almost none) and supplies vitamin A and some of the B vitamins. The following list will help you select cheeses that are best for your diet, taking into consideration calories, fat, and calcium content.

Fruit is a delicious complement to cheese and provides important vitamins and minerals. Eating fruit as a snack is another opportunity to include fiber in your diet, and the energy-producing natural-sugar carbohydrates are digested and absorbed into your bloodstream quickly. Keep an apple or orange in your desk drawer and bring a piece of cheese from home. Below are some fruits that rank especially high in nutrients. Note that while dried fruits are good sources of vitamins

Cheese (1 oz.)	Calories	Fat (g.)	Calcium (mg.)
Cheddar	114	9.4	204
Gouda	101	7.78	198
Gruyère	117	9.17	287
Mozzarella	80	6.12	147
Mozzarella, part skim	72	4.51	183
Muenster	104	8.52	203
Neufchatel	74	6.64	21
Swiss	107	7.78	272

and minerals, they are high in natural sugars and calories. They should be eaten in moderation.

Vitamin A:	Apricots (raw and dried), cantaloupe, nectarines, peaches, prunes, watermelon
Vitamin C:	Grapefruit, oranges, strawberries, tangerines, tomatoes
Potassium:	Bananas, dried apricots, raisins
Thiamine and iron:	Dates, dried fruits, raisins, prunes

Other suggestions for snack foods that are rich in nutrients include peanut butter and whole wheat crackers, popcorn, raw vegetables (you can wrap them in thin slices of lean meat for added protein), nut and raisin mixtures, yogurt, graham crackers or bread sticks, and fruit and vegetable juices.

Snacks can be easily incorporated into a

Instead of	Calories	Substitute	Calories	Calories Saved
Apple pie, 1 piece (⅙ of 9″ pie)	345	Apple, raw	70	275
Cheesecake (2″ piece)	200	Graham crackers, 2	110	90
Chocolate bar (1.3 oz.)	210	Banana	90	120
Chocolate chip cookie	80	Vanilla wafer	20	60
Chocolate cake with icing (2″ piece)	445	Sponge cake (2″ piece)	120	325
Cola drink (12 oz.)	150	Grapefruit juice (6 oz.) with seltzer water (6 oz.)	75	75
Doughnut, jelly	180	Raisins (1 oz.)	107	73
Fudge (1 oz.)	115	Tangerine	40	75
Ice cream (4 oz.)	150	Low-fat yogurt (4 oz.)	75	75
Potato chips, 10	115	Popcorn (1 cup)	50	65

weight control program. Many women find that if they save one part of a meal to be eaten later as a snack, their diet stays intact without their feeling hungry or deprived. Additionally, several "mini-meals" throughout the day supply a steady input of calories that keep your blood sugar level stable and decrease cravings for refined sugars.

Sodium content is a factor that should be taken into consideration when selecting any food or beverage. High sodium intake has been linked to many health problems, including high blood pressure and water retention. While sodium is vital to your body for normal metabolic functions, most people consume far too much. The generally accepted daily intake of sodium is 1,100 to 3,300 milligrams, and the average American consumes two to four times that amount.

The easiest way to reduce sodium intake from snacks is to avoid items such as potato chips, corn chips, and pretzels unless you can find unsalted brands. Many manufacturers have recently introduced no-salt or low-salt items. Watch for the calorie counts on these products, though, since the oil used for frying can make them undesirable for dieters.

While sugar-free and caffeine-free soda solves the calorie and caffeine problems of regular soda, a twelve-ounce can contains about 40 mg. of sodium. Clearly, two or three sodas over the course of an afternoon can shoot your sodium consumption up. Seltzer water or low-sodium club soda mixed with a fruit juice is a more nutritious, energy-boosting drink. Cranberry, orange, and grapefruit juices make particularly tasty mixers and are great thirst quenchers.

Items low in refined sugar, salt, and fat are the ideal for snacks, but there may be times when a candy bar is what you really want. A sensible food plan is one that enables you to eat practically anything within moderation. Constantly denying yourself a piece of candy or a pastry that is truly desired is the most likely way to set up an eating binge. Refined sugars can be included in a normal diet but not in excess. All types of foods can be a part of your eating plan if they are budgeted day by day. But it is important for your health that essential nutrients provided from the basic food groups are not eliminated to allow for the extra calories of "treats."

When selecting snack items throughout your day, the above list can help you make the best choices. It offers suggestions for substituting lower-calorie items for standard snack fare.

Brown-Bagging

There are days when an impending deadline means working through lunch. On those occasions, lunch is generally something sent in from the local fast-food restaurant. When there is not much time for a meal, this does not mean that the quality of your food has to diminish in proportion to the time you have to eat. With a little foresight and a few minutes of preparation time, you can pack a lunch at home and assure yourself of nutritious and tasty food on those "no time for lunch" days.

Brown-bagging has caught on with many busy executive women as a way of ensuring that they will eat well even when demanding schedules leave few options for noontime meals. In fact, the term "brown-bagging" may soon become passé, as manufacturers are now producing elegant lunchboxes that far surpass brown paper bags aesthetically and functionally; many of these lunchboxes have waterproof compartments for salads or other messy foods.

If fast food is a temptation on those hectic days, be aware that you can easily consume over 1,000 calories by downing a cheeseburger, French fries, and a soda. In addition, the fats and sodium in this kind of meal are excessively high and fiber is almost nonexistent. While a coffee-shop sandwich may provide more nutrients, most restaurants use too much mayonnaise for sandwich spreads such as chicken or egg salad. This could be adding hundreds of extra calories to your meal.

Bringing lunch from home must satisfy two criteria for it to be of value to busy working women: it has to be fast, and it has to be uncomplicated. The thought of a brown-bag lunch does not have to be depressing, nor does the food have to be boring, standard lunchbox fare. The following tips will broaden your thoughts about brown-bagging with new ideas for great lunches!

- When making a tossed salad do not add the dressing; wait until you are ready to eat. Dressing added early in the day means a soggy salad by noon.
- Watch salt intake. Substitute herbs, spices, and even low-salt mustards to replace salty condiments.
- Your brown-bag menu should emphasize nutrients and fiber, including items from the four basic food groups to give you an edge on energy for the afternoon.
- Select exotic vegetables and fruits to include in your meals. Liven up your lunch with the vibrant colors and interesting textures and flavors of different foods. Try a kiwi fruit, new varieties of apples, or even slices of papaya for a change. Vegetables like jicama, water chestnuts, and rutabaga add unusual tastes to ordinary salads.
- Leftovers from previous nights' dinners can be combined with whole grains or pastas to make interesting salads or sandwich fillings.
- Use lots of sprouts for garnishes; these are

high in nutrients. Alfalfa and mung bean sprouts are available at most vegetable markets.

- Canned tuna is a good source of protein and easy to prepare for lunch. Purchase water-packed, low-sodium brands for calorie savings and reduced salt intake.

One of the best options for brown-bag lunches is a sandwich. Sandwiches are fast and simple to prepare, can be eaten easily, and the variety is almost endless. Included here are recipes for a week's worth of sandwich fillings that can be used on any kind of bread, though pita bread is recommended. Pita is a Middle Eastern bread with a pocket for the filling. Pita bread is available in whole wheat and with sesame seeds—making it more interesting than the standard two slices of regular bread.

Pita Bread Stuffers

Each of the following pita sandwiches is under 400 calories. Combine them with a piece of fruit for dessert and you have a well-balanced, nutritious lunch.

■ FARMER CHEESE AND VEGETABLES ■

4 ounces farmer cheese or low-fat cottage cheese
¼ cup chopped vegetables (carrots, green pepper, cucumber, cabbage, mushrooms, alfalfa sprouts)

Seasonings to taste: dill, celery seed, pepper
Lettuce leaves

Mix cheese with vegetables and seasonings, place lettuce in pita bread, and stuff pita with filling.

■ TUNA CURRY ■

3 ounces tuna fish (water-packed, low-salt)
¼ apple, chopped
1 tablespoon raisins
1 tablespoon walnuts, chopped
1 teaspoon mayonnaise
¼ teaspoon curry powder
Lettuce leaves

Mix tuna with chopped apple, raisins, walnuts, and mayonnaise. Add curry powder and blend well. Stuff pita with lettuce leaves and tuna mixture.

■ TANGY TOFU SALAD ■

Tofu, or bean curd, is a soybean product high in protein and low in fat and calories. (And it has almost no cholesterol!) It is an extremely versatile food, taking on the flavors of items mixed with it, and can be used in main courses, side dishes, soups, and even desserts. Tofu can be found at most natural foods stores and at many grocery and produce stores.

4 ounces tofu, chopped
¼ cup grated vegetables (carrots, red cabbage, scallions, green pepper)
1 teaspoon lemon juice
2 teaspoons mayonnaise
  Cayenne pepper to taste
  Lettuce leaves
  Alfalfa sprouts for garnish

Mix tofu with vegetables, lemon juice, and mayonnaise. Add cayenne pepper. Place lettuce in pita and stuff with tofu salad.

For an authentic Middle Eastern sandwich, stuff your pita with tabooli. Tabooli is a salad made with bulgur, a parboiled, dried, cracked-wheat grain. High in protein and fiber, tabooli makes a nutritious salad by itself as well as a sandwich filling. Bulgur cooks very quickly—simmer it for fifteen minutes and it is ready. To save time in the morning, make a large amount of bulgur one evening and use it throughout the week. You can purchase packaged bulgur at most grocery stores or buy it in bulk from natural food stores.

▪ TABOOLI ▪

Add 1 cup bulgur to 2 cups of boiling water and simmer until all the liquid is absorbed (about 15 minutes). After draining the cooked bulgur (squeeze out any excess water), add the following ingredients:

¼ cup vegetable oil
¼ cup fresh lemon juice
2 medium tomatoes, finely chopped
1 cup chopped fresh parsley
1 cucumber, peeled and finely chopped
1 bunch scallions, finely chopped
  Freshly ground black pepper to taste

Mix all ingredients with cooked bulgur and chill. Refrigerated, tabooli can be stored for up to two weeks.

▪ TABOOLI AND CHEESE SANDWICH ▪

½ cup prepared tabooli
1 slice cheddar cheese
  Lettuce leaves

Place lettuce leaves and cheese in pita bread and stuff with tabooli.

▪ CHICKEN AND TABOOLI ▪

This is a great way to combine leftovers. Mix tabooli with chicken or another lean meat from a previous night's dinner. Add whatever vegetables are in the refrigerator and you have a tasty, nutrient-rich noon meal.

½ cup prepared tabooli
2 ounces cooked chicken, chopped
  Chopped vegetables, if desired
  Lettuce leaves

Mix tabooli with chicken and vegetables and stuff into pita bread with lettuce.

Eating Out— How to Dine Right at Any Restaurant

The business meal has become standard in the work life of the professional woman. As a tradition of good will and public relations, business lunches and dinners are often the time when deals are closed and agreements confirmed. But while dining out might be beneficial to one's career, it can become a waistline disaster and health problem if restaurant meals become a series of caloric overindulgences.

Restaurant menus are designed to tempt customers, and it is easy to throw caution to the wind and select the special of the day, the house salad dressing, and the chef's pièce de résistance dessert. Once in a while, splurging is fun, an opportunity to enjoy foods that are not a regular part of your daily eating plan. But if you dine out frequently, it's important to follow guidelines for watching weight control, cholesterol level, and fat intake. You must know how to read a menu with an eye to good nutrition.

Extra calories—from the moment you sit down to a restaurant meal you are confronted with foods and beverages packed with unnecessary calories. The bread basket and butter dish are the first items placed on the table and then you are asked for your cocktail order. Within the first five minutes it is possible to consume over 400 calories with one gin and tonic (175 calories) and a buttered roll (235 calories)!

While it is possible to request that the bread basket be removed, it is not the optimal action if you are entertaining business clients. If they want bread and butter, then you are better off practicing some discipline and self-restraint. Your best bet is to select bread items that are lower in calories, and skip the butter or use it sparingly. Compared to the above-mentioned buttered roll, a breadstick (40 calories), RyKrisp (23 calories), or melba toast (18 calories) is a better choice.

In the not so distant past, not ordering an alcoholic beverage was considered a breach in dining-out etiquette, and refusing a celebratory drink somehow put a damper on the party. Fortunately, attitudes have changed and club soda, seltzer water, and mineral waters are popular alternatives to alcohol. Served with a wedge of lime or a lemon twist, these drinks are refreshing, thirst-quenching, and calorie-free.

When you do want an alcoholic drink, consider ordering a wine spritzer. A mixture of white wine and club soda, a six-ounce spritzer has only 50 calories. Even a glass of regular wine (about 100 calories) beats the calories of mixed drinks.

Once you are ready to order your meal, follow these guidelines to help you make the best choices nutritionally and calorically.

- Choose fish, poultry, or veal as an entrée. They have less fat and calories than dark or red meats such as duck, pork, lamb, and beef. While organ meats such as beef liver are a good source of iron, they should not be eaten more than once or twice a week because they are exceptionally high in cholesterol.

- When ordering an entrée, do not hesitate to ask your waiter how the item is prepared. Restaurants frequently list selections with names that really do not describe the cooking method. Simple preparation techniques, such as broiling, boiling, or grilling, usually mean that the entrée will be a calorie saver. Avoid anything that is fried or in a heavy sauce or gravy, as it will add extra fat. For instance, broiled flounder with lemon is 150 calories, while frying will double the calories. If the entrée comes with a sauce, ask that it be left off or served on the side.

- Appetizers are a great way to subdue your hunger and at the same time bypass the bread basket. A selection that will require lots of chewing and takes time to eat is a good choice. For instance, an artichoke is a satisfying, low-calorie start to any meal and is a source of fiber and potassium. Other wise selections are leafy salads and seafood cocktails. Again, order sauces, dressings, or cocktail dips on the side. Soup is another suggestion that can be particularly advantageous for women watching their weight. The length of time it takes to eat soup helps control appetite.

- Be sure to ask how vegetables will be served or you may be confronted with boiled greens drenched in a rich sauce. Request that your vegetables be steamed if possible, and not prepared with butter. Potatoes, contrary to popular belief, are not fattening. It is the oil used in frying or the butter or sour cream added to baked potatoes that makes them high in calories. A plain baked potato is only 90 calories, and a tablespoon of cottage cheese or yogurt can be a healthy substitute for high-fat sour cream.

- There may be times when you are served a meal and no options are offered—for example, at a convention banquet or press conference luncheon. While some of the foods may not be the wisest choices nutritionally, you can make the best of the situation. When you are given an entrée that is fatty or laden with sauce, discreetly remove the fat or skin and scrape the sauce to the side. Also, there is no rule that says you must finish everything on your plate.
- Keep a list of the restaurants you know that cater to special requests or offer entrées suitable for calorie watchers. Put the list on a rolodex card so it is handy when you are asked to suggest a restaurant for a business meeting.

ETHNIC AND SPECIALTY RESTAURANTS

Do you resign yourself to extra calories when dining at an Italian restaurant because of the rich pastas and heavy entrées? Do you flinch at the thought of French food because it will ruin your diet? Does a meal at a Mexican res-

taurant or Chinese food make you hesitate because of the fried specialties, added salt, or MSG? Ethnic restaurants do not have to be diet disasters or an invitation to high blood pressure. It is possible to eat right at a variety of restaurants and enjoy many selections while keeping to a balanced food plan.

Chinese

Chinese restaurants are a good choice for health-conscious diners because just about everything is cooked to order, thereby maximizing freshness and nutrients. But selecting low-calorie menus can be a challenge because so much of Chinese food preparation involves frying. Most chefs will comply with special requests to omit monosodium glutamate, limit soy sauce, and decrease the oil used in stir-frying. When Chinese food is simply prepared, highlighting delicate or spicy flavors, it can provide a satisfying, healthful meal.

Appetizers such as wontons, shrimp toast, dumplings, spare ribs, and egg rolls are the items we so closely identify with Oriental cuisine. While you may be tempted to begin a meal with an assortment of these foods, keep in mind that you can easily consume a large portion of your calorie quota with them. A single fried wonton has over 50 calories, and it is nearly impossible to eat just one. The rest of the above-mentioned items range from 76 calories for a fried dumpling to 140 calories for an egg roll.

Instead of choosing an appetizer, a better

	Best Choice	Second Choice	Avoid
SELECTIONS	Chicken, fish, vegetable dishes	Shellfish, beef	Duck, pork
PREPARATION	Clear chicken broth, garlic, scallions, vegetables, ginger sauce	Brown bean sauce, soy sauce, peanuts	Oyster sauce, sweet and sour sauce, cream sauce
** MENU LISTINGS	Steamed Chicken with Wine (1 cup meat) 315 calories	Chicken with Chinese Vegetables (1 cup meat) 675 calories	Sweet and Sour Chicken (1¼ cup meat) 1163 calories
	Steamed Fish with Ginger (1 lb. fish) 376 calories	Shrimp with Black Bean Sauce (1 cup shrimp) 465 calories	Shrimp in Lobster Sauce (12 shrimp) 1286 calories
	Beef with Mushrooms (8 oz. beef) 567 calories	Beef with green pepper/ mushrooms/pea pods/ sauce) (8 oz. beef) 907 calories	Beef Lo Mein (with oyster sauce) (8 oz. beef, 1 cup noodles) 1095 calories

*Charts courtesy of International Paper Company's Health Fitness Center.
**Menu listings and calorie values reprinted by permission of the Berkeley Publishing Group from *The Complete Calorie Counter for Dining Out* by K. F. Ernst. Copyright 1981 by K. F. Ernst.

bet would be to order a lower calorie soup (and request that the crispy fried soup noodles not be brought to the table). Bean curd soup is the best choice at only 40 calories for an average bowl. Egg drop and wonton soup with soft, not fried, noodles are both under 100 calories. Many of the thicker soups, such as hot and sour, are over 200 calories because of the cornstarch that is used liberally as a thickener.

When ordering an entrée, your wisest choice nutritionally and calorically is a chicken or fish dish that is prepared with a minimum of oil. Skip the sweet and sour sauces or you will add nearly 750 extra calories to one portion. Recommended entrées include those that are prepared with vegetables—for instance, sliced chicken and broccoli, shrimp with water chestnuts, or steamed fish with black beans. If you prefer your food spicy, request that hot peppers or a small amount of Szechuan hot oil be added to the dish.

Fried rice should be avoided unless you are looking for the fastest way to add extra calories to your diet. Fried rice has over twice as many calories as its boiled counterpart and is laden with MSG, soy sauce, and salt. One-half cup of white rice is 100 calories and provides a nice balance to fiery entrées. If you have the option of substituting brown rice for white rice, you will be getting a generous supply of B vitamins, which dehulled white rice lacks.

Exotic vegetables are one of the special treats of Oriental cooking. Bok choy, pea pods, Chinese cabbage, straw mushrooms, and bamboo shoots comprise the vegetarian dish "Buddha's Delight," a low-calorie, high-fiber entrée. For added protein, request that slices of bean curd be mixed with the vegetables.

Desserts are usually limited to fruit or ice cream. While one scoop of ice cream is a reasonable 150 calories, dieters would do better to choose the fruit and a fortune cookie (only 30 calories each!)

French

The French coined the term <u>haute cuisine</u>, and their food ranks among the best of gourmet offerings. Its delicacy and presentation are hard to surpass, and a meal at a French restaurant promises to be something special. Unfortunately, it is the sauces—hollandaise, béarnaise, and béchamel, to mention a few—that create high-calorie, high-fat dishes. When served without butter, cream, or mayonnaise-based sauces, the basics of French cooking—fish, veal, chicken, and vegetables—are wise diet choices.

Salads are a wonderful start or finish to any French meal. Several salads are usually listed on the menu, offering a choice of interesting greens and vegetables. Endive, for example, is a type of chicory with long, whitish leaves and a thicker texture than most salad lettuces. Low in calories and a good source of vitamin A, endive is often paired with watercress, and together they make a nutrient-rich and visually pleasing first course.

Appetizers at French restaurants are varied and range from low-calorie items such as consommé and broiled grapefruit to selections such as pâté and rich onion soup with bread and melted cheese that should not be ordered regularly. Liver pâtés are very high in fat and cholesterol and not recommended for dieters. Vegetable pâtés, although made with cream and butter, are a better choice. They have a texture similar to liver pâté but contain less fat.

Quiche lorraine is a French specialty that

FRENCH

	Best Choice	Second Choice	Avoid
SELECTIONS	Veal, fish, chicken, frog legs	Shellfish, lamb, ham, pork	Brains, liver, duck, goose
PREPARATION	Tomato sauce, mushrooms, garlic, vegetables, brown sauce, grapes	Cheese, butter, almonds, cherry or orange sauce, breaded	Cream sauce, hollandaise, bacon
MENU LISTINGS	Truite (trout) au Vin Blanc (in white wine) (6 oz.) 495 calories	Truite (trout) au Bleu (boiled, vinegar/butter) (6 oz.) 636 calories	Truite (trout) au Hollandaise (6 oz.) 902 calories
	Veau (veal) Fricadelles de Niçoise (tomato/onion/ brown sauce) (7 oz.) 614 calories	Veau (veal) Escalope de Anglaise (breaded/parsley/ lemon/butter sauce) (7 oz.) 706 calories	Veau (veal), Côtes de, aux Herbes de Provence (with herbs/hollandaise sauce) (2 small chops) 863 calories

has become a favorite of Americans. A pie made with a filling of eggs, cream, cheese, and bacon, quiche is not the best selection for anyone on a strict weight control diet. But an appetizer-size portion of quiche with a salad could be a reasonable lunch choice.

The safest guideline to follow when ordering a meal is to request that sauces be served on the side. This means everything from a la carte vegetables to entrées featuring cream or fruit sauces. Do not hesitate to ask for details on the preparation of menu listings. Poultry, veal, and seafood items are low in calories when they are prepared simply—i.e., broiled, poached, or cooked in a light wine or tomato-based sauce. Entrées such as Sole Véronique (sautéed with grapes), Truite Amandine (trout with slivered almonds), or poached salmon with vegetables are delicious meals that won't sabotage weight control. Even rack of lamb is acceptable if it is trimmed of all fat before roasting.

Choices that are particularly unwise include duck, because it is very fatty and is frequently glazed with a sweet sauce that makes it a double disaster. Sweetbreads should also be avoided, as they are extremely high in cholesterol and often prepared with cream.

While chocolate mousse at over 400 calories a portion is better left unordered, the French are masters at creating wonderful fresh fruit desserts that can be guilt-free choices. Poached pears or sliced fruit with a light dousing of Cointreau or Grand Marnier are delicious, satisfying, and low-calorie.

Contrary to popular belief, Italian food does not have to present a dieter's dilemma. In fact, the staples of this cuisine are actually the elements of any sensible food plan—plain pasta, vegetables, chicken, veal, and fish. The problem arises when rich sauces, heavy creams, and butter are added. Generally, Southern Italian-style cooking is heavier than Northern Italian. The Southern specialties frequently use sausage and beef and include parmigiana preparations that are made with rich tomato sauce, breading, and cheese. Northern dishes emphasize lighter fare such as primavera (vegetable) sauces for pasta and delicately prepared entrées with lemon sauces or oil-free marinara (spicy tomato-based) sauce.

One of the hardest temptations to resist at any Italian restaurant is the delicious crusty bread. If you cannot restrain yourself to one slice with just a light spread of butter, immediately order an appetizer to take the edge off your hunger. Salad with dressing on the side, melon (request it without prosciutto), or steamed mussels are low-calorie yet satisfying foods to start your meal.

Attitudes toward pasta mirror the misconception many people have about potatoes. Pasta and potatoes are not high-calorie foods —they only become fattening when butter, oil, or cream is added. One cup of plain spaghetti has just 155 calories and almost no fat. When prepared with a light tomato sauce or a sprinkling of Parmesan cheese, calories are kept to a minimum without sacrificing taste.

Another Italian favorite is risotto, a special

	Best Choice	*Second Choice*	*Avoid*
SELECTIONS	Chicken, fish, veal, pasta	Shellfish, pasta	Beef, sausage, pork
PREPARATION	Wine, tomato, mushrooms, onions, lemon, broiled, marinara, primavera	Butter, oil, breaded	Parmigiana, meat sauce, cream sauce, anchovies, fried dishes
MENU LISTINGS	Baked Chicken (with prosciutto/garlic/wine) (8 oz. with bone) 460 calories	Sautéed Chicken (with butter/wine/floured) (8 oz. with bone) 575 calories	Chicken Parmigiana, (breaded chicken with mozzarella/tomato sauce) (8 oz. with bone) 1012 calories
	Shrimp Marinara (6 shrimp) 240 calories	Shrimp Scampi (oil/garlic) (6 shrimp) 293 calories	Shrimp Parmigiana (mozzarella, tomato sauce) (6 shrimp) 469 calories
	Linguini with Red Clam Sauce (2 cups pasta) 589 calories	Linguini with White Clam Sauce (2 cups pasta) 708 calories	Fettuccine Alfredo (cream/butter/Parmesan) (2 cups pasta) 786 calories

Milanese rice dish. While plain rice works well in a diet, risotto is made with substantial amounts of butter and Parmesan cheese. Parmesan cheese is very high in sodium, and the combination of high salt and high calories makes risotto a less than preferred choice.

Entrées such as veal piccata, chicken Marsala, and fish marinara-style reflect the subtlety of finely prepared Italian food and are good selections for diet-conscious women. If these dishes are accompanied by fried vegetables (fried zucchini is popular), request that a more simply prepared vegetable be substituted if possible. When no substitutions are allowed, let the vegetable be served with your meal only if you can limit yourself to one or two bites. Otherwise, tell your waiter to hold the vegetable and order a salad instead.

Italian desserts are renowned, but they are best refused because the pastries, cheesecakes, and cream desserts are high in calories, sugar, and fat. Fresh fruits served without a cream topping are a lighter, healthier way to conclude your meal. But if your resolve falters, share a rich dessert rather than eating the entire portion yourself. The best alternative, however, is a cup of cappuccino—espresso served with steamed milk and topped with a dusting of cinnamon (many restaurants offer decaffeinated cappuccino).

Japanese

Japanese food is the ultimate for healthful, low-calorie restaurant dining. The preparation style, often focusing on raw fish and fresh vegetables, makes selecting items for a meal an easy task. There is also a variety of good choices in cooked foods for diners who have not acquired a taste for raw fish.

The best start to a Japanese meal is soup. Clear soup with scallions or miso (a product derived from soybeans) soup is only about 50 calories for a one-cup serving. Other possibilities are cucumber salads served with a light lemon sauce or bean curd and seaweed,

	Best Choice	Second Choice	Avoid
SELECTIONS	Raw fish (squid, tuna, octopus, bass, shrimp), cooked fish	Chicken, beef	Pork, duck
PREPARATION	Sushi and sashimi preparation, grilled	Soy sauce, baked, grilled, fried tempura-style	Sukiyaki
MENU LISTINGS	Assorted Raw Fish (4 oz.) 120 calories	Shrimp Tempura (3 large shrimp) 315 calories	Butanabe (pork casserole) (8 oz. pork) 900 calories
	Grilled Tuna (4 oz.) 178 calories	Chicken Teriyaki (4 oz.) 389 calories	Sukiyaki Beef (8 oz. beef) 849 calories

which is very low in calories and high in nutrients. Vegetables served with a ginger sauce are also a sensible and tasty choice, but make sure that the vegetables (usually eggplant, spinach, or squash) are broiled or lightly steamed. Some restaurants tend to sauté vegetables in excessive amounts of oil, making them an undesirable selection.

Sushi and sashimi are the mainstay of most Japanese restaurants. Sushi is raw fish, vegetables, or an egg mixture placed on vinegared rice or wrapped in seaweed and rice. Sashimi consists of slices of raw fish usually accompanied by white rice. Both sushi and sashimi are excellent low-calorie sources of protein. Four ounces of sashimi is about 120 calories (without rice), and an average serving of sushi is 400 calories. Raw fish is always served with a garnish of fresh sliced ginger, and hot mustard and soy sauce on the side for making a dipping mixture. While the calories in the soy sauce are negligible, the high salt content of this condiment should limit its use.

In cooked foods, Japanese specialties include fish soup casseroles (yosenabe), lightly batter-fried vegetables and shrimp (tempura), and beef and chicken dishes (sukiyaki, which is sautéd, and teriyaki, which is grilled). The soup casseroles tend to be the lowest in cal-

ories because there is very little fat. Tempura when prepared well should not be greasy, because it is fried quickly and drained well. But if you are counting calories, it is better to skip fried foods completely. Sukiyaki and teriyaki recipes both use ample amounts of soy sauce, and sukiyaki generally includes suet and monosodium glutamate. You can request that these ingredients be reduced. An eight-ounce portion of sukiyaki beef is over 800 calories, making it a poor choice for the dieter; the same size portion of beef teriyaki is a better selection at about 400 calories.

Desserts are not a problem at most Japanese restaurants. Fresh sliced pineapple and melon wedges are popular offerings and a good ending to lunch or dinner. Do try to refuse the plum wine that is frequently offered at the end of a meal to diners compliments of the management. It is the calorie equivalent of a sweet liqueur, and several sips will add an extra 100 calories.

Mexican

Eating out at a Mexican restaurant does not have to constitute the demise of a sensible food plan. If visions of tacos and enchiladas make you think you have to discard notions of good nutrition, then it is time to put these fears to rest. The basic foods of Mexican cooking—chicken, corn, beans, and tomatoes—are not a dieter's downfall. Rather, it is the frying that adds fat and calories, plus the addition of sausage and lots of cheese to many dishes.

Immediately after you sit down at the table, the first matter at hand is deciding what to drink. A beverage other than water is usually essential to counteract the effects of the fiery jalapeño peppers and hot chilis. Club soda or seltzer with lemon or lime will cool your palate without adding any calories. If you want to indulge in an alcoholic drink, you might try such Mexican favorites as a margarita (tequila/Triple Sec/lime), piña colada (rum, cream of coconut, pineapple juice), or sangria (red wine/brandy/Curaçao/lemon/orange juice/sugar/sliced fruit). Calorically, the best choice is sangria, with 150 calories per four-ounce glass compared to 255 calories for a piña colada and 215 calories for a margarita. Margaritas are generally served with a coating of salt on the rim of the glass. Order yours without the salt!

MEXICAN

	Best Choice	Second Choice	Avoid
SELECTIONS	Chicken, vegetable, or bean dishes	Cheese	Beef
PREPARATION	Onion, sherry, garlic, tomato, pepper	Butter, cheese, chili sauce	Oil, sour cream, chocolate, nuts
MENU LISTINGS	Pollo en Salsa Verde—chicken in green sauce (green tomatoes/chilis/onion/garlic/coriander/sherry) (8 oz. with bone) 486 calories	Chicken in red chili sauce (chilis/onion/garlic/stock) (8 oz. with bone) 552 calories	Mole Verde—chicken in green chili sauce (green tomatoes/green peppers/onion/pumpkin seeds/coriander/oil) (8 oz. with bone) 711 calories
	Taco (chicken with chilis/onion/tomato/lettuce) 175 calories	Taco (cheese with chilis/sour cream/tomato/lettuce) 188 calories	Taco (beef with cheese/onions/lettuce) 231 calories
	Tostadas (chicken with onion/tomato/lettuce/chili sauce) 264 calories	Tostadas (chicken with guacamole/lettuce/tomato sauce) 310 calories	Tostadas (beef with refried beans/chilis/lettuce/tomato/sour cream) 458 calories

Crisp-fried tortilla chips with chili dip are usually provided as an appetizer compliments of the restaurant. At 11 calories per chip, a handful can easily add up to over a hundred calories in no time. While the chili dip is reasonably low-cal, the other favorite dip, guacamole (a mixture of avocado, tomato, onion, chilis, lemon, garlic, and oil), is about 170 calories per one half cup. Avocado is a rich source of vitamin A and potassium but is high in oil (and fat), making it an unwise choice for dieters. Better selections for appetizers include tossed salad, bean salad in a vinegar marinade, or seviche (marinated fish).

Tacos, enchiladas, burritos, and tostados all use tortillas made of corn or wheat flour as the base for various fillings. A taco is a fried corn tortilla shaped into a shell and stuffed with ground beef, chicken, cheese, or refried beans and sour cream. The chicken taco is the best choice, as it is the lowest in fat and calories (about 175). Enchiladas are soft tortillas rolled around one of the above mixtures, while tostados are fried flat tortillas upon which toppings are placed. Burritos are wheat tortillas that are rolled around a filling, sometimes fried and served with hot sauce. To reduce fat and calories, the unfried tortillas are the best selections. Sausage fillings should be avoided as well as thick layers of melted cheese. Sour cream is best scraped to the side if you are dieting.

Other possibilities for entrées include a variety of chicken and fish dishes prepared in a green sauce (green tomatoes, chilis, garlic, and onions). These range from 300 to 500 calories per serving. It is best to avoid fried beef and foods prepared in a sour cream or sweet sauce.

A staple of most Mexican cooking is refried beans and rice, and they accompany many entrées. Moderate amounts of beans and rice can be included in a sensible eating plan, but restaurant portions tend to be huge. The refried beans should certainly be limited because the additional frying makes them about 170 calories per half-cup. You can order plain beans as an alternative.

Desserts at most Mexican restaurants are usually very sweet or fried and are best bypassed. If slices of fresh mango or papaya are available, they make a wiser choice to complete your meal.

Seafood and Steak Houses

Seafood and steak restaurants can be safe choices when entertaining business associates because generally there are no surprises. You know that the menu will be predominantly fish or beef with a chicken entrée to satisfy those who do not eat red meat or who dislike seafood. The challenge is to select an entrée that will not be too high in fat or cholesterol. It is also important to take into consideration portion size, as ample quantities tend to be characteristic of these restaurants.

Appetizers at fish and steak restaurants provide a wide range of options. Low-calorie pos-

	Best Choice	Second Choice	Avoid
SELECTIONS	Halibut, whitefish, flounder, swordfish, bluefish	Scallops, shrimp, mackerel, snapper, salmon, sardines	Lobster, breaded or frozen seafood
PREPARATION	White wine, lemon, smoked, stewed, broiled, baked	Butter, breaded	Deep-fried, cream sauces
MENU LISTINGS	Whitefish (smoked) (6 oz.) 260 calories	Snapper (broiled or baked with butter) (6 oz.) 398 calories	Sole (fried) (6 oz.) 441 calories
	Flounder (filet) (broiled or baked in white wine) (6 oz.) 242 calories	Mackerel (filet) (broiled with butter) (6 oz.) 402 calories	Lobster Newburg (butter/egg yolk/sherry/cream) (1½ cups) 728 calories
	Steamed Scallops (7 large) 224 calories	Scallops (breaded/broiled) (7 large) 413 calories	Fried Scallops (7 large) 595 calories

sibilities (under 100 calories) include melon, a seafood cocktail, or consummé. Cream soups and bisques should be avoided, as they are over 250 calories per serving. While six oysters on the half shell are a very reasonable 90 calories, when they are prepared with butter, bacon, cheese, and bread crumbs as in Oysters Rockefeller they are nearly 600 calories!

A tossed salad is a good start to any meal —it is high in fiber, low in calories, and rich in nutrients. Beware, though, of the temptation to overindulge at salad bars, which are popular at many seafood and steak restaurants. The array of items offered can be overwhelming, and there is a tendency to sample a bit of everything. Skip the mayonnaise-based salads and stick with lettuce and vegetables. Also, choose a light vinaigrette instead of a thick creamy dressing.

Fresh fish is the perfect choice for health-conscious and weight-conscious diners. It is very low in calories and fat and is an excellent source of protein. Preferred methods of preparation are broiled (without butter!), baked, or poached using wine, lemon, or spices. Frying nearly doubles the calories of any fish, and tartar sauce adds an extra 75 calories per tablespoon. While shellfish is a bargain calorically, it is extremely high in cholesterol. For example, eight ounces of lobster is only 200 calories but it has 450 mg. of cholesterol, compared to 100 mg. for eight ounces of most fresh fish. Additionally, shellfish have a high iodine content, which many women find contributes to skin problems.

The key to selecting a beef entrée is to look for a lean cut that has no visible fat, such as London broil. Large amounts of marbled fat make many cuts of beef tender, but they also make them high in calories. While a T-bone steak may "melt in your mouth," a less tender cut that has been marinated to reduce toughness is a better choice. If you do select a cut of meat with visible fat, carefully trim it. When ordering your entrée, select a smaller portion—the four-ounce filet mignon, for example, instead of the restaurant's ten-ounce strip sirloin luncheon special. You will save calories, reduce your fat intake, and not return to your office feeling that you have overeaten.

	BEEF		
	Best Choice	**Second Choice**	**Avoid**
SELECTIONS	Lean cuts	Top or bottom round, flank, sirloin tip	Organ meats, cuts with visible fat, T-bone
PREPARATION	Grilled	Broiled	Roasted
MENU LISTINGS	London Broil (8 oz.) 445 calories	Porterhouse (lean) (8 oz.) 506 calories	Porterhouse (with fat) (8 oz.) 1054 calories
	Filet Mignon (8 oz.) 468 calories	Rib Steak (lean) (8 oz.) 565 calories	Sirloin (with fat) (8 oz.) 878 calories
	Sirloin (lean) (8 oz.) 470 calories	Rib Roast (lean) (8 oz.) 547 calories	Rib Roast (with fat) (8 oz.) 998 calories

Cottage or French fries and onion rings often accompany steak orders. If possible request a baked potato and forgo the onion rings for an unfried green vegetable. Again, the less oil you consume the better your diet and your health. Rice is usually served with fish, and along with a vegetable it provides a well-balanced meal.

Fresh fruit is the optimal choice for dessert, but in most seafood and steak restaurants you can be tempted by an array of cakes, pies, and cheesecake. Portions are generally huge, and a slice of one of these desserts could easily total over 400 calories. If temptation wins, request extra forks and "persuade" your dining companions to help you out.

CHAPTER EIGHT

At-Home Dining

It is 6:30 P.M., you have just gotten home, and you are tired and hungry. Sound familiar? The first matter at hand is what to eat for dinner that won't require hours of preparation in the kitchen. Are there options for meals that can be quick, easy, and nutritious? Indeed there are. Whether you are taking charge of dinner for a family or just for yourself there are lots of short-cuts, time-savers, and fast-cooking entrées that can be used to create a well-balanced meal and make your life easier.

Today's working woman has a number of possibilities to consider for the final meal of the day. Eating out is one alternative that solves the question of preparation. But after a long day at the office, you may opt for heading home, kicking off your shoes, and relaxing over a meal in your own kitchen. It may also be the more practical and economical choice if there is a family to be fed.

The most reasonable solution to dinner at home is a meal that can be put on the table in less than thirty minutes. Just by knowing that it will not be hours before you eat, it is possible to muster the energy to create a well-balanced meal that is both tasty and nutritious. And many women find that preparing dinner is a relaxing way to relieve the pressures that build up over the workday.

Meals at home can be accomplished in one of three ways—cooking from scratch, using canned or frozen foods, or purchasing take-out items from specialty stores. Each option provides specific advantages. Take-outs are convenient, though they can be costly.

Frozen foods are easy, but often high in sodium and saturated fat. Doing the cooking yourself means a little more foresight in planning a menu, but it can be the least costly and you can create reduced-calorie and low-salt menus of your choosing.

The secret to cooking quick meals is organization and planning. Use these tips suggested by the New York Heart Association in their Culinary Hearts Kitchen Course on how to make meals in a hurry:

Consider your budget.

In many recipes, chicken or turkey cutlets can be substituted for veal to save food dollars. Meatless dishes are also an excellent choice to reduce meal costs. When combined properly, vegetable proteins will provide the protein equivalent of animal foods.

Consider food preferences.

It is important to experiment with new tastes and new food combinations, but if you dislike tofu or your children will not eat broccoli, then limit recipe experimentation to foods that are appealing.

Modify recipes.

Review your favorite recipes to determine what changes can be made to reduce preparation and cooking times.

Stock required ingredients.

Read recipes thoroughly before beginning your preparation. Develop a list of ingredients that you use frequently and stock them in your pantry for quick meal preparation.

Saving Time

The woman of the eighties has an unprecedented array of kitchen equipment that can reduce the time involved in meal preparation. It is important to be familiar with your appliances so you can use them to their fullest capacity. While many gadgets are useful, take into consideration the time it will take to clean them. If you are using a food processor for one slicing task, it will probably take more time to clean it than to slice the food yourself. Weigh the labor-saving time of the appliance against its clean-up time.

Many kitchen tasks can be done in advance, reducing preparation and cooking time. Here's how:

1. Decide which part of your recipes can be prepared in advance.
2. Vegetables and fruits can be cleaned, dried, and bagged in advance of cooking, but they should not be cut. Nutrients are lost once produce is cut and not eaten immediately.
3. Whole grains such as brown rice, barley, or bulgur can be prepared in large quantities, refrigerated, and used throughout the week. Simply portion out the necessary

DINNER #1

Spinach Salad
Veal Piccata
Boiled Red Potatoes
Broccoli Spears
Fresh Strawberries

amount each evening and reheat.

4. Meats and poultry can be thinly sliced in advance for skillet and stir-fry cooking. Partially freeze chicken and beef to make slicing easier. Roasts can be cut into smaller quantities for faster cooking.

5. Prepare your own frozen dinners. Freeze single portions of entrées and vegetables in aluminum trays and you will have home-cooked meals that only need to be oven-warmed.

One of the most valuable techniques for quick preparation is stir-frying. It is a fast cooking method that uses a minimum amount of hot oil to cook foods in just minutes. Ingredients are sliced or diced and then tossed vigorously and continuously in a heavy skillet or large wok. The hot oil seals in the juices and preserves color, texture, and flavor. Each ingredient has its own cooking time, so tougher items are added first and more tender foods added at the end.

The following menus provide you with a week's worth of dinners that can be prepared in under thirty minutes. The recipe for each meal's entrée is included.

▪ VEAL PICCATA ▪

Serves 4
Calories per serving: 275

8 thin slices of veal (about ¾ pound)
  Salt and pepper to taste
2 tablespoons margarine
¼ cup fresh lemon juice
¼ cup chopped fresh parsley

1. Lightly pound pieces of veal between two sheets of wax paper or foil with the flat side of a meat pounder, cleaver, or large knife.
2. Sprinkle veal with salt and pepper.
3. In a large skillet, melt the margarine. Sauté the veal for 20 to 30 seconds over high heat. Turn and cook for an additional 15 seconds. Remove veal from skillet and place on a warm platter.
4. Add lemon juice and parsley to skillet. Heat and pour sauce over veal.

DINNER #2

Tossed Green Salad
Eggplant Parmigiana
Spinach Noodles
Fresh Pears

DINNER #3

Lettuce Wedges
Broiled Fish with Dill and Scallion Sauce
Steamed Carrots
Fresh Orange Slices

▪ EGGPLANT PARMIGIANA ▪

Serves 4
Calories per serving: 265

2 small eggplants (about 1 pound total)
8 ounces prepared tomato sauce with herbs
    (purchase natural brands without added
    sugar, starch, or preservatives)
6 ounces low-fat mozzarella cheese, thinly
    sliced
3 tablespoons grated Parmesan cheese

1. Trim ends from eggplant and cut into 1½-inch
   slices.
2. Broil eggplant slices on both sides until brown.
3. Remove eggplant from broiler and place in
   baking dish. Cover with tomato sauce, top with
   slices of mozzarella cheese, and sprinkle with
   Parmesan.
4. Bake at 350 degrees for 15 minutes.

▪ BROILED FISH WITH DILL AND SCALLION SAUCE ▪

Serves 4
Calories per serving: 275

4 fish filets (flounder, sole, or turbot), each about
    ⅓ to ½ pound
2 tablespoons margarine
2 tablespoons lemon juice
1 tablespoon chopped fresh dill
1 tablespoon chopped scallions
¼ teaspoon black pepper

1. Preheat the broiler to high.
2. In a small saucepan, melt margarine and add
   lemon juice, dill, scallions, and pepper.
3. Arrange filets in a broiling pan and brush with
   lemon, margarine, and herb sauce.
4. Broil fish about 3 inches from heat source for 5
   to 8 minutes, depending on thickness of fish.
   Baste once.

DINNER #4

Raw Vegetables with Vinaigrette Dressing
Linguine with Clam Sauce
Green Beans and Mushrooms
Cheese and Apples

DINNER #5

Sliced Tomatoes
Oriental Chicken with Vegetables
Rice with Sliced Almonds
Sliced Fresh Peaches

▪ LINGUINE WITH CLAM SAUCE ▪

Serves 4
Calories per serving: 365

2	tablespoons margarine
1	small clove garlic, finely chopped
1	tablespoon flour
1	cup clam juice
¼	cup chopped fresh parsley
	Pepper to taste
½	teaspoon dried thyme
1½	cups minced clams, fresh or canned
1	pound linguine, cooked and drained

1. In a saucepan, melt the margarine, Add garlic and cook for 1 minute over moderate heat. Stir in the flour and cook for 2 minutes, stirring constantly. Add the clam juice and stir until thickened.
2. Add the parsley, pepper, and thyme. Simmer gently for 10 minutes, stirring occasionally. Add minced clams and cook only until clams are heated.
3. Serve over linguine.

▪ ORIENTAL CHICKEN WITH VEGETABLES ▪

Serves 4
Calories per serving: 260

1	pound boneless chicken
2	tablespoons vegetable oil
½	cup shredded red cabbage
2	cups chopped broccoli
1	cup sliced mushrooms
1	cup snow pea pods
	¼-inch slice of ginger root
2	tablespoons soy sauce (sodium-reduced soy sauce can be used if desired)
½	teaspoon pepper
1	teaspoon cornstarch

1. Cut chicken into 2-inch slices. Set aside.
2. Heat 1 tablespoon of the oil in skillet or wok. Add cabbage and broccoli and ¼ cup water. Stir-fry for 2 minutes.
3. Add mushrooms and pea pods and stir-fry for 1 minute.
4. Put vegetables in a bowl and set aside.
5. Add remaining oil to skillet, add ginger, and stir. Add chicken and stir-fry for 4–5 minutes. Add soy sauce and pepper.
6. Combine vegetables with chicken mixture and add cornstarch dissolved in 1 teaspoon of water. Simmer for 1 minute. Serve with rice.

Frozen Foods

On evenings when convenience is the priority or you are eating alone and do not feel like cooking, frozen foods can be the answer. The days of frozen products emphasizing foods that were heavy, fatty, and salty are past. No longer are you restricted to a limited choice of greasy fried chicken or entrées laden with soupy gravy and accompanied by soggy French fries. Frozen food manufacturers have responded to consumer demand for high-quality convenience products and developed lighter, more nutritious, and more flavorful fare.

Everything from appetizers and entrées to side dishes and desserts are now available at grocery stores throughout the country. Frozen foods are not only an acceptable alternative to cooking, but they can even be more nutritious in certain instances. For example, some vitamins in vegetables have a natural tendency to deteriorate when exposed to light or heat. A quick-frozen vegetable that is kept in the freezer until cooking may be more nutritious than a fresh vegetable that has been shipped, stored in a supermarket bin, and then refrigerated at home for a few days before cooking.

Quality frozen dinners—or "gourmet frozen meals," as manufacturers like to refer to them —have been marketed toward people who do not have the time to cook fancy meals. The entrées include such specialties as chicken Cordon Bleu, sirloin tips with mushroom gravy, lobster Newburg, and beef Stroganoff, to mention a few. Weight-conscious consumers have also been targeted with single-serving entrées that are under 300 calories and full-course dinners that range from 300 to 500 calories. Lean cuts of beef, chicken, and filets of fish are combined with special low-fat sauces and seasonings to create main courses that are appetizing and filling without being high in calories.

It is important, though, to check the package for sodium content, because it may be higher than desirable. Cholesterol content is also listed for many of the frozen dinners, thus making it helpful for individuals who are modifying their dietary intake of cholesterol.

Many frozen food manufacturers have replaced the tin trays of their products with containers that can be used in microwave ovens. This is an added convenience factor for women who do not want to wait the requisite forty-five minutes to cook frozen dinners.

Take-Out Foods

One of the easiest ways to cope with dinner is to bring it home with you. Throughout the country, specialized gourmet shops are catering to customers who want precooked entrées to take out. These prepared foods can range from simple fare such as broiled chicken and meatloaf to fancier items like pasta with pesto sauce and stuffed veal. Generally, you can expect to pay premium prices for these foods (pastas can range from four to six dollars a pound, while some seafood items can hit a high of twenty dollars a pound), but ingredients are usually top quality.

The main concern with take-out foods is the unknown quantity of butter, oil, and salt used in the preparation. If your diet requires low-salt or reduced-calorie menus, the gourmet shops may not be for you. Some stores, however, will cater to special requests. Regular customers are cultivated by many of the gourmet shops, and it is in their best interest to satisfy you. For example, they might prepare a pasta sauce with less oil and salt on request or create a dessert with reduced sugar.

Both frozen foods and take-out specialties can be integrated into a well-balanced diet. It is important to incorporate additional items from the four basic food groups with these convenience products to ensure that a meal provides maximum nutrients and fiber. Include a tossed salad and some whole grain bread to your prepared entrée and you have a quick, easy, and nutritious dinner.

Traveling— Meals in the Air and Out of Town

Eating right during business trips can be a challenge to even the most experienced traveler. Skipped breakfasts, too many elaborate meals, and the problem of where to eat dinner confront many women when they are in a new city on business. When you include the issue of airline meals, your concern with eating well actually starts before you arrive at your destination. Business travel does not have to mean that good nutrition must be sacrificed while you are away. With minimal planning and a little foresight you can guarantee that the meals you eat will be well balanced, nutritious, and satisfying.

In the Air

If you are an airplane traveler who stocks up on candy bars before departure to be sure you will have something satisfying to eat in-flight, your days of chocolates and nut rolls as substitute meals may be over. As one airline spokesperson said, "The passenger has never had it so good." Meal options for travelers are more extensive than ever, and the variety of selections is bound to please even the most particular passenger.

In addition to their regular meals and snacks, special meals are now available on nearly all major airlines. The offerings are extensive—from low-calorie, low-carbohydrate, and low-cholesterol to diabetic, vegetarian, and kosher. Some airlines also have menus featuring seafood, salad, or sandwich items that can be ordered as an alternative to the regular fare.

Many of the special meals are more appealing to travelers who prefer a lighter selection and want to avoid the extra calories that are found in some meat entrées, sauces, and pastry desserts of the standard menus. While all the airlines strive for well-balanced meals that include the four basic food groups, frequently more fresh vegetables, fruits, and whole grains are used in the special menus. Additionally, when fewer processed foods are a part of your meal, sodium intake is reduced.

Airlines are making every effort to cater to passengers' special needs and have enlisted the services of dieticians to ensure that particular dietary requirements can be satisfied. If you want a special meal for reasons of health, religion, or personal preference, all you have to do is let the airline know your needs when you make your reservation. Each airline differs on the amount of advance notice it requires —anywhere from six to thirty-six hours. It is also recommended that you reconfirm your order prior to the flight.

The following list provides a sample of the variety of special meals offered by several domestic and international airlines.

AMERICAN AIRLINES

Dietary meals are available on breakfast, brunch, lunch, dinner, and snack flights. The minimum notice required for specially ordered meals is six hours. Kosher lunch or dinner requires twelve hours notice. Selections include:

Bland-soft
Diabetic
Kosher
Low-calorie
Low-carbohydrate
Low-cholesterol
Low-sodium
Vegetarian (lacto-ovo or strict)

A special American Traveler Menu is also available on brunch, lunch, and dinner flights in place of regular meals. Selections include:

Chef's salad
Fruit salad
Quiche
Seafood platter
Seafood cassolette
Roast beef and Swiss cheese sandwiches
Reuben Sandwich
Hamburger

KLM ROYAL DUTCH AIRLINES

Dietary meals are available on transatlantic and long-haul flights for breakfast, lunch, and dinner. Requests for special meals must be made not later than thirty-six hours before departure. Selections include:

Child's meal
Diabetic
Gluten-free
Hindu

Kosher
Liquid
Low-calorie
Low-cholesterol
Low-fat
Low-protein
Moslem
No-salt
Seafood
Semi-fluid
Vegetarian

TRANS WORLD AIRLINES

Dietary meals are available on breakfast, lunch, dinner, and snack flights. Special meals must be ordered twenty-four hours in advance. Selections include:

Child's meal (lunch and dinner only)
Cold seafood (lunch and dinner only)
Low-calorie
Low-carbohydrate
Low-cholesterol
Low-sodium
Hindu
Kosher
Moslem
Vegetarian

UNITED AIRLINES

Dietary meals are offered for all meal flights, but must be ordered at least twenty-four hours in advance. Selections include:
Bland
Child's meal

Diabetic
Fruit plate
Hypoglycemic
Kosher
Low-calorie
Low-cholesterol
Low-fat
Low-sodium
Vegetarian

Even though most airline meals offer moderate portions of entrées, side dishes, and desserts, an average coach-class meal can total about 800 calories. Women who want to ensure they won't be tempted by sugary desserts or extra fats will find that the special reduced-calorie meals will suit their needs, as they range from 290 to 425 calories (varying from airline to airline). It is interesting to note that the strict vegetarian or low-sodium meals served by some airlines can actually be lower in calories than the low-cal meal. For example, one airline's reduced-calorie menu consisting of chicken with lemon, broccoli, tomato and lettuce, melba toast, and fresh fruit is 429 calories. This airline's low-sodium meal of chicken with cranberry glaze, cauliflower and green beans, tomato wedges, and fresh fruit totals 331 calories, while the vegetarian meal, which includes a stuffed pepper, salad, crackers, and fruit, is 359 calories.

All airlines offer a range of beverages— soda, juice, coffee, tea, and club soda as well as wines and liquors. Certain liquids have a particular effect on the body which should be taken into consideration. As discussed earlier, the humidity level of pressurized cabins is so low that it is important to prevent dehydration by drinking plenty of fluids throughout the flight. Fruit juice and water are the best for quenching thirst and replenishing body fluids.

Caffeinated beverages can have a diuretic effect; they tend to drain more water from the body than they add. So it is best to limit the amount of coffee, tea, and cola you drink while flying. As an example, for every cup of coffee you drink your body can lose up to one and one-half cups of fluid. A better selection for a hot drink is herbal tea or a cup of hot water with freshly squeezed lemon.

Alcohol's dehydrating properties make it an unwise choice during flights, but also keep in mind that a drink's effect is twice as potent at 5,000 feet above sea level than on the ground. If you choose to drink an alcoholic beverage, it is wise to limit the amount.

While the airlines are now providing passengers with meals that are nutritious and appealing, if you prefer to forgo airline food you can bring aboard some nonperishables like fruit, cheese, crackers, and vegetables. Either way you can ensure that your business trip gets off to a good healthy start!

Out of Town

Eating right while you are out of town means following many of the suggestions offered in Chapter 7, "Eating Out," but traveling makes good nutrition more difficult because all meals are "out." Add the problems of erratic hotel room service, hectic schedules, and lots of fancy restaurant meals and it is obvious that healthful dining takes some extra effort. Once again, though, by identifying potential nutritional setbacks you can take steps to counteract them.

Early morning meetings or pre-dawn departures can present a problem with regard to breakfast. If you want to grab a quick bite before leaving your hotel and cannot spend extra time waiting at the hotel coffee shop, the apparent alternative is room service. Unfortunately, room service does not start until 7 A.M. at some hotels. This means that unless there is particularly speedy service, it is unlikely that your breakfast will be delivered before 7:30. If you are scheduled for an 8 A.M. appointment somewhere else, you may opt simply to skip breakfast.

Many hotels are now making an effort to cater to the business traveler and have instituted round-the-clock room service and other amenities to satisfy meal needs at all times. If early meetings are a standard part of your travel schedule, you might want to book reservations only at hotels that provide twenty-four-hour room service. Some hotels have perfected breakfast room service by letting you place your order the evening before. For example, at the Fairmont Hotel in Denver, a hotel guest hangs a card on the doorknob of her room at night specifying the time breakfast is to be delivered and noting her choices from the menu. Breakfast arrives promptly at the requested time along with the morning newspaper.

An additional aid is a small refrigerator that some hotels supply upon request. This ensures that you can keep a convenient supply of energy foods like yogurt and cheese or other nourishing snacks. When your accommodations do not include a refrigerator and room service is limited, the most convenient solution other than eating out is to provide your own breakfast. As with brown-bagging on the plane, taking along several items requires minimal effort. A few pieces of fruit, some bread, muffins, or crackers, and a small, portable electric cup to heat water for coffee or tea can guarantee that you won't start a busy day on an empty stomach.

The opportunity to eat at restaurants for lunch and dinner throughout a business trip is sometimes viewed as an excuse to overindulge and throw diet caution to the wind. If you are continuously wined and dined while out of town, it is not unlikely that you could return home with some extra pounds: It is possible, though, to eat a variety of different foods and make certain splurges without gaining weight. The following suggestions can help you enjoy your out-of-town meals without sacrificing diet and nutrition sense.

1. Visiting different areas of the country enables you to sample regional specialties. While you might not take the time to prepare unusual vegetables, salads, or entrées at home, an out-of-town restaurant gives you the chance to try new dishes. Concentrate on selecting a variety of foods that provide a well-balanced meal.

2. If you have been on a diet prior to your trip, the most realistic approach while traveling is simply trying to maintain your weight. Don't put pressure on yourself to lose pounds during the trip. You can continue to be prudent in your meal choices, but give yourself some leeway to try new foods.

3. When you know that dinner will be an elaborate meal, plan for it by curtailing your caloric intake earlier in the day. Eat a light breakfast and lunch and "save up" calories so you can indulge guilt-free in the evening.

4. When lunch and dinner are both going to be full-course meals, decide in advance what you will eat so as not to be tempted to eat everything. For example, limit yourself to an appetizer and entrée at lunch and at dinner plan to have the entrée and dessert.

5. If you require a particular dietary menu, select a hotel where you know your special needs can be accommodated. For instance, three major hotel chains—Marriott, Stouffer's, and Hilton—have incorporated lighter selections into their menus. Marriott has designed a menu program called "Good for You" which has been approved by the American Heart Association. It offers health-conscious travelers well-balanced meals that are low in cholesterol and fat. The "Good for You" menu highlights a variety of breakfast, lunch, and dinner selec-

tions that where appropriate feature items prepared with margarine, no additional salt, and cholesterol-free egg products.

Women traveling alone often find that dinner poses a problem. Unfortunately, many women who dine alone at hotel restaurants have had unpleasant experiences where the maître d' or waiter gave them less than satisfactory service. A single woman may often be seated at a table in a corner and given poor treatment.

Hotel chains are becoming savvy to the problems women encounter and are attempting to reeducate their employees. Both Hyatt and Sheraton hotels have made changes in their dining rooms to accommodate women dining alone. The Hyatt has put single tables in more pleasant locations in its dining rooms, and the Sheraton now has instituted "captain's tables" at which single diners, male and female, can be seated together if desired.

Room service is of course an option if eating alone in a restaurant makes you feel uncomfortable. But there are many pleasures that dining alone can offer. After a hectic day of meetings and appointments, being served dinner in an attractive restaurant can be a chance to unwind and relax. In fact, a couple hours by oneself can be a luxury, particularly for the woman whose private time is limited. You can take all the time you want to consider the menu and then select a special meal to savor as you reflect on the events of your day.

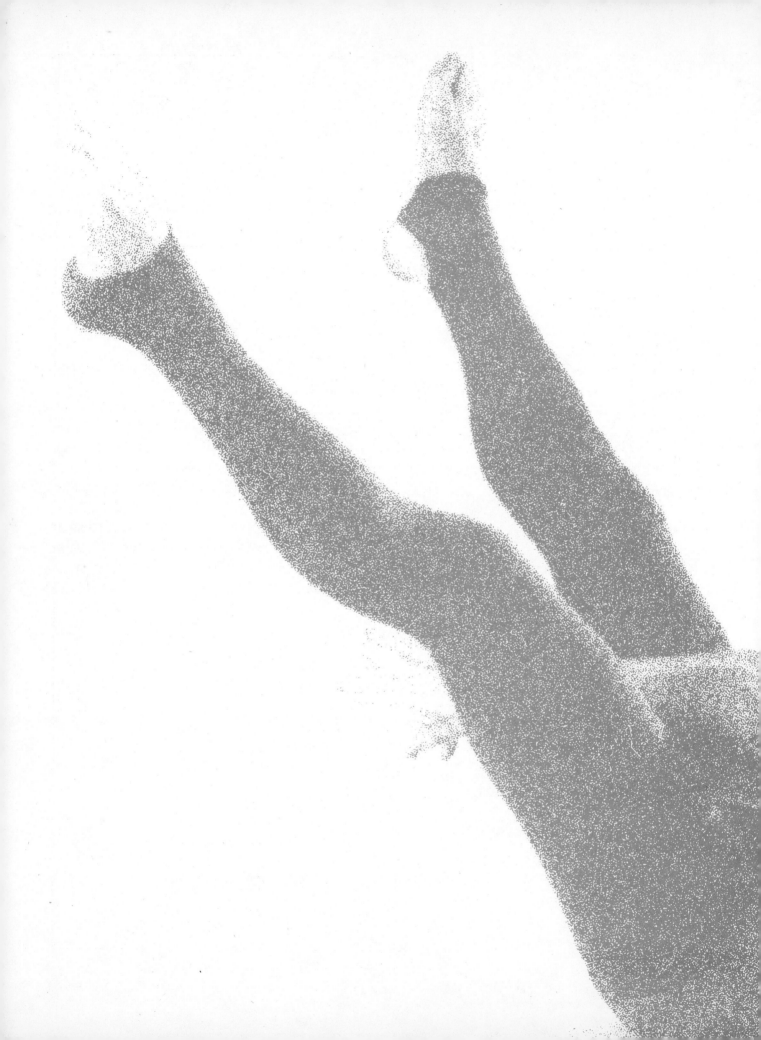

PART III

Stress

CHAPTER
TEN

Stress
and
the
Working
Woman

Stress. It is the topic of the eighties and a significant concern of the working woman. Today's woman takes on many pressures as a professional. As women rise in the ranks of the work force, the stress that in the past was the cause of health disorders traditionally associated with male executives is now affecting females. While equality in salary, position, and authority are the right of all, clearly the effects of stress are an undesirable accompaniment.

What is stress, and what does it do to us? Stress is the reaction of the body or the mind to physical and emotional strain. Stress can be the force against you, or it can be your resistance to the force. The stress reaction is of major concern to the medical profession because it has been implicated in many health problems.

The stress reaction is best exemplified in what is known as the fight-or-flight response. When a situation poses a threat to life or limb, the body responds by supplying extra energy to spur physical action. After the energy is released, the body returns to normal. Our primitive ancestors handled threats by naturally completing the fight-or-flight cycle; a caveman who encountered a wild animal invading his den would either hurl a rock at the intruder or run for protection. The energy that was produced for survival was a life-saving mechanism expended physically by using muscular action to fight or flee.

Today the complete fight-or-flight response is cut short. While we do not encounter wild animals in the workplace, the metabolic reaction of the body to anxiety, tension, or pressure is the same as the life-saving response. The body prepares for physical action, but the energy is not released. Energy that is not discharged causes the body to react adversely.

We cannot eliminate stress, but we can learn to recognize it and manage it. This chapter provides the tools to define stressors that affect you and offers guidelines that can put you in control.

Physical Effects of Stress

Consider stress and the physiological reaction as it might occur in an office setting.

Emily is a reporter for a major metropolitan newspaper. It is 3:30 P.M. and she is working on a half-finished story for a 5 P.M. deadline.

"My telephone rings and suddenly I am faced with a newsbreaking event that must be covered immediately. No sooner do I put the phone down than three more calls come in for me. To make things even more intense my editor appears, with whom I have a strained relationship. He announces that my last two stories were unsatisfactory and sarcastically asks if I value my job.

"I feel like my heart is racing. I want to give this editor a torrid comment and a good punch. I value my job, though, so I say and do nothing."

Here is what is now happening in Emily's body:

1. Her heart is pumping harder and faster, her blood sugar level is rising rapidly.
2. The rate and volume of respiration and oxygen consumption are increasing.
3. Adrenaline is being produced in large amounts.
4. Blood pressure rises to help increase circulation.
5. Senses are heightened.
6. Muscles are tensing, ready for action.
7. Nerves and glands are aroused in the brain and in the spinal cord to stimulate various organs.

Emily's body is in a heightened state of readiness to take physical action. If she needed to fight or run for her life, she is prepared with extra energy and stamina. This response has been triggered by her reaction to the editor, but the energy will not be expended. The torrid comment and punch are repressed, and Emily stays in control by clenching her fists and biting her lip.

When this kind of energy is not discharged, the body channels it inward, affecting the nervous system and various organs. While human beings have a substantial capacity to withstand stress, chronic fight-flight responses that are quelled take a toll that is recognized in stress's contribution to a variety of ailments. Stress is an aggravator of existing health problems and a major reason for the increased use of tranquilizers (and over-the-counter drugs). Stress is implicated in all the following health problems.

Stress Signals Inventory*

Stress-Related Illnesses and Disorders

Hypertension
Ulcers
Backaches
Asthma
Heart disease
Allergic reactions
Insomnia
Headaches
Acne
Depression

Illnesses Aggravated by Stress

Multiple sclerosis
Diabetes
Genital herpes
Cystitis
Rheumatoid arthritis

While the capacity to withstand stress varies with individuals, there are common physiological signals that indicate stress. These signals are significant because frequently we do not realize that we are under stress. Certain physical, emotional, or behavioral changes are your clues that stress is making its impact. Understanding how and when stress affects you is the first step in learning how to counteract and manage it effectively.

The following inventory will help you survey your personal stress signals. Do you experience any of these symptoms?

PHYSICAL SIGNALS

Skin oiliness
Hands cold
Hands sweaty
Feet cold
Feet sweaty
Burping
Gassiness
Need to urinate
Diarrhea
Tight or tense muscles
Acid stomach
Palpitations
Face flushes
Face feels hot
Hands shake
Shallow, rapid breathing
Shortness of breath
Pain in neck or lower back
Dryness of the throat and mouth
Headaches
Premenstrual tension or missed periods
Exhaustion
Elevated blood pressure

EMOTIONAL SIGNALS

Boredom, dullness, and lack of interest
Depression
Listlessness

* Adapted from Occupational Stress Conference sponsored by the U.S. Dept. of Health, Education and Welfare, Los Angeles, November 3, 1977.

Feeling of being fatigued
Feeling of unreality, weakness, and fear
Inability to concentrate
Urge to cry or run or hide
General irritability
Feeling of hyperexcitation or mania
Nightmares
Feeling that something is going to go wrong
Feeling invaded, resentful, or defensive
Feeling of apathy
Feeling powerless or hopeless
Feeling loneliness

BEHAVIORAL SIGNALS

Bite your nails
Pull your hair
Scratch your body
Grind your teeth
Stuttering or other speech difficulties
Increased smoking
Increased use of drugs or alcohol
Decreased or increased eating
Increased tendency to move without
   reason
Insomnia
Accident proneness
High-pitched nervous laughter
Trembling or nervous tics
Impulsive behavior
Holding on to something tightly
Yelling or screaming at someone else
Wagging your legs when crossed
Increased swearing
Withdraw or isolate oneself
Loss of enthusiasm/humor

Sources of Stress

Sources of stress can be divided into two categories—major life events and everyday common occurrences. While both are sources of strain, psychologists have not determined which has a greater impact on the stress response. Some believe that the relentless strain caused by daily irritations—missing the bus, for example—can affect a person more significantly than a major life change such as divorce or changing jobs.

We often think of stress events as being tragedies, but they may also be experiences that bring success or happiness into your life. Change in itself can produce stress.

The following Social Readjustment Rating Scale is designed to help you predict the likelihood of stress affecting your health within the next two years. Your susceptibility to illness increases proportionately to the amount of stress in your life, psychological and physical. It is important to realize that while the scale gives an indication of your predilection to illness, you can take precautions to counteract the possibility of adverse health change.

Circle the point values for the life events that have happened to you in the last year, then total them.

The Social Readjustment Rating Scale*

Life Event	Mean Value
1. Death of spouse	100
2. Divorce	73
3. Marital separation	65
4. Jail term	63
5. Death of close family member	63
6. Personal injury or illness	53
7. Marriage	50
8. Fired at work	47
9. Marital reconciliation	45
10. Retirement	45
11. Change in health of family member	44
12. Pregnancy	40
13. Sex difficulties	39
14. Gain of new family member	39
15. Business readjustment	39
16. Change in financial state	38
17. Death of close friend	37
18. Change to different line of work	36
19. Change in number of arguments with spouse	35
20. Mortgage over $10,000	31
21. Foreclosure of mortgage or loan	30
22. Change in responsibilities at work	29

Life Event	Mean Value
23. Son or daughter leaving home	29
24. Trouble with in-laws	29
25. Outstanding personal achievement	28
26. Spouse begins or stops work	26
27. Begin or end school	25
28. Change in living conditions	24
29. Revision of personal habits	24
30. Trouble with boss	23
31. Change in work hours or conditions	20
32. Change in residence	20
33. Change in schools	20
34. Change in recreation	19
35. Change in church activities	19
36. Change in social activities	18
37. Mortgage or loan less than $10,000	17
38. Change in sleeping habits	16
39. Change in number of family get-togethers	15
40. Change in eating habits	15
41. Vacation	13
42. Christmas	12
43. Minor violations of the law	11

*Reprinted with permission from Psychosomatic Research, Volume 11, Thomas H. Holmes and R. H. Rahe, "The Social Readjustment Scale," Copyright 1967, Pergamon Press, Ltd.

TOTAL SCORE

Less than 150   You have a low (about one in three) chance of having a serious health change for the worse in the next two years. Your level of resistance is probably high.

| 150–300 | Your chance of having a serious health change in the next two years is moderate (about 50–50). Your level of resistance is borderline. |
| 300 + | Your chance of having a serious health change in the next two years is high (from 50 to 90 percent). Your level of resistance is low. |

In addition to these life events, everyday pressures at work, commuting, the noise of public transportation, lines at the bank, or a rude salesperson can push you to the brink. Identifying the stressors in your life establishes an awareness that can help you change the experience or affect how you relate to it. You can design a stress map that will distinguish the things that trigger anxiety and tension for you, some within and some outside your control.

As an example, the following stress map was completed by Margaret, a forty-two-year-old public relations executive who is married and has two children, ages sixteen and twelve. The arrows indicate how stressful Margaret perceives the factors she has listed, the arrows closest to her signifying greatest stress.

Margaret's stress map reveals that her stressors are closely balanced between those over which she has some control and those that are outside her control. Living in the city, the economy, the health of her parents, weather conditions, and her staff's other work obliga-tions are sources of stress over which Margaret has no power to influence. So what can she do when she becomes tense and anxious about these situations? While these stressors automatically trigger a physiological response, Margaret can learn to program a response that counters the physical reaction. This programmed response can be achieved through relaxation techniques that calm the body and establish an emotional balance; they enable an individual to physiologically remain calm by increasing body temperature and improving blood flow to the extremities. This provides additional energy to cope rationally and intelligently.

The relaxation techniques are just as valuable for stressors that are within one's control. By remaining calm, Margaret can analyze the particular stress, prioritize her goals, and channel her energy into creative skills that will improve the quality of her life. By rationally surveying a situation that creates inner conflict, she can work on developing alternatives that would be more rewarding. (Creative problem solving, described later, outlines the process for making changes.)

You can design a stress map to identify sources of stress in your life. Using a blank sheet of paper, follow the format created for Margaret on page 160 and consider both stressors within and outside your control.

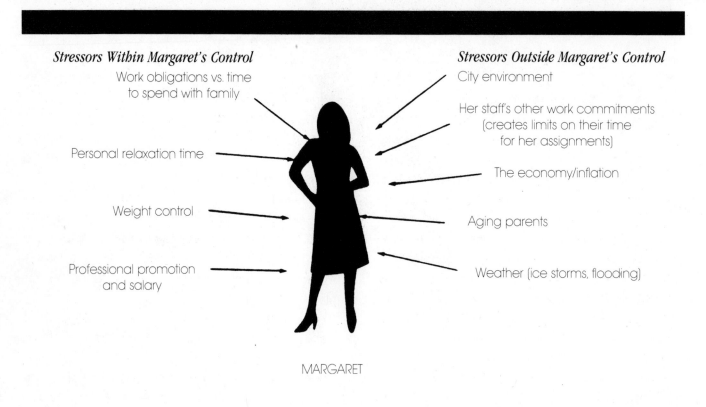

Stressors Within Margaret's Control

Work obligations vs. time to spend with family

Personal relaxation time

Weight control

Professional promotion and salary

Stressors Outside Margaret's Control

City environment

Her staff's other work commitments (creates limits on their time for her assignments)

The economy/inflation

Aging parents

Weather (ice storms, flooding)

MARGARET

Type A and Type B Personalities— Which Are You?

Behavioral characteristics have been studied as a factor in individuals' responses to stress, and it has been determined that certain personalities may set the stress response in motion more frequently than others. Two categories, Type A and Type B, have been designated as defining the personalities. Each personality type has its own set of actions, attitudes, and outlooks, and these characteristics influence reactions to everyday events and life changes. Type A is described as the compulsive, overly active individual who is at greater risk for disease than the Type B person, who is a more relaxed, easygoing individual. The stress threshold for these types differs, and tolerance and recovery from stress are affected as well.

Type A personalities push themselves to the limit. They are intense individuals who are hard-driving and highly achievement oriented. The Type A person is very competitive, demands control, sets unrealistic deadlines, and puts undue pressure on herself and others. Vacations are truly stressful times for these individuals because they cannot relax or slow down. Frequently, Type A's will bring work on vacations (if they take time off) and may cut the vacation short to get back to the office. They exhibit all the characteristics of the "workaholic."

Conversely, while Type B personalities can be hard workers, they do not exhibit the extreme behavior of Type A. They are not as preoccupied with time and do not become as impatient as their counterparts. This is not to say that Type B's do not set or meet deadlines, but they view them realistically. Type B enjoys leisure time and schedules vacations regularly. This personality creates a balance for herself emotionally, professionally, and personally by putting her work into a realistic perspective.

These questions can help you determine your behavior type.

1. Are you unaware of objects around you, at the office, at a friend's house, or in a new environment?
2. Do you take work home from the office at least twice a week?
3. Do you get impatient and upset if you have to wait in line because you feel you should be doing something more productive?
4. Do you always eat, talk, and walk rapidly?
5. Do you finish other people's sentences for them?
6. Do you usually try to do two or more things at the same time?
7. Are you obsessed with material gains?
8. Have you not taken a vacation in the last twelve months?
9. Do you ignore fatigue if it interferes with work?
10. Do you feel driven to succeed?
11. Do you feel guilty if you are not working?
12. Do you tend to blame others if something goes wrong?

All of the above behavior is representative of the Type A personality. If you answered yes to three or more of the questions, it is an indication that your behavior makes you more stress prone and the likelihood of your falling ill is greater.

Type A behavior has been studied extensively by psychologists and medical specialists to determine its effect on health. Although there is controversy over the implication of Type A behavior as a factor in heart attacks, there is concurrence that compulsive, hard-driving behavior contributes to the stress response. Being able to relax is one of the essentials of stress resistance, and Type A's, who cannot unwind and escape work, may have lower resistance. It has been recognized that it is not the amount of stress that determines if you become ill but rather how you handle the stress. Dissipating stress by doing something else increases your chances of staying healthy.

Type A personalities who do want to make changes in their behavior might find it helpful to focus on relaxation. By consciously learning to slow down through specialized techniques, the Type A woman may be able to transfer the serenity and calm achieved through relaxation to other behavior areas. Scheduling leisure activities as regular appointments may be another way to encourage diversion initially. While it is difficult to make behavioral changes, decreasing tension that is caused by stress is a positive beginning. Ultimately, habitual patterns that are of a negative nature may be transformed into more productive actions for a healthier life style.

Stress Management and Techniques for Stress Survival

Life is stressful. To cope with the pressures of daily living at work and at home, a woman must take care of herself and give herself permission to spend time to take care of herself. If stress gets "the better of you," neither your body nor your mind will function at its optimal level. Ideally, most of us would like to find a technique for removing the sources of stress in our lives. Unfortunately, many of the day-to-day stressors, ranging from deadlines to commuting, will always be there. Since it is impossible—and undesirable—to remove all sources of stress, one solution to the problem lies in developing skills to offset its effects.

Coping Skills

We all use a variety of methods to relax—talking to a friend, listening to music, taking a bath. These activities affect the body and mind by helping relieve tension. The bath relaxes the muscles, the music lets the mind focus on sounds, and talking to another person can help to work out a problem.

Sometimes activities that are associated with relaxation actually have the opposite effect. Frequently, such an activity—for example, a cigarette to steady the nerves or a cup of coffee to calm down—becomes habitual and activates the stress response. Both nicotine and caffeinated beverages act as stimulants; they arouse the central nervous system, not quiet it. In analyzing the kinds of relaxation techniques you use to cope with stress it's possible to identify habitual patterns that have negative effects.

The following questions can help you survey your present methods of dealing with stress at work. What do you do to relax when you feel tense, anxious, or under pressure on the job? Do you:

- take a tranquilizer?
- leave the work area for a few minutes?
- smoke a cigarette?
- exercise during lunch hour?
- have a cup of coffee, a soda, or a vending machine snack?
- meditate?
- talk to a co-worker or call a friend?
- have an alcoholic drink at lunch or after work?
- take a headache remedy?
- do some tension-releasing movements at your desk?

If you use tranquilizers, cigarettes, coffee, or alcoholic beverages frequently, your method of relaxing is harmful to the body. As mentioned, caffeine and nicotine stimulate the body, and this results in a draining of important nutrients from the system. If you choose to take aspirin be sure to read the label; many aspirin products contain a high content of caffeine. Tranquilizers and alcohol are an energy drain, and because they are depressants, they are a way of avoiding rather than facing the source of your problem. If drugs or drinking have become a coping tool for you, then it's important to seek professional counseling.

Exercise, meditation, talking with a friend, and getting out of the work area are methods that calm and energize. They provide you with resources, internal and external, that help you cope with pressure. If the mind can relax and escape the source of stress for even a short time, it is possible to reapproach a problem with renewed strength and mental clarity.

Developing Stress Resistance

Your body has a great reserve of energy and strength that can respond to resist stress. Often we take our bodies for granted. Only during times of illness or injury do we truly appreciate the value of good health and a strong body.

Staying healthy takes commitment, discipline, and time, but it is energy well directed because ultimately you are the winner. What you do for your body will pay off in vitality and stamina to live life to its fullest and prevent you from succumbing physically or mentally during times of stress.

Developing resistance is a three-part program that involves rest, exercise, and nutrition. Each component is a crucial element to good health and together they create a total package of strength and energy that equals resistance.

REST

Try functioning at your top level when you have not had a good night's sleep. You feel groggy, listless, lethargic. Add any extra pressures and it is easy to fall prey to stress. Adequate rest and regular sleeping patterns can give you the reserves to start each day with energy and a centered state of mind to withstand workday problems.

There is no absolute number for the exact amount of sleep each person requires, but most need between six and eight hours. While inadequate rest is depleting to the body, too much sleep is an indication that something is wrong. Sleep can be used as an escape, a way of withdrawing. If you are sleeping over nine hours every night, it is important to consider what you may be trying to avoid and understand the source of your problem.

Bouts of insomnia and restlessness can also be indicative of unresolved issues that need to be analyzed. Tension or anxiety can keep your mind so intent on problems that you are unable to fall asleep or sleep peacefully. If falling asleep is difficult because you feel too keyed up to rest, relaxation techniques can help ease tension by redirecting your focus. Meditation, yoga exercises, and relaxation methods facilitate a feeling of calm and decrease muscular tension. Using these techniques before going to bed can help you ease into sleep comfortably and easily.

Sleeping problems sometimes occur as the result of habits that are disruptive to rest. Active exercise or consuming large quantities of food late in the evening will disrupt your sleeping pattern. Vigorous exercise before bed will keep you up because it energizes the body and makes you feel too lively to sleep. If you want to exercise in the evening, stretching exercises or yoga postures will be more conducive to a good night's rest.

A heavy meal before bedtime will interfere with your sleep, as your digestive system will be active when your body wants to rest. Ideally, you should allow four to six hours for food to digest before you go to bed.

While large quantities of food are not recommended before sleeping, small amounts of certain foods can actually help induce sleepiness. Tryptophan is an amino acid found in protein foods that raises the level of the brain chemical serotonin. Serotonin is a neurotransmitter that causes sleepiness and also acts as an antidepressant. Foods containing tryptophan that will help combat mild insomnia include turkey and warm milk. In a New York Times article entitled "How Diet Can Affect Mood and Behavior" (November 18, 1982), health writer Jane E. Brody cites studies on the effects of tryptophan by Dr. Ernest Hartmann, a sleep specialist at Tufts University School of Medicine, and Dr. Harris Lieberman, a psychologist at the Massachusetts Institute of Technology. Their research indicates that eating foods containing tryptophan before bedtime can be an aid to sleep without the side effects of barbiturates and other sleep-inducing drugs.

Tryptophan is also available in tablet form.

Taken regularly about one hour before bedtime (with Vitamin B₆ to assist utilization), it can be a nonaddictive sleeping aid.

EXERCISE

Exercise and stress have an interesting connection because stress often attacks areas of the body that are weak. While stress may not cause the weakness, a vulnerable area seems to flare up under stress. A healthy body, and that means strong bones, toned muscles, and mobile joints, is your best resistance against the effects of stress.

Unfortunately, exercise is not a priority in the lives of many busy professionals whose days are filled with deadlines, meetings, and decision-making. While you would not consider breaking an appointment with your attorney or accountant, the time set aside for exercise often falls to the bottom of the list of priorities. Intention to exercise is admirable, but it means nothing if you do not follow through with regularity in an exercise regimen.

When the body is treated with care and is exercised regularly, it works for you, not against you. Flaccid muscles, poor circulation, and weight problems can aggravate a range of ailments associated with stress. Seventy-five million Americans in the work force suffer from lower back pain, and muscle deficiency is the prime contributing factor.* Exercise is critical in providing your body with strong resources against the stresses of daily life.

* from the President's Council on Physical Fitness

Exercise can be the panacea for a tense executive who works under continual pressure. The fight-or-flight response that triggers a surge of adrenaline in the body does not have an opportunity to discharge itself in the workplace. When energy that is released in the body to prepare it for physical action is contained, muscular tension and psychological strain result. One of the most constructive ways of dispelling this energy is through exercise. The excess adrenaline is expended through muscular activity, which then allows the body to relax.

Frequently women say that they are too tired to exercise. By the end of the day they feel exhausted and have enough energy only to get themselves home. The idea of exercise seems punishing. It's important to state some of the benefits of exercise to clarify any misconceptions.

1. Exercise gives you energy. Exercise is one of the most significant energy boosters because it dissipates the mental weariness that people often mistake for physical fatigue. At the end of a long day, you will find that after engaging in physical activity for as little as several minutes you will feel as though you have gotten a "second wind." The increased oxygen intake and improved circulation as a result of the movement gives you energy to spare. When you are exhausted after exercising, it is a true physical exhaustion that feels good. This type of activity several hours before bedtime can also help you sleep better.

2. Exercise is an antidepressant. When you

exercise vigorously your body releases a chemical called beta-endorphin. Endorphins are mood elevators. Beta-endorphin creates a sense of euphoria and can affect a person's emotional state significantly. People who feel anxious become less tense, depressed individuals feel more cheerful, and angry people become less hostlie. Any kind of aerobic activity will stimulate the production of beta-endorphin, and it's practically guaranteed that you will feel better after exercising. It is the release of beta-endorphin that also accounts for the "runner's high" to which dedicated joggers become addicted.

3. Aerobic exercise has a positive effect on cardiovascular function. In recent years women have begun to fall victim to heart disease at an earlier age. Heart attacks used to occur infrequently in premenopausal women. Since the great influx of women into the work force, job-related stress is thought to be a contributing factor in the increase in heart disease and hypertension in this group. Exercise is a key element in making the heart work more efficiently. Increased activity will lower the resting heart rate, improve the cardiovascular system, and boost the body's oxygen intake.

Premenopausal women, because of their higher levels of the hormone estrogen, have higher levels of HDL2 than men. This is a high-density lipoprotein that breaks down fat. Research studies conducted by Josef R. Patsch, a medical professor at Baylor College of Medicine in Houston, indicate that increased HDL2 levels can prevent the buildup of fat in the arteries that leads to heart attacks. In menopausal and postmenopausal women, the levels of HDL2 are significantly lower and the built-in protection against clogged arteries has diminished. Exercise increases the level of HDL2, thus affording greater protection against heart disease.

4. Exercise is a weight control aid. Obesity is a problem that affects millions, and it is no secret that a contributing factor is a sedentary life. Many weight problems develop not because of overeating but as the result of a lack of activity. Exercise burns up calories and helps the body stabilize at a proper weight.

People often eat excessively when they are anxious or depressed. In these situations the stomach is not regulating hunger, an emotional state is affecting food intake; the food serves to gratify unmet needs. Exercise is a constructive channel for those emotions. In addition to its antidepressant effect, activity will enhance your physical image and ultimately your self-image.

NUTRITION

Stress takes its toll in ways that can be quite subtle. When you are under strain, the stress response calls upon the body's reserves of many vitamins and minerals. As these reserves are depleted, the body's resistance to infection and illness is lowered. It is crucial to prepare your body to handle stress so that your chances of remaining physically healthy are high. The best guarantee for resistance is a well-balanced diet that provides you with adequate amounts of complex carbohydrates, protein, and fats. Refined carbohydrates, excessive fats, and sugar are the body's enemies—the fuel for stress to ravage the body.

In our fast-food culture there is always the temptation to grab a quick snack for a meal. Sweets, caffeinated drinks, and fried foods are the typical between-meal "pick-me-ups," and many convenience foods are nutritionally deficient and full of chemicals. What options are available to women who are always on the go? As with sleep and exercise, good nutrition can be an integral part of your life style if you make it a priority. It does mean using forethought and not opting for the handy snack machines at the office or skipping a meal if you are busy.

Set aside time for breakfast and lunch and you will find that your blood sugar does not fluctuate dramatically, causing great shifts in energy levels. Digestion improves when you eat slowly, and time set aside for a meal can be a chance to unwind as well. Food is your body's fuel, and you owe it to yourself to eat properly.

In times of stress you might want to consider adding a daily vitamin supplement. Vitamin C, B vitamins, and pantothenic acid (a part of the vitamin B complex) are drained from your system when stress is high, and caffeine, nicotine, and sugar also deplete the body of these nutrients. Since these vitamins are all water-soluble they are not stored by the body and must be replaced continually. As a precautionary measure, "stress vitamins" can help your body cope during times of added stress. These extra stores of vitamins B and C will contribute to your system's ability to remain in balance under stress.

Counteracting Workday Stressors

Creative problem solving is a way of thinking that can be useful in every area of life. Instead of problems being viewed as obstacles that are unsolvable, they are seen as challenges that can be surmounted. This kind of thinking requires an ability to objectively consider a situation and recognize that there are a number of choices that provide various benefits.

The process involves developing a series of questions that encourage you to understand the nature of the stressful problem, the options that are available to you, and the ramifications. The technique divides a problem into components and helps you consider alternatives in a rational, balanced manner. By using this deliberate approach, emotions that are heightened under stress are not given as great an opportunity to influence actions.

Using the following questions, employ the process to consider pressures you encounter daily at home and at work.

1. What is the specific problem?
2. What effect is the problem having on me, and what changes do I desire?
3. What alternatives are available to me?
4. What will be the effect of these alternatives?

Write down your responses, which will help you clarify your thoughts. It is surprising at times how writing something down helps get to the core of a problem. This process puts you in command to make a decision that is based on evaluation and foresight.

Consider the case of Susanna, who is a thirty-two-year-old public affairs director for a mid-sized corporation:

Susanna's problem:
There are constant deadlines that I am having difficulty meeting, and my work demands are overwhelming. I can never get enough accomplished because my work load exceeds the normal workday. Phone calls continually interrupt me, and I rarely have a block of time to concentrate on a major project. I always stay late just to catch up with each day's routine work. I am involved in so many projects at once that my desk overflows with papers, mail, and research information. I feel that I have to handle all the projects myself because I don't have confidence in other staff members.

The problem's effect:
I am physically tense, mentally drained, and my personal life is suffering because I don't have the time, energy, or stamina to do anything but work. When I leave the office I worry about unfinished projects and cannot even enjoy the few hours I have away from my job. I haven't taken a vacation in over one year —it takes too much effort to go away.

The changes that are desired:
I want to have more energy and feel more in control. I want to enjoy my friends and family and spend more time with them. I want a "normal" life that is balanced between work and play.

What alternatives are available to Susanna to establish a work life that won't monopolize her to the extent of destroying her personal life, physical health, and mental well-being? There are several options she can exercise if she closely examines the working environment she has created for herself:

1. Delegating work. Susanna feels compelled to handle all projects. This is impractical and unrealistic. She needs to learn how to delegate different aspects of a project to other staff members. By dividing the work among employees she could ease her work load.

In learning to delegate, it is also important for Susanna to understand her own reasons for trying to be a "superwoman." Feelings of insecurity and fear of failure are often at the core of perfectionism. It is possible to suppress these feelings by becoming so immersed in work that there is little time for reflection. Understanding her motives would be helpful in breaking a pattern that may be unconscious.

2. Establishing priorities. A sense of organization and ranking each project's importance facilitate the work process. Making lists and writing down the successive tasks to accomplish a goal would force Susanna to clarify the process into workable components. This kind

of organization would also aid her in delegating specific jobs.

Understanding and integrating the principles of time management would help Susanna to organize her responsibilities and priorities most effectively. Reading a good book on the subject would help her develop guidelines and specific strategies for efficient use of time.

3. Recognizing one's capacity. As important as it is to delegate work and establish priorities, it is also critical to learn how to say no. Susanna overextends herself by taking on new projects when previous commitments have not been fulfilled. She needs to regularly assess her work load and recognize that it is impractical to undertake more work when the deadline for a current commitment is imminent.

4. Limiting interruptions. Phone calls, staff meetings, and individual consultations are disruptive to getting a job done. Susanna would profit by setting aside a time period when she handles calls and appointments and establishing another block of time that is not to be interrupted. She might also consider an occasional work-at-home day. These alternatives provide opportunities for steady concentration.

5. Making time for leisure. Susanna has to begin incorporating other activities into her life. Her inability to free herself from work is unhealthy and ultimately counterproductive because "burn-out" is inevitable. Some physical activity would provide a release from her workday tension, and it would be an opportunity to build in recreational time with friends. At first Susanna may find that she schedules time for "fun" with the same determination with which she approaches her work life. Eventually a balance between the two will create a personal vitality that she currently lacks.

Any one of the five options will provide Susanna with a more reasonable outlook and better organized methods. By instituting all the suggestions, she should be able to achieve the changes she desires. Delegation, establishing priorities, recognizing personal capacities, limiting interruptions, and including leisure time would provide a sensible and well-organized plan for working more efficiently and exerting control over situations. She could ultimately achieve a better and more satisfying use of work hours that would create more time and energy for personal life. Additionally, by revamping her work style she would be able to schedule vacations more frequently and with less anxiety.

What causes stress in one woman may not set off a similar response in another. Individuals react differently to similar situations, and stress responses are the result of a number of personal factors. The following list of common workday stressors can help you identify situations that may trigger a stress response. The number and variety of job features that are stress-producing would seem endless. In addition to those listed, try to think of any other situations that create personal anxiety and tension for you.

STRESSFUL JOB FACTORS

Job security
Sudden increase in overtime hours
Too much work
Too little work
Poor work conditions
Difficulty with work relationships
Work crisis
Lack of esteem
Lack of recognition
Excessive travel
Poor salary
Lack of opportunity

Just as too much work creates tension and anxiety, too little work can also be a cause of stress. Extremes of any sort are uncomfortable for most people. A balance between work pace and work load is important for job satisfaction and productivity.

Career development is an issue that affects much of the female work force. Anxiety over opportunities for advancement as well as the emotional strain resulting from being overlooked for a promotion have been related to job stress and various health problems.

Additionally, a lack of respect, lack of involvement, or lack of power can be extraordinarily frustrating for most workers. This is a particularly familiar situation for many women, even those in high-level positions. A woman who attains an executive-level title in name only can feel tremendous hostility when she is not taken seriously. The uphill battle takes its toll in stress.

Support Systems

One of the most critical factors in dealing with stress and coping with problems is the support of family and friends. Isolation and loneliness increase the ill effects of stress, whereas a support system provides strength and resiliency. As children we relied on parents, siblings, and best friends to help us through difficult times and to share in the successes of our lives. It is important to retain a network of this sort in adulthood for emotional sustenance.

Many people feel that adulthood implies an ability to stand on your own without need for others. There are individuals who feel they can't share their fears or concerns with anyone—it would be a sign of weakness and evidence of failure. Communication is a vital factor in dealing with stress, and human beings need social support and communication for survival.

A support network can exist in the workplace, and during times of stress you may find that a co-worker's friendship and empathy can help you cope.

PROFESSIONAL COUNSELING

Personal insights are valuable for handling stress, but there are times when solutions are not evident. It may be that one particular problem creates frustration or that a variety of factors are affecting you emotionally. At this stage it can be helpful to seek outside counseling with a professional who can help you work through a specific problem or a period of difficulty.

Many people associate counseling with psychological therapy lasting for years. But many psychologists, psychiatrists, and therapists have developed short-term techniques that promote rapid change through cognitive therapy, assertiveness training, ego supportive therapy, and behavioral techniques. Many of the programs are geared specifically for people seeking symptom relief as their sole form of therapy or for individuals who use short-term therapy in conjunction with other therapies.

Some individuals feel hesitant about seeking the help of a therapist because they associate psychotherapy with severe mental disorders. Psychotherapy and psychiatry are broad-based fields and cover a range of techniques for assisting people with a variety of problems.

As there is medical aid for physical problems, there is psychological assistance for the issues that trouble the mind. You consult your physician when you are ill or have an injury. You should feel the same freedom to contact a specialist for stress or anxiety disorders. The specialist's goal is to help you overcome specific difficulties that stand in the way of optimal functioning, and you should not underestimate the effects of stress on your health.

Relaxation for Stress Management

Learning to relax is at the core of stress management. In some cases we have the control to change external circumstances and cancel out the stress-producing factors, but at other times it is necessary to find internal resources to manage stress. It is through relaxation that individuals can acquire the ability to effect physiological changes in the body and offset the stress response.

In 1971 Herbert Benson, a research physician at Harvard University Medical School, recognized that a well-structured relaxation period could help physiological and psychological functioning. Benson's studies identified the specific elements required for a "relaxation response" and proved that they could provide an antidote to tension. The four basic components necessary to facilitate the relaxation response are: (1) a quiet environment; (2) a comfortable position; (3) a receptive attitude; and (4) a phrase, word, or image that promotes a supportive, relaxed feeling.

By using these elements, Benson found, an individual could make herself feel more serene, centered, and confident. Just as the stress response is automatic, so is the relaxation response. It is a programmed reaction that counters physiological stress and helps to put a person in control.

Physiologically, relaxation affects the body in many ways. Oxygen consumption decreases, as does blood pressure, blood lactate levels, carbon dioxide, the rate and volume of respiration, and the heartbeat rate. Additionally, there is an increase in skin temperature and brain alpha waves. Essentially, the response of the body to relaxation techniques is almost the opposite of what occurs during the fight-or-flight response.

The relaxation response will effectively diminish anxiety and tension and enable an individual to regain a state of equilibrium physically and mentally. A relaxation method performed on a daily basis for about twenty minutes can be used as a preventive measure against the stress response, and is useful for improving work efficiency and productivity.

There are several techniques that can be employed—all result in the relaxation response. Every individual is unique. A particular relaxation exercise may work more effectively for some people than others. Be patient in exploring the various relaxation methods until you find the one that works for you.

RELAXATION TECHNIQUES

Begin by giving yourself permission to take the time to relax. Recognize that you deserve this time, for you must direct your energies toward achieving a state of physical and mental calm. You might want to set aside a regular time period each day that you devote to the technique in addition to using it when stress mounts. It can be done at home or at work.

Consider the elements that Benson stated as prerequisites for a relaxation response:

A quiet environment—Find a place where you will be undisturbed. Although this can be difficult, try to make sure you will have time to be by yourself. If you are at work and need to relax, close the door to your office, put the phones on hold and instruct your secretary or support staff that your office is off-limits for a certain time period. At home make sure you unplug the telephone.

A comfortable position—Loosen constricting clothing and remove your jewelry. Find a position where the body is supported without muscular tension. This can be achieved by either sitting back in a comfortable chair or lying on your back on a firm surface. For additional comfort on your back, place a cushion or pillow under the knees to prevent any strain on the lower spine.

A receptive attitude—Receptive means being open to the relaxation experience. Stop thinking. If thoughts come into your mind, let them pass through. Do not become frustrated if you begin concentrating on a problem or thought. Let the mind focus if it has to and then let go of the thought.

A phrase, word, or image that promotes a supportive, relaxed feeling—Focus your attention on something that will limit interference from other thoughts. For example, attention could be centered on an image of the ocean if that represents tranquility to you. Some people find that words such as "peace" or "light" help lull them into a restful state.

DIAPHRAGMATIC BREATHING

Have you noticed that when you are scared, anxious, or tense your breathing becomes rapid and shallow? This is one of the body's reactions during the fight-or-flight syndrome. As the breathing rate becomes faster and faster, taking in less oxygen per breath, the heart correspondingly works harder and beats faster. Additionally, if you observe your body's reactions during the stress response, you will notice that your muscles have become more constricted. Diaphragmatic breathing can help you control your oxygen intake and muscle tension. (The diaphragm is a muscle located between the lungs and the stomach. When you take a deep inhalation that fills the bottom of the lungs with air, the diaphragm expands, causing your abdomen to protrude.) By consciously monitoring your breathing, you have the ability to increase oxygen in the body, influence the heart rate, and release tension.

Sitting or lying down in a comfortable position, begin by closing your eyes and studying your breathing. Are you inhaling and exhaling through your mouth? When you inhale do you lift your shoulders? Does your stomach tighten as you inhale? Diaphragmatic breathing enables you to bring maximum oxygen into your body.

1. Inhale deeply through your nose. Nasal breathing helps filter the air and control oxygen intake. As you inhale concentrate on letting the muscles of the body relax. You do not need to use your shoulders in order to breathe. They will rise slightly, which is normal, but they should not be lifting and dropping excessively on each inhalation/exhalation.

2. Let the air fill the bottom of the lungs first (the diaphragm now expands with this deep inhalation), then the middle of the lungs (the rib cage area), and finally the top of the lungs (the upper chest area). When you inhale using the diaphragm you will know if you are breathing properly if the abdomen expands. As the breath fills the upper chest you will notice that the collarbone rises.

3. When you reach your full inhalation, hold your breath for a count of three and then begin a controlled exhalation through the mouth. The exhalation should be done with the same attention given to the inhalation. Begin by allowing the collarbone to lower, then expel the air from the top of the lungs (upper chest), the middle of the lungs (rib cage), and the bottom of the lungs (the diaphragm contracts and the abdomen pulls inward). The breath should be one continuous flow from inhalation to full exhalation.

4. To gain maximum relaxation from diaphragmatic breathing it is recommended that you make the exhalation twice as long as the inhalation. For example, you can in-

hale to the count of four, hold the breath for three, and exhale to the count of eight.

Diaphragmatic breathing can be practiced anytime during the day and should be done for a minimum of several minutes. You can use this breathing exercise for energy when you are fatigued or to establish a state of tranquility under stress.

DEEP MUSCLE RELAXATION

Many people complain of muscular problems. Tense shoulders, stiff necks, tight back muscles, eye strain, even cramped fingers, can be the effect of stress on the body. Progressive deep muscle relaxation is a technique developed by Edmond Jacobson, a Chicago physician, in which one consciously tenses muscles, then releases them to induce relaxation. By completely scanning the body to relieve muscular tension, you not only feel relaxed but energized as well.

The optimal position for deep muscle relaxation is lying flat on your back on a firm surface with feet about eighteen inches apart. The exercises can also be done seated if you are sitting on a chair that provides support for the entire body. Begin by removing your shoes and closing your eyes. (Initially allow about twenty minutes for the complete series. As you become familiar with the process, select those exercises that apply to your tension areas.)

1. Focus your concentration on the right leg. Lift the leg 6 inches off the floor and tense the leg muscles by flexing the foot and curling the toes. Hold the muscles tight for 8 seconds and then abruptly release them. The leg should become limp immediately and drop to the floor. Roll the leg from side to side to release any residual tension. Leave the leg in this relaxed position and forget about it as you continue to relax other body areas.

2. Repeat the same instructions for the left leg.

3. Lift the right arm 6 inches off the floor or chair arm and tense it completely by curling the fingers in a fist and tightening the lower arm and bicep. Hold the muscles in this state of tension for 8 seconds and then abruptly release them. The arm should be completely limp and drop immediately. Roll the arm from side to side, wriggle the fingers, and then forget about them.

4. Repeat the same instructions for the left arm.

5. Tighten the buttocks muscles by squeezing them together—this should make the hips rise. Hold the muscles for 8 seconds and then release them. The hips will drop back to the floor. Let them relax and then forget about them.

6. Inhale through the nose and push the abdomen out. The belly should expand like an inflated balloon. Hold this position for 8 seconds without moving. Next, open the mouth and exhale by letting the air gush

out as the stomach deflates and returns to its normal size. Now forget about the stomach.

7. Inhale again and this time expand the chest to its fullest breadth. Hold for 8 seconds. Open the mouth and exhale completely, letting the air gush out as the chest collapses. Resume normal breathing and forget about the chest

8. Round the shoulders forward toward the chest and then lift them toward the head. Try to touch the shoulders to the ears and hold that position for 8 seconds. Let the shoulders completely release. Shrug them slightly if there seems to be any residual tension. Now forget about the shoulders.

9. Tilt the head slightly back so that the chin is jutting up. Concentrate on trying to tense the throat and the back of the neck. Hold for 8 seconds and release. Roll the head from side to side if you feel any discomfort. Let the head slide back to its original position and forget about the neck.

10. Pinch the muscles of the face together by tensing the muscles around the lips and pursing them up toward the nose. At the same time squeeze the eyes and push the eyebrows down by tensing the forehead muscles. Hold this position for 8 seconds and release.

11. Stretch the mouth, tongue, eye muscles, and cheeks by opening the mouth and stretching the tongue over the bottom lip toward the chin. At the same time open the eyes and look upward at your eyebrows. Let the nostrils flare as you hold this position for 8 seconds. Release immediately, let the muscles go slack, and forget about the face.

12. Now, with the muscles in a state of relaxation, mentally scan each body area. If you become aware of muscular tightness, concentrate on the area and try to induce the tension to dissipate. Use soothing images to encourage letting go.

13. Once the body is relaxed, concentrate on the breath. Imagine that each breath is bringing fresh energy into the body. Be aware of the calm of the inhalation and exhalation and notice how the mind can relax as well as the body.

14. When you are ready to come out of deep relaxation begin by gently moving your fingers, hands, and arms. Next, wiggle the toes and rotate the legs inward and outward. Let your head roll from side to side and finally open your eyes. If you have been lying down, slowly roll to your side and sit up.

Deep muscle relaxation is an energizing way to begin your day relaxed, refreshed, and tension-free. The technique is also useful for countering stress and can be done prior to a speaking engagement, staff presentation, or any other situation that causes you anxiety. Additionally, deep muscle relaxation is helpful for sleeping problems. Done before going to bed, the exercises can release tension and help the mind relax.

AUTOGENICS

"Autogenous" is defined as self-generated or self-generating. Autogenic relaxation is a kind of self-hypnosis that is achieved by instructing your body to let go of tightness and constriction. You give your body directions about how it should feel and the result is reduced muscle tension and mental relaxation. The process is simple and the benefits invaluable for managing stress.

The words "heavy" and "warm" convey the feeling of relaxation for most people. If a limb of the body feels heavy, then it is submitting to gravity and not holding tension. (For some people, once the tension is released a lightness replaces the heavy feeling.) Warmth elicits a sense of calm and peacefulness. In fact, contrast this to the common phrase "cold and clammy" that describes the hands of a person who is anxious or scared.

Begin the autogenic exercises by sitting in a comfortable position or lying on the floor. Close your eyes and tell yourself that you are relaxed and tension will be leaving the body.

1. Slowly repeat the phrase "My right arm and hand are heavy." Continue to recite the phrase until you feel the effect—a heaviness in that arm and hand.
2. Repeat the phrase for the left arm and hand, the right leg, and the left leg.
3. Once all your limbs feel heavy continue the exercise by repeating the phrase "My right arm and hand are warm." Repeat the phrase for the left arm and hand, the right leg, and the left leg. To enhance this image it sometimes helps to imagine that your heart heats the body by sending warm blood through the limbs to the body's extremities.
4. Next, use the same process for the abdomen, back, and neck. If you find it difficult to experience heaviness in these body areas, simply focus on the warmth phrase.
5. Finally, repeat to yourself that you feel relaxed and free of tension. Enjoy this state of peacefulness and the effect it has on you physically and mentally.
6. Prepare to come out of autogenic relaxation by gradually moving and stretching your arms and legs. Think about opening your eyes and then open them slowly.

As you become proficient with autogenics, you can do the exercise with your eyes open. This can be helpful, for instance, if you are in a meeting and anxious about a presentation. Autogenic relaxation is also a useful aid for counteracting insomnia. Reciting the phrases before bed can put you in a relaxed state ready for sleep.

BIOFEEDBACK

Biofeedback differs from other relaxation techniques, in that instruments are used to give you information about the level of tension in your body. It is a method of relaxation that involves control over bodily functions that previously had been thought of as involuntary. By regulating these functions you can consciously make yourself relax. The advantage of a biofeedback machine is its ability to give you an immediate reading on the level of stress that is affecting your body and tell you if you are being successful in reducing anxiety.

There are two steps in the biofeedback process: (1) identifying the fact that tension is affecting the body and (2) your efforts to release that tension. Biofeedback equipment monitors a variety of body signals: skeletal muscle tension, skin temperature, sweat gland activity, brain waves, and heart rate. Increased levels of activity for all these physiological functions mean that you are being affected by stress. The equipment gives you auditory or visual signals indicating the extent of the stress.

For example, using an electromiogram (EMG) machine that records muscle tension in the forehead, an individual who feels calm and relaxed will hear a steady rhythmic click from the machine. If a stress-producing thought is introduced, the machine will respond by clicking with an increased tempo signifying greater muscle tension. As relaxation is restored, the EMG clicks will return to a slow, steady beat.

To reduce the clicks emitted by the equipment, you must put your body into a relaxed state. The relaxation can be achieved through diaphragmatic breathing, deep muscle relaxation, autogenics, or by just letting your mind drift. You are controlling the stress response by creating the relaxation response. Biofeedback makes you aware of what is happening in your body and helps you counteract stress or potential stress-causing situations.

After learning to reduce tension using the biofeedback equipment, you become sensitized to your body's signals and can achieve the same relaxation results without the machinery. Biofeedback has been effective in treating a variety of stress-related problems, including tension headaches and migraines, muscle spasms, circulatory disorders, and colitis.

Biofeedback training is taught by many practitioners throughout the country and is even provided by some corporations to help their employees cope with stress. Equipment has also been developed for biofeedback monitoring at home.

CHAPTER TWELVE

On-the-Job Tension-Releasing Exercises

During the average working day, a variety of physical discomforts beset many people in addition to the strain of stress-related problems. While stress and pressure can make muscles tense, the body is also affected by a work life that is primarily sedentary. Muscles and bones are designed to be used and when they're not, the body rebels with stiffness, cramps, or tightness. The mind and body are connected and when one is not functioning properly, the other is affected. Just as emotional stress can create tense muscles, a body that is tense can distract your mind.

Millions of Americans suffer from lower back pain, and a sedentary job combined with poor posture is a factor contributing to this problem. Incorrect body alignment creates a chronic strain on the muscular-skeletal system, and years of improper posture at your desk can cause an abnormal curvature of the spine. When body alignment is distorted the result can be pain, physical tension, and costly medical bills.

If you sit for extended periods of time, slump over a typewriter, hold a telephone receiver between your head and shoulder, or do considerable reading, your body will likely feel the uncomfortable effects of being confined to a desk. But relief is possible; specific physical movements can loosen stiff joints, release cramped muscles, and even strengthen abdominal muscles.

When pressures mount on the job, the best thing you can do is to make certain that you are working most productively with energy and stamina. If tight muscles are causing discomfort, it is important to release the physical tension. The following series of exercises has been designed to help you beat the strains and pains of a desk job. The exercises take only a few minutes and can be done anytime. Select individual exercises for particular problem areas or do the entire series to dissipate fatigue and tension.

1. Eye Movements

Cause for eye strain: Lengthy periods of reading, particularly under fluorescent light

The following movements exercise and relax the eye muscles. They tone the optic nerve, increase circulation, and generally improve eyesight.

1. Keeping the head stationary, move the eyes up and down as far as possible without strain. Repeat 10 to 15 times, then close the eyes and relax.
2. Moving the eyes horizontally, look to the far right. In a straight path of vision, glide the focus to the far left. Repeat 10 to 15 times, then close the eyes and relax.

Cause for stiffness: Holding the telephone receiver between your head and shoulder

A speaker phone is an ideal piece of equipment to prevent the strain many people develop from holding the telephone incorrectly. If you are unable to have a speaker phone, then it is important to break the habit of propping the receiver on your shoulder. When you do find yourself falling into the old pattern, use this exercise to stretch contracted muscles.

1. Tilt head to the right as if "listening" to shoulder with right ear.

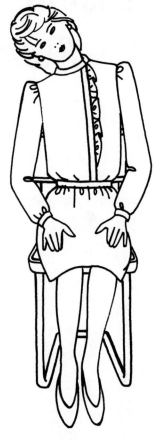

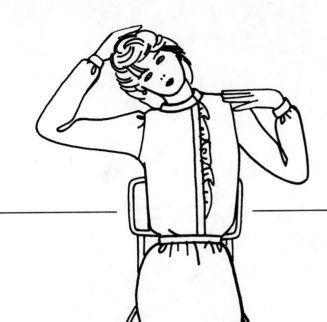

3. Head and Neck Massage

Cause for stiffness: Lack of mobility and stress

The neck is the first place most workers will feel tense. Massage can break up the muscle tension and create an energy flow that makes you feel more alert and relaxed. It is also helpful in relieving headaches.

1. Using the fingertips, gently press into the base of the neck (where neck and shoulder blades meet).
2. Making small circular motions, work fingers up the neck to the hairline.
3. Gently press fingertips along the hairline to ears.

Repeat as necessary.

2. Place right hand on top of head and left hand on left shoulder. Inhale.
3. Exhale and use hands to apply gentle pressure to head and shoulder. This pressure will help stretch and lengthen neck muscles. Reverse and tilt head to left.

Repeat as necessary.

4. Shoulder and Arm Stretch

Cause for tightness: Long periods of sitting and poor posture

The muscles in the shoulders and upper arms tense up if you work at a desk or over a typewriter for hours. Opening the shoulder area with a stretching movement and lengthening the tricep muscles can make you feel more comfortable.

PART I

1. Wrapping arms around chest, hook fingers under the shoulder blades. Inhale.
2. On the exhalation, gently pull the shoulder blades as though you are trying to increase the width of your back.

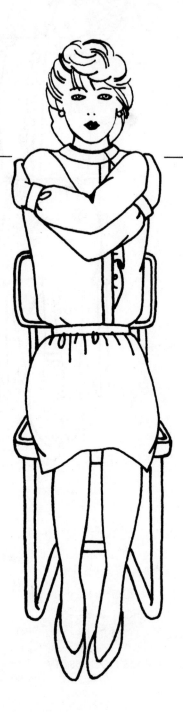

PART II

1. Lift arms above head, cross forearms, and hold on to elbows.
2. With gentle pressure, push elbows behind head. You will feel a stretch in the triceps.

Repeat both parts 4 times or more as necessary.

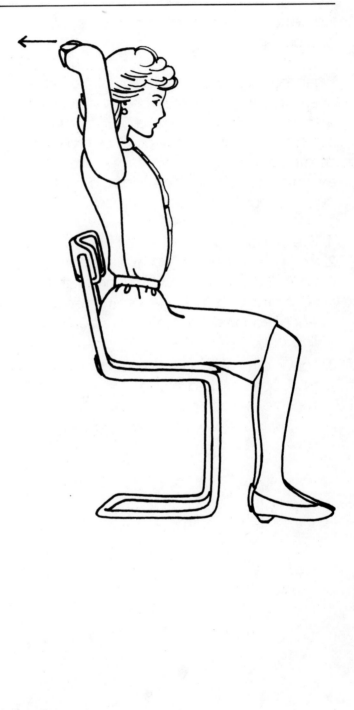

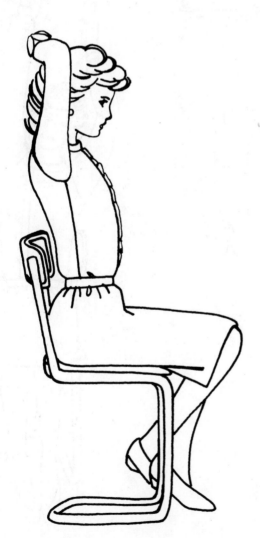

5. Torso Lengthener

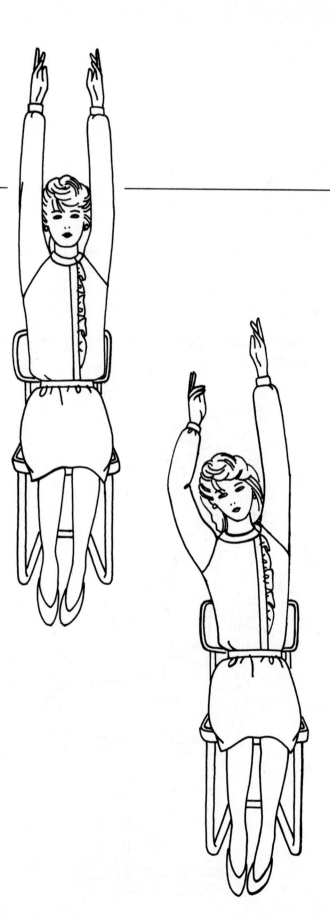

Cause for discomfort Long periods of sitting and poor posture

When the torso is curved over a desk the entire chest area is compressed and this interferes with proper breathing. It is difficult to get as much oxygen into your lungs as normal, and as a result energy level is affected. This torso exercise expands the chest and rib cage and puts the body into proper alignment.

1. Stretch both arms above the head.
2. Imagine you are climbing a ladder and grabbing on to the rungs. Reach with the right arm and then the left 8 times. With each reach you should feel the body getting longer.
3. Lower arms and prepare to go back to work. Do <u>not</u> slump into your previous position. The exercise has increased the length of your torso—keep that upright position.

6. Spinal Curve and Arch

Cause for back problems: Most backaches are the result of weak abdominal muscles and back muscles that lack flexibility.

Sitting contributes to the problem if the stomach muscles are flaccid and not providing adequate support for the back. The spinal curve exercise makes you use the abdominal muscles and also stretches the muscles in the back. The arch expands the chest and gives you added mobility in the upper spine.

PART I. SPINAL CURVE

1. Drop head and let chin rest on chest. Roll down the back, articulating each vertebra until you reach the tailbone. Let arms hang at your sides.
2. Pull the stomach in and keep the abdominal muscles activated. This action is the impetus to return to an upright position. Roll up.

PART II. ARCH

1. In your upright position lift the chest and tilt the chin toward the ceiling.
2. Slightly arch the upper back by imagining you are bending backward over a huge beachball. Only the upper back is involved —the arch should not extend to the lower spine.
3. Return the body to an upright position.

Repeat both parts 3 times.

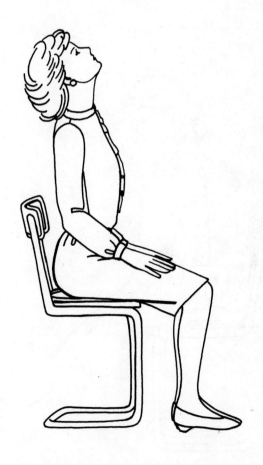

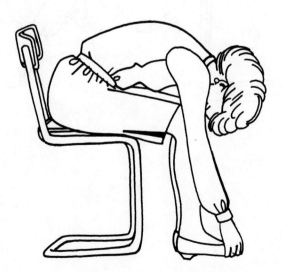

7. Calf Stretch and Hamstring Lengthener

Cause for tension: High-heeled shoes cause the leg muscles to contract and tighten.

These stretches will increase flexibility and are particularly useful if you have been sitting for a long period.

PART I. CALF STRETCH

1. Sitting on the edge of a chair, extend legs on floor in front of you.
2. Flex feet up to the ceiling and hold for several seconds.
3. Point toes to the floor.

PART II. HAMSTRING STRETCH

1. With feet flexed as in the calf stretch above, drop the body over the legs. Depending on your flexibility, hold on to the back of the knees, calves, or ankles. Make sure the head is dropped and the chin is resting on the chest. Hold for 10 seconds.
2. Return to initial position.

Repeat both parts 4 to 8 times.

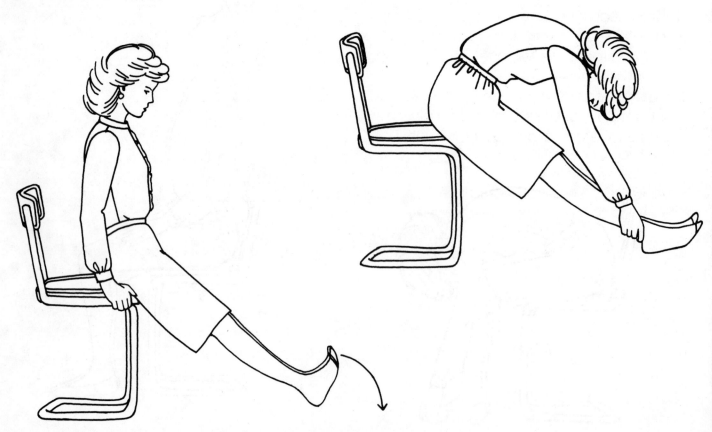

Anytime Tension Releasers

There are times when it may seem inappropriate to you to do any kind of physical exercise that would relieve tension. During the course of a board meeting or in the middle of an intense discussion with a prospective client you would probably feel very foolish if you started stretching your arms above your head. And no doubt your colleagues would question your credibility after seeing such a display. Indeed, certain movements are best done in the privacy of one's office, but you do have options for public situations.

There are some physical gestures that are acceptable behavior during the course of daily interaction. These are usually movements that we do intuitively to release tension, though we might be unaware that we are even moving the body. By being aware of these motions, you can consciously use them (without embarrassment or strange stares) when you are feeling tense.

All of the following movements can be done standing or sitting. They are part of the normal repertoire of body movement and can be repeated several times to relax tense muscles.

Shoulder Shrugs

These motions will release tension in the shoulder and neck area.

1. As you inhale, lift the shoulders toward the ears.
2. Exhale and let the shoulders drop completely.

Variation: Lift and drop each shoulder separately.

Limb Shaking

If you have a tendency to clench your fists or tense the fingers under pressure, this movement will release energy and loosen the muscles.

1. Shake the right hand back and forth from the wrist.
2. Move the forearm from the elbow and include it with the wrist shake.
3. Now add the upper arm and shake the entire arm from the shoulder.

Repeat with the left arm.

This exercise can be adapted for the legs. Begin by shaking the ankle and foot, add the lower leg, and finally shake the entire leg from the hip joint.

Joint Flexibility

Moving the joints helps increase circulation and is particularly important for the wrists and ankles.

WRIST

1. Holding the right wrist in the left hand, make circles by rotating the hand outward.
2. Reverse and make inward rotations.

Repeat with the left wrist.

ANKLE

1. Place the ball of the right foot on the floor and lift the heel.
2. Pressing into the ball of the foot, move the ankle in a circular motion outward.
3. Reverse and make inward circles.

Repeat with the left ankle.

Face Flexibility

Pursed lips and a clenched jaw are a giveaway that you are reacting to tension. These movements will relax the face.

1. Open the mouth slightly and move the jaw from side to side.
2. Yawn (fake it if you're not tired) to stretch the mouth, cheeks, and jaw.

Neck and Spine Twist

When tension builds in the neck and back, the best release is a gentle twist that stretches the muscles.

1. Turn the head slightly from side to side.
2. Increase the turning movement by looking behind you.
3. Increase the range of motion by twisting from the waist.

PART IV

Services

Making Your Life Run More Smoothly

One of the most treasured commodities for working women is time. Extra time is a priceless gift and one that is savored. When a day is jam-packed with work and personal obligations it seems there are never enough hours to accomplish everything. While no magic solution exists for injecting a twenty-fifth hour into the day, there are ways of maximizing your use of time. Dozens of services are available that essentially buy you time by making your life easier. They facilitate a variety of tasks and help you coordinate and manage your responsibilities with greater ease.

Your Wardrobe

Although clothes do not make the person, in today's business world the image that you project through your appearance strongly influences how you are perceived. What is the "executive look"? According to Susan Dresner, a New York City wardrobe consultant, "what distinguishes a person in a position of power and authority is his or her sense of quality." She explains,

> While proponents of the "dress for success" school (who are mostly men) advise the business uniform—conventional suiting in somber shades of blue and grey with a simple blouse—career women do not have to limit themselves to tame, colorless, noncommittal clothes.
>
> Women who have secured a relatively high position or work in a more creative field can wear more feminine, individually-styled

apparel. What is important is that no outfit should attract more attention than what you are saying or doing. Avoid tight and above-the-knee skirts, revealing necklines, sheer blouses, jeans and heavy, jangling jewelry. Additionally, trendy "costumes" and worn, ill-fitting or cheaply-made garments do not make a professional statement.

In Ms. Dresner's book, Managing Your Business Image: A Practical Guide to Personal Style, she recommends the following guidelines for developing a wardrobe:

Rule 1. Don't confuse quality with fashion. Quality is long-lived and classic while fashion is whimsical and often exaggerated. Don't go after "designer" labels thinking that you are automatically buying quality. It is no insurance of fine cloth and cut.

Rule 2. Don't confuse quality with price. The price of a garment is triggered by not only its manufacturing cost but what the market will bear. If a particular style or designer is "in," the price shoots up.

Rule 3. Select the hallmarks of excellence.
a. Quality fabrics (e.g. weight, closeness of weave, softness of finish). Natural fibers (silk, cotton, linen, wool) are far superior to man-made ones. They breathe, and therefore have the ability to drape better, last longer and bounce back to their original shapes after each wearing.
b. Superb cut in the shaping and drape of a garment.
c. Hand-tailoring or partial hand work.

Rule 4. Avoid the purely functional. A wardrobe composed solely of good, serviceable clothes can be tiresome and ineffectual. Don't be afraid to experiment and to reveal sparks of your personality.

Rule 5. Never sacrifice comfort for style. To perform at your best, you want to feel comfortable in your clothes. Never compromise when it comes to fit, and dress in a way that is natural to you.

Rule 6. Be moderate in all things. Balance the timeless with the contemporary; your own special look within the context of the business setting; your wardrobe investment with your career perspective.

Generally, the particular type of attire most suitable to you depends upon four factors:

• The specific industry and company in which you work
• The "style" of your division or department
• Your current position and, equally as important, the next position you want
• Your body type and coloring *

With these factors in mind, your next step is shopping and developing an awareness of the services available to facilitate wardrobe building. Shopping takes time, energy, and foresight to coordinate and accessorize outfits. Some women find shopping enjoyable, while to others it is an unavoidable chore. If shop-

* Reprinted with permission, Managing Your Business Image: A Practical Guide to Personal Style by Susan Dresner, 1983.

ping is a tiresome task for you, the following aids can make your life easier. And even if shopping is your idea of a good time, certain services can complement your efforts.

PERSONAL SHOPPERS

Many women are reluctant to ask for help regarding their wardrobes because they feel they should already know how to dress their best. But with the array of styles and fabrics and the cost of clothing, deciding what is most appropriate, becoming, and sensible budget-wise can be confusing. One of the most helpful services to a busy executive is a personal shopper. This consultant can provide the expertise to help you look your best by developing a well-integrated style of dressing that is right for you.

In selecting a personal shopper, find a consultant who can provide a variety of services. For example, Dresner's New York–based firm, Successful Ways & Means, starts with an extensive personal profile encompassing a client's professional needs, career aspirations, and private life. This is followed by an at-home wardrobe analysis. Then specific strategies for achieving the look you want and an annual wardrobe budget are developed, highlighting what you need to buy and how much you can expect to spend. The company scouts stores and arranges shopping trips to specially selected shops. Finally, they assemble a wardrobe diagram/travel planner that coordinates all separates and accessories into well-planned ensembles.

The value of a consultant's skill is an asset to the busy woman in ways that extend beyond the time-saving advantage:

1. You will spend less time deciding what to wear each day because a coordinated wardrobe eliminates trying to figure out how to create ensembles from separates.
2. You can do a lot more with less since you will own a versatile and distinctive wardrobe that will look good for years to come.
3. You can be more confident about your appearance, assured that your clothing is appropriate and comfortable.
4. You will ensure that your wardrobe will not lag behind your career advancement.

IN-STORE SHOPPING SERVICES

Many large department stores as well as specialty shops have created in-house resources for clothing and accessory consultations. The range of services is quite broad—from a single consultant who advises customers free of charge to a specialized staff that provides extensive personal service for a minimal fee.

Many of the stores will do your shopping for you. You make an appointment with one of their consultants, who takes your fashion profile and makes notes on what you need—the item, style, color, size, fabric, and price range. You can then request that the consultant make selections for you to consider on your next visit to the store or you can "work the floor" with the consultant.

One well-known service is "Macy's By Appointment" (MBA for short), available in Macy's East Coast, Florida, and Texas stores. They help customers find a single special item or update an entire wardrobe. The service is complimentary and is available in the evenings and on the weekends, which makes it ideal for the working woman. The MBA consultants keep a record of your selections on file so they can help you build and coordinate your wardrobe as desired.

The particular needs of the executive woman have been addressed by Saks Fifth Avenue through a program initiated in 1980 called "The Executive Service." This service was specifically created for the woman whose schedule is demanding and for whom time is at a premium. Based on a limited, private membership concept that requires an initial fee of $50 for a twelve-month subscription that can be renewed yearly, the service is available at selected stores throughout the country.

The Saks service offers a number of unique features that make it appealing to the business woman, including:

1. An initial visit with a personal shopping consultant to discuss your designer preferences, favorite colors, and information as to what you already own. With this material on file, the consultant can have what you are looking for ready for your consideration when you arrive for an appointment, or you can tour the store together. A private fitting room is also reserved for your use.
2. Simply by telephoning, you can request a consultant to update your wardrobe without your having to come to the store, and same-day delivery service can be arranged.
3. A consultant will remind you of birthdays and anniversaries if desired and will do the necessary shopping for you if requested.
4. Other features include priority service on alterations, special billing arrangements for separate home and office accounts, light snacks, a receptionist to take your phone messages while you are in the store, plus special arrangements for additional requested services.

SPECIALTY SHOPS

Just as an executive woman has a personal banker and broker, the specialty shop is a personal clothier geared to successfully dressing the career woman. Whether you believe that you must conform to a masculine dress code and require strictly tailored, classic clothing or feel that you can look businesslike and feminine with softer-looking garments, there are shops that cater to your particular needs. If you do not have the time to search racks of clothes in pursuit of the ideal suit or a blouse to match an outfit, specialty stores can simplify your life.

Many of the executive apparel stores specialize in custom-made items as well as carrying their own ready-to-wear lines. Some will also order ready-to-wear designs for women who do not conform to stock size or who prefer a different fabric. Additionally, many carry evening wear, sportswear, and accessories, resulting in one-stop shopping.

The personal attention offered by specialty stores makes them particularly appealing. Their staffs recognize the time limitations of their clients and will often provide private appointments outside of regular store hours to accommodate a customer's schedule. Many also keep a file on each client and a record of purchases to facilitate the client's wardrobe coordination.

Personal Helpers/Facilitators

Your niece's wedding is this weekend and you haven't had time to buy a gift. A last-minute trip abroad has just been scheduled and your passport has expired. You are giving a cocktail party in honor of a colleague, but work has you swamped with little time for preparations. There are myriad problems that can suddenly pose a problem for busy women. Too much to do and not enough time. If you are confronted with specific tasks that can be delegated, then your solution may be just a phone call away.

Party planners, gift shoppers, people who will wait for you (for example, stand in line for licenses, process registrations, wait at your home for the refrigerator repairman), and even information resources that can tell you everything from where to get a handbag repaired to the best Mexican restaurant in town, are available in many cities. The variety of personal services available is so extensive that you can probably find someone who will handle any type of task.

While these services exist throughout the country, often the biggest problem is simply finding out about them. Many of the "personal helpers" are individuals who have started their own businesses and, as sole proprietors, are not listed in the telephone business pages. Word of mouth is frequently the way these entrepreneurs secure new clients, so your best bet is to ask colleagues if they are familiar with anyone who provides the services you require.

The individuals/companies who do advertise tend to use publications that have a wide readership throughout a specific metropolitan area. City magazines such as The Washingtonian (Washington, D.C.), "D" (Dallas), New York Magazine, Los Angeles Magazine, St. Louis Magazine, and Miami Magazine, to mention only a few, contain classified ads listing personal services.

Business Accessories

Organization is a key element in running your professional life as smoothly and effectively as possible. If you have been scribbling notes on scratch pads and on the backs of envelopes, you can probably recall the many times those notes were lost. If you have ever pulled a crumpled business card out of your wallet to hand to a client, you were embarrassingly aware of not making a good impression professionally. The accessories you select for your work life should serve two functions—enhance your productivity and highlight an executive image through their style and quality.

No longer is the working woman limited to items specifically geared to the male executive. You now have a wide choice of handsome, functional pieces to serve nearly every conceivable need. Everything from a six-year planner booklet with monthly calendars and note pages to a briefcase organizer that includes writing pads, pockets for a calculator and business cards, plus several zippered compartments, are on the market for the female professional. Many of the products are well-designed record keepers, useful in analyzing work efficiency as well.

Whereas coordinating business accessories in the past tended to be rather haphazard, recently designers have developed lines exclusively for working women. For example, "Executive Organizers," by international designer Nicolai Canetti, is a complete line of accessories for professionals which were created with several factors in mind. They are light, streamlined, and highly functional.

Other manufacturers who have geared their products to combining efficiency with aesthetics include Buxton, Executive ScanCard Systems, Royce, Personal Resource Systems, and Day-Timers, to mention just a few. Many working women have commented that these products improve personal and organizational productivity dramatically even among the most organized.

Catalog Shopping

The development of catalogs for almost every kind of product has become a growing industry in the eighties. Never before has shopping by mail been so accessible. For the busy woman, catalog browsing can be a time-efficient method of surveying a variety of items, and its at-home convenience makes it one of the most appealing shopping techniques.

From food and furniture to clothing and computers, catalogs can be the answer to facilitating purchases for yourself as well as gifts for others. It is an easy but still personal way of choosing presents for all occasions and can be particularly helpful during the holiday season. Many catalog companies also provide toll-free customer relations lines to answer questions and handle complaints.

Some direct-mail companies have specifically addressed the needs of working women through catalogs that specialize in career clothing. Many of the catalogs also assist in wardrobe management by featuring clothing that is styled and color-coordinated to illustrate a variety of possibilities for maximizing a wardrobe.

In addition to convenience, the beauty of catalog shopping is the variety of choices provided that may not be available in certain regions of the country. Without leaving your home you have the opportunity to purchase items that normally might be inaccessible. For example, one-of-a-kind items that are made and sold in a small New England town can be enjoyed by consumers from all states via catalogs.

While shopping by catalog can be a busy woman's salvation, it is important to avoid the pitfall of placing an order with an unreliable company. By checking a few details you can reduce the possibility of any difficulties:

1. If a company is unfamiliar to you, check with the Better Business Bureau in the town where the company is located or with the Federal Trade Commission in Washington, D.C., to find out if there are any complaints on file against the firm.
2. Always read the details and fine print in the catalog order form, and familiarize yourself with the refund/return policy.
3. Keep a record of your order—both the date of the order and the method of payment. American companies are legally required to respond to an order within thirty days by sending the merchandise, writing a letter explaining the delay, or refunding your payment. If service is unsatisfactory you should inform the Better Business Bureau.

4. If you select a catalog item that is to be sent as a gift directly to the recipient, send a note to the recipient notifying him or her that a package will be arriving. This will ensure that should the item not be delivered, you will be alerted and can take appropriate action.

Perhaps the ultimate in "at home" convenience is shopping via computer. With a personal computer, the executive woman has a storehouse of products at her fingertips. One of the most extensive programs available is a nationwide electronic purchasing center called Comp-U-Star from The Source, a computer information and communication service. With an input of over 50,000 name-brand items, it enables you to comparison-shop by manufacturer, model number, and price. Additionally, the best price is calculated for you automatically, including delivery charges. Further information about The Source can be obtained from most computer dealers or by calling them toll-free at 1-800-336-3366 (in Virginia, 1-800-572-2070).

You Deserve to Be Pampered— Tips on Feeling Good

In addition to services that eliminate specific aggravating or time-consuming obligations for you, many personal care services are available that can make you feel terrific. When life gets complicated there is a tendency to reduce the time spent on personal well-being. While it may seem that services to pamper the body are luxuries, their value extends beyond the physical. When you do things "just for you," it is a statement that you deserve time for yourself and are worth it. Feeling good about yourself is one of the best strategies for staying fit and living life to the fullest.

Spas

Taking time out to reenergize and "de-stress" is essential. It can be accomplished in many ways, but perhaps the ultimate is getting away from it all by going somewhere or doing something that offers an escape from the tensions and pressures of everyday life. Personal services designed to help you look and feel your best are the ideal for a rejuvenating and energizing lift—physically and mentally.

The special quality that draws so many people to spas is the focus on services that pamper the body. Skin care, massages, herbal wraps, whirlpools, saunas, and Jacuzzis can be enjoyed daily by guests. Nail and hair care specialists are also available. In addition to these services, the emphasis on nutrition at many spas is renowned. Guests who come to shape up and slim down can choose from a variety of diet plans ranging from gourmet calorie-reduced menus to vegetarian meals to partial-fast juice diets. Generally the emphasis is on decreasing the intake of sodium, saturated fats, and refined sugar and highlighting foods rich in vitamins, minerals, and fiber.

A stay at a spa that is geared toward fitness is not only an opportunity for the executive woman to unwind from the responsibilities of "real life," but also a chance to make exercise, good nutrition, and health her primary focus. Many spas offer a variety of regimens that provide numerous options for sports activities, weight control plans, fitness programs, and even stress management training.

While you can opt for a more passive regimen and limit exercise activity, the special attraction of many spas is the emphasis on physical activity. Comprehensive exercise programs, including classes in yoga, dance, calisthenics, and aerobics, are usually held continuously from early morning to early evening and are complemented by swimming, hiking, tennis, racquetball, horseback riding, and even martial arts.

At one time most spas were located on the West Coast and in the Southeast (warm weather providing an obvious appeal). However, in recent years noted spas have been established in nearly every region of the country. The following list is a guide to some of the best spas in the United States. All will send brochures, rate information, and detailed descriptions of their fitness and diet programs upon request.

MIDWEST

The Kerr House
17605 Beaver Street
Grand Rapids, Ohio 43522
(419) 832-1733 or (419) 255-8634

Oasis Spa
French Lick Springs Golf and Tennis Resort
French Lick, Indiana 47432
1-800-457-4042

The Spa at Olympia Resort
1350 Royal Mile Road
Oconomowoc, Wisconsin 53066
1-800-558-9573

NORTHEAST

International Health and Beauty Spa
   at Gurney's Inn
Old Montauk Highway
Montauk, New York 11954
(516) 668-2345 or (212) 895-6400

New Life Health Spa
   Summer Address:
Liftline Lodge
Stratton Mountain, Vermont 05155
(802) 297-2600 or 1-800-223-9832

   Winter Address:
Prospect Reef Resort
P.O. Box 104
Road Town
Tortola, British Virgin Islands
1-800-223-9832

SOUTHEAST

Bonaventure Inter-Continental Hotel and Spa
250 Racquet Club Road

Fort Lauderdale, Florida 33326
(305) 389-3300 or 1-800-327-8090
(in Florida, 1-800-432-3063)

Sea Pines Behavioral Institute
Sea Pines Resort
Hilton Head Island, South Carolina 29928
(803) 671-6181

The Spa at Palm-Aire
2601 Palm-Aire Drive North
Pompano Beach, Florida 33060
(305) 972-3300 or 1-800-327-4960

SOUTHWEST

Canyon Ranch Spa
8600 East Rockcliff Road
Tucson, Arizona 85715
(602) 749-9000

Maine Chance
5830 East Jean Avenue
Phoenix, Arizona 85018
(602) 947-6365

The Phoenix
111 North Post Oak Lane
Houston, Texas 77024
(713) 680-1601

WEST COAST

The Golden Door
P.O. Box 1567
Escondido, California 92025
(619) 744-5777

La Costa Hotel and Spa
Costa del Mar Road
Carlsbad, California 92008
(619) 438-9111

The Oaks at Ojai
122 East Ojai Avenue
Ojai, California 93023
(805) 646-5573

The Palms
572 North Indian Avenue
Palm Springs, California 92262
(619) 325-1111

The Spa at Sonoma Mission Inn
P.O. Box 1
Boyes Hot Springs, California 95416
(707) 996-1041 or 1-800-358-9022
(in California, 1-800-862-4945)

Salons

When a ten-day, week-long, or even three-day spa retreat is not possible, some of the same pampering and service are available to you at many local beauty salons. The psychological value of a facial, massage, haircut or styling, manicure or pedicure can be the panacea to a difficult day.

An additional plus of these services is their long-lasting effects. A professional facial provides the deep cleansing, specialized masks, and individualized care that can be the key to achieving and maintaining healthy skin. It can also help alleviate the blemishes that even mature women may experience as a result of stress. Many of the salons also offer lessons in makeup application and guidelines on how to streamline your daily makeup routine.

Chipped nail polish or an unbecoming

hairstyle does not fit the image of an executive woman. To look their best and maintain a professional image, most women find they need a weekly manicure and a haircut once every six to eight weeks. But trying to schedule appointments on the spur of the moment can be unsuccessful. You might find it helpful to arrange a series of standing appointments with your favorite stylists. This is a way to guarantee that your particular nail and hair care specialists will be available and that you have booked the appointment into your schedule.

Some salons offer special half and full days of beauty treatments during which a variety of services are provided for you. Similar to a one-stop shopping trip, these beauty packages enable you to take care of several personal needs at one time. The convenience makes it ideal for the busy woman who does not have the time or energy to find various specialists around town.

Excellent salons can be found in nearly every city. The following firms are renowned for their beauty packages as well as single services. Their salons, located in cities throughout the United States, cater to professional women, and are a boon to the traveling executive who finds herself in an unfamiliar city and wants the assurance of top service from reputable specialists.

ELIZABETH ARDEN SALONS

The Elizabeth Arden Salons offer a number of beauty services including face treatments, makeup applications, makeup lessons, exercise instruction, massage, waxing treatments, manicures, pedicures, hair styling, and hair coloring. Their beauty packages are:

Maine Chance Day $160
Exercise, steam cabinet, massage, hair styling, manicure, pedicure, face treatment, daytime makeup, plus a light lunch. Approximately 5 hours.

Miracle Morning $110
Massage, hair styling, manicure, face treatment, daytime makeup. Approximately 4 hours.

Visible Difference Day $115
Face treatment, hair consultation and styling, manicure, makeup application and lesson. Approximately 4 hours.

P.M. Pick-Me-Up $42
Massage and steam cabinet. 90 minutes.

Elizabeth Arden Salons are located in:

Beverly Hills, California
434 North Rodeo Drive
(213) 273-9980

Chevy Chase, Maryland
5225 Wisconsin Avenue N.W.
(202) 362-9895

Chicago, Illinois
717 North Michigan Avenue
(312) 266-5750

Coral Gables, Florida
340 Miracle Mile
(305) 445-5443

Dallas, Texas
The Galleria
13350 Dallas Parkway, Suite 1685
(214) 458-8888

New York, New York
691 Fifth Avenue
(212) 407-7900

Palm Beach, Florida
351 Worth Avenue
(305) 655-7270

Phoenix, Arizona
Biltmore Fashion Park
24th Street and Camelback Road
(602) 956-1500

San Francisco, California
230 Post Street
(415) 982-3755

Southampton, New York
(June-September)
14 Main Street
(516) 283-0871

Surfside, Florida
9592 Harding Avenue
(305) 865-3586

Washington, D.C.
1147 Connecticut Avenue N.W.
(202) 638-6212

GEORGETTE KLINGER SALONS

At the Georgette Klinger Salons services include facials and specialized skin treatments, scalp treatments, massage, manicures, pedicures, makeup lessons and applications. Their beauty packages are:

Full Day of Beauty $200
  Facial, massage, scalp treatment, manicure, pedicure, makeup lesson, light lunch. Approximately 6½ hours.
Half Day of Beauty $105
  Facial, choice of body massage or scalp treatment, makeup lesson.

Georgette Klinger Salons are located in:

Bal Harbour, Florida
Bal Harbour Shops
9700 Collins Avenue
(305) 868-7516

Beverly Hills, California
312 North Rodeo Drive
(213) 274-6347

Chicago, Illinois
Water Tower Place
835 North Michigan Avenue
(312) 787-4300

Dallas, Texas
The Galleria
13350 Dallas Parkway
(214) 385-9393

New York, New York
501 Madison Avenue
(212) 838-3200

Palm Beach, Florida
Esplanade
150 Worth Avenue
(305) 659-1522

CHRISTINE VALMY SALONS

The Christine Valmy Salons services include facial treatments, eyelash and eyebrow treatments, makeup lessons and applications, waxing treatments, massage, manicures, and pedicures. Complete corrective facial treatments start at $30 to $60. A beauty package they provide is called the Valmy Day. It is $160 and includes a facial and skin treatments, body massage, manicure, pedicure, makeup lesson, and eyebrow shaping, plus lunch. It takes approximately six hours.

The Christine Valmy Salons are located in:

NORTHEAST

Boston, Massachusetts
114 Newbury Street
(617) 266-1221

Natick Towne Mall
Route 9 and Speen Street
(617) 235-7575

Forest Hills, New York
107-27 71st Avenue
(212) 793-0222

Greenvale, New York
82-6 Glen Cove Road
(516) 484-0160

Manhasset, New York
1360 Northern Boulevard
(516) 627-7067

Massapequa, New York
4131 Merrick Road
(516) 541-8130

New York, New York
767 Fifth Avenue (GM Plaza)
(212) 752-0303

153 West 57th Street
(212) 581-9488

Paramus, New Jersey
409 Bergen Mall Shopping Center
(201) 843-4180

Philadelphia, Pennsylvania
Rittenhouse Regency Hotel
225 South 18th Street
(215) 546-5660

Pittsburgh, Pennsylvania
One Oxford Centre
301 Grant Street
(412) 471-1300

Stamford, Connecticut
100 Grey Rock Place
Stamford Town Center
(203) 327-2640

Washington, D.C.
70 Woodmont Avenue
Bethesda, Maryland
(301) 652-3840

SOUTHEAST

Fort Lauderdale, Florida
3307 N.E. 33rd Street
(305) 565-6500

WEST

Houston, Texas
2630 Sage Road—Galleria West
(713) 840-8888

Las Vegas, Nevada
157 The Fashion Show
3200 Las Vegas Boulevard South
(702) 369-8411

Midland, Texas
39 Plaza Center
(915) 683-9891

Scottsdale, Arizona
4400 North Scottsdale Road
(602) 994-8584

WEST COAST

Beverly Hills, California
9675 Wilshire Boulevard
(213) 273-3723

Marina Del Rey, California
562 Washington Street
(213) 821-8892

San Francisco, California
77 Maiden Lane
(415) 986-8377

Torrance, California
24450 Hawthorne Boulevard
(213) 373-0792

OTHER

Anchorage, Alaska
3700 Old Seward Highway
(907) 563-4142

Tokyo, Japan
Patio Building 7F 13-23
03/408-3651

Toronto, Ontario, Canada
11 Hazelton Avenue
(416) 964-6216

When last-minute engagements necessitate a quick hair styling, makeup application, or manicure and it is impossible to get an appointment with your regular stylist, an alternative is available in many cities. There are a number of salons that now feature "instant services"—no appointments are required and the emphasis is on taking care of a client's needs as quickly as possible. Generally, these salons advertise no-frills service, meaning that the range of hair, skin, and nail treatments is limited. For example, the stylists will specialize in haircuts, sets, and blow-drying, but will not do hair coloring.

These services frequently are budget savers, many of the charges being about ten percent less than regular salon services. The savings is possible because the client makes certain accommodations. While no appointment is needed, services are provided on a first-come, first-served basis. You may have to wait a short time for an available stylist or manicurist, although turnover is quite rapid. Also, since no appointment is made with a particular stylist, it is likely you will have a different person working on you each time.

Some of the most extensive fast services for working women have been designed by Glemby. Its "Super Saver Services" in over 150 salons in the United States and Canada cater to women who are "on the go." Glemby has geared itself toward a new technology of quicker services and haircuts that can be done in minimal time. In addition, permanent waves are available without appointments. For the nearest Glemby Super Saver Salon in your area, call (800) 821-7700; in Hawaii, (800) 821-3777.

At-Home/In-Office Services

The ultimate in personal care services is the hair stylist or makeup specialist who comes to you. A growing cadre of beauty experts are now providing house calls or office visits to busy women whose schedules place limits on salon appointments. When you are going straight from the office to an evening event, the convenience of an in-office visit from a beauty stylist who will touch up your hair and makeup can help you feel and look your very best.

Many of these "on call" beauty experts work in a number of capacities for their clients. Not only are they available for creating a special look for a variety of occasions—from corporate events to weddings to photo sessions—they also provide consultation services. One New York hair and makeup specialist, Ouidad Wise, instructs her clients on how to apply makeup to best effect, offers advice on the most useful products to purchase, and designs a personalized makeup chart with guidelines on application and color choices. Of her home/office visits Ms. Wise says, "For the busy executive you cannot top the convenience and privacy of a personalized makeup and hair session. Women also find that a private appointment is doubly instructive for understanding how to use makeup and hair styling to accentuate facial structure."

Often the biggest challenge in securing the services of a traveling beauty specialist is simply finding out who will make house/office calls. Sometimes the hair stylists and beauty specialists at various salons will travel to their clients if requested, so it is worth checking this possibility. Otherwise, a phone call to a local photographer or modeling agency is a good method for acquiring names of recommended specialists who come to clients.

Massage

When the opportunity to schedule a massage is possible, many women will jump at the chance, while others will not consider the idea at all. For some, massage suffers from a tarnished reputation because it is associated with unprofessional practitioners. However, when performed by a qualified masseur or masseuse, massage is a therapeutic technique for easing tension out of the body. It is not only one of the most effective ways of relaxing tight muscles but also a wonderful remedy for a tired body and spirit.

A variety of massage and bodywork therapies are practiced by specialists throughout the country. Swedish massage, shiatsu, the Alexander Technique, and the Feldenkrais Method are some of the most widely known techniques. Generally, a session runs from thirty minutes to one hour and prices are based on the length of the session.

Many massage practitioners are trained at specialized institutes that grant certificates or licenses. In determining the qualifications of a massage therapist, it is important to ask questions about the person's training and experience and to request references. A reputable practitioner will provide this information willingly.

If finding a massage therapist is difficult, there are massage training centers that can offer referrals for certified specialists in your area. The following centers will also provide information on their respective techniques.

The American Center for the Alexander
  Technique, Inc.
142 West End Avenue
New York, New York 10023
(212) 799-0468

The American Massage Therapy Association
P.O. Box 1270
Kingsport, Tennessee 37662
(615) 245-8071

The Feldenkrais Guild
P.O. Box 11145
Main Office
San Francisco, California 94101
(415) 550-8708

Muscular Therapy Institute, Inc.
910 West End Avenue
New York, New York 10025
(212) 866-2069

Shiatsu Education Center of America
52 West 55th Street
New York, New York 10019
(212) 582-3424

At-Home Pampering

In addition to the numerous personal services you can acquire from specialists, there is nothing like going home knowing that you have provided special luxuries there for yourself. At the end of a long day, certain indulgences at home can ease away stress and renew energy.

Treating yourself to a long luxurious bubble-bath can be the cure for tired muscles as well as a balm to the senses. In fact, rather than a luxury, a leisurely bath can be considered a necessary means for relieving tension and stress. Ten to twenty minutes in a warm tub can simulate some of the effects of isolation tanks (completely enclosed tanks that cut off all external stimuli in which you float in water made highly buoyant with Epsom salts). By turning off the lights you can let your mind drift as the warm water soothes aching muscles. You may even want to light a scented candle to enhance the calming experience.

A variety of special salts, gels, and oils are available that can heighten the relaxing effects of your bath as well as acting as skin-softening agents. One common household product, baking soda, is an inexpensive yet highly effective skin conditioner. Half a cup of baking soda added to your bath will leave your skin feeling naturally smooth, soft, and clean. A number of bath products are specifically formulated to pamper the skin and muscles. For example, the Kneipp Corporation has created six different bath oils based on herbal extracts that can counteract specific stresses and strains of everyday life. Using rosemary, camomile, juniper, and extracts of hops, wintergreen, spruce, and pine, their Bath Botanics can help calm, revitalize, and unwind a tired body after a hectic day.

For a more invigorating experience, a shower with a water massage attachment can relieve aching neck, shoulder, and back muscles, Using a loofah in place of a washcloth can also stimulate the skin. If you need a real wake-up sensation, finish your shower with a bracing blast of cold water.

One of the best ways to conclude any bath or shower is wrapping yourself in a large, fluffy bath sheet or a luxurious terry cloth robe. Follow up with a rich moisturizing body lotion and a splash of cologne and you will feel like a guest at a spa in your own home!

In Closing . . .

As a career woman you have accepted the challenges and responsibilities of being a professional in the working world of the 1980s. The information in The Executive Body provides you with the resources and tools to realize your full potential. Fitness is your personal foundation for achieving and maintaining the most satisfying work life and home life. Here's to your life of happiness, success, and health!

For Further Reading

Judy Alter, Surviving Exercise (Boston: Houghton Mifflin, 1983).

Judy Babcock and Judy Kennedy, The Spa Book (New York: Crown Publishers, 1983).

Herbert Benson, The Relaxation Response (New York: Avon, 1975).

Jane Brody, Jane Brody's Nutrition Book (New York: W. W. Norton & Co., 1981).

Martha Davis, Elizabeth Robbins Eshelman, and Matthew McKay, The Relaxation and Stress Reduction Workbook (Oakland, Calif.: New Harbinger, 1982).

Susan Dresner, Managing Your Business Image: A Practical Guide to Personal Style, 1983. Available from Successful Ways & Means, 36 West 89th Street, New York, N.Y. 10024. The cost is $6.50 plus $1.50 postage and handling.

K. F. Ernst, The Complete Calorie Counter for Dining Out (New York: Jove, 1981).

Mary Fiedorek and Diana Lewis Jewell, Executive Style —Looking It...Living It (Piscataway, N.J.: New Century Publishers, 1983).

John D. Kirschmann, Nutrition Almanac (New York: McGraw-Hill, 1973).

Charles Kuntzleman, Diet Free (Emmaus, Pa.: Rodale, 1982).

Alan Lakein, How to Get Control of Your Time and Your Life (New York: Signet/New American Library, 1974).

Martin Shaffer, Life After Stress (Chicago: Contemporary Books, 1983).

Stephanie Winston, Getting Organized (New York: Warner Books, 1980).

Hotels and Motels with Sauna/Spa Facilities*

* Courtesy of American Hotel and Motel Association

ALABAMA

Olympia Spa
Golf and Country Club
U.S. Highway 231 S
Box 6108
Dothan, AL 36302
(205) 677-3321

Grand Hotel
Highway 98
Point Clear, AL 36564
(205) 928-9201

ARIZONA

Best Western Canyon Squire Inn
Highways 64 & 180
P.O. Box 130
Grand Canyon, AZ 86023
(602) 638-2681

Rio Rico Resort Hotel
Calabasas Rd. & I-19
Box 2050
Nogales, AZ 85621
(602) 281-1901

The Adams Hotel
Central & Adams
P.O. Box 1000
Phoenix, AZ 85001
(602) 257-1525

Howard Johnson's Caravan Inn
3333 E. Van Buren
Phoenix, AZ 85008
(602) 244-8244

Pointe Resort
7677 N. 16th St.
Phoenix, AZ 85020
(602) 997-2626

Rodeway Inn-MetroCenter
10402 N. Black Canyon
Phoenix, AZ 85021
(602) 943-2371

Sheraton Greenway Inn
2510 W. Greenway Rd.
Phoenix, AZ 85023
(602) 993-0800

Hospitality Inn-Scottsdale
409 N. Scottsdale Rd.
Scottsdale, AZ 85257
(602) 949-5115

The Inn at McCormick Ranch
7401 N. Scottsdale Rd.
Scottsdale, AZ 85253
(602) 940-5050

The Registry Resort
7171 N. Scottsdale Rd.
Scottsdale, AZ 85253
(602) 991-3800

Fiesta Inn
2100 S. Priest Dr.
Tempe, AZ 85282
(602) 967-8809

ARKANSAS
Fairfield Bay Resort and
    Conference Center
P.O. Box 3008
Fairfield Bay, AR 72088
(501) 664-6000

Red Apple Inn & Executive
    Conference Center
Eden Isle Highway 110
Heber Springs, AR 72543
(501) 362-3111

CALIFORNIA
Quality Inn/Anaheim
616 Convention Way
Anaheim, CA 92802
(714) 750-3131

San Luis Bay Inn
Avila Rd.
Avila Beach, CA 93424
(805) 595-2333

Rio Bravo Tennis Ranch Resort
11200 Lake Ming Rd.
Bakersfield, CA 93306
(805) 366-3251

Berkeley Marina Marriott
200 Marina Blvd.
Berkeley, CA 94710
(415) 548-7920

Beverly Wilshire Hotel
9500 Wilshire Blvd.
Beverly Hills, CA 90212
(213) 275-4282

Quail Lodge
8205 Valley Greens Dr.
Carmel, CA 93923
(408) 624-1581

Eureka Inn
Seventh & "F" Sts.
Eureka, CA 95501
(707) 442-6441

Hacienda Inn
2550 W. Clinton Ave.
Fresno, CA 93705
(209) 486-3000

Erawan Garden Hotel
76-477 Highway 111
Indian Wells, CA 92260
(714) 346-8021

Registry Hotel
18800 MacArthur Blvd.
Irvine, CA 92715
(714) 752-8777

Royal Inn
7830 Fay Ave.

La Jolla, CA 92037
(714) 459-4461

Summer House Inn
7955 La Jolla Shores Dr.
La Jolla, CA 92037
(714) 459-0261

Hacienda Hotel
525 N. Senulveda Blvd.
El Segundo
Los Angeles, CA 90245
(213) 615-0015

Westwood Marquis Hotel
930 Hilgard Ave.
Los Angeles, CA 90024
(213) 208-8765

Hilton Inn Resort
1000 Aguajito Rd.
Route 1
Monterey, CA 93940
(408) 373-6141

Sheraton Newport
4545 MacArthur Blvd.
Newport Beach, CA 92660
(714) 833-0570

Sheraton Universal Hotel
30 Universal City Plaza
North Hollywood, CA 91608
(213) 980-1212

Canyon Hotel Racquet/Golf Resort
2850 S. Palm Canyon Dr.
Palm Springs, CA 92262
(714) 323-5656

International Hotel Resort
1800 E. Palm Canyon Dr.
Palm Springs, CA 92262
(714) 323-1711

Sheraton Plaza Palm Springs
400 E. Tahquitz-McCallum Way
Palm Springs, CA 92262
(714) 320-6868

SPA Hotel and Mineral Springs
100 N. Indian Ave.
Palm Springs, CA 92262
(714) 325-1461

El Rancho Racquet Resort Hotel
1029 W. Capitol Ave.
Sacramento, CA 95691
(916) 371-6731

Half Moon Inn
2303 Shelter Island Dr.
San Diego, CA 92106
(714) 224-3411

Hyatt San Jose
1740 N. 1st St.
San Jose, CA 95112
(408) 298-0300

Santa Barbara Inn
435 S. Milpas
Santa Barbara, CA 93103
(805) 966-2285

Sheraton Santa Barbara
  Hotel & Spa
1111 Cabrillo Blvd.
Santa Barbara, CA 93103
(805) 963-0744

Coto de Caza
22000 Plano Trabuco Rd.
Box 438
Trabuco Canyon, CA 92678
(714) 586-0761

COLORADO
Lazy H Guest Ranch
P.O. Box 248
Allens Park, CO 80510
(303) 747-2532

Aspen Square
617 E. Cooper Ave.
Aspen, CO 81611
(303) 925-1000

The Gant
610 West End
Aspen, CO 81611
(303) 925-5000

The Broadmoor Hotel
Lake Ave and Lake Circle
Colorado Springs, CO 80901
(303) 634-7711

Colorado Springs Hilton Inn
505 Pope's Bluff Trail
Colorado Springs, CO 80907
(303) 598-7656

Four Seasons Motor Inn
2886 S. Circle Dr.
Colorado Springs, CO 80906
(303) 576-5900

Copper Mountain Resort
  Association
P.O. Box 1
Copper Mountain, CO 80443
(303) 668-2882

Denver Hilton Hotel
1550 Court Place
Denver, CO 80202
(303) 893-3333

Executive Tower Inn
1405 Curtis
Denver, CO 80202
(303) 571-0300

Stapleton Plaza Hotel
  and Athletic Center
3333 Quebec St. Stapleton Plaza
Denver, CO 80207
(303) 321-3500

Stouffer's Denver Inn
3203 Quebec St.
Denver, CO 80207
(303) 321-3333

Western Motor Inn
4757 Vasquez Blvd.
Denver, CO 80216
(303) 534-8553

Tamarron
P.O. Box 3131
Durango, CO 81301
(303) 247-8801

Longs Peak Inn and Guest Ranch
Longs Peak Rt 1
Estes Park, CO 80517
(303) 586-2110

Holiday Inn on Lake Dillon
Exit 203 on I-70
Frisco, CO 80435
(303) 668-5000

Holiday Inn
755 Horizon Dr. I-70 and
  Airport Exit
Grand Junction, CO 81502
(303) 243-6790

Keystone Resort
P.O. Box 38
Keystone, CO 80435
(303) 321-1802

Pagosa Lodge
US Highway 160 W.P.O. Box 245
Pagosa Springs, CO 81147
(303) 264-2271

The Crestwood
P.O. Box 5460
Snowmass Village, CO 81615
(303) 923-2450

The Crest Resort Hotel
250 S. Frontage Rd.
P.O. Box 1928
Vail, CO 81657
(303) 476-1676

Marriott's Mark Resort
715 West Lionshead Circle
Vail, CO 81657
(303) 476-4444

Mountain Haus at Vail
292 E. Meadow Dr.
Vail, CO 81657
(303) 476-2434

CONNECTICUT
Showboat Inn
500 Steamboat Rd.
Greenwich, CT 06830
(203) 661-9800

Sheraton Hartford
315 Trumbull St.
   at Civic Center Plaza
Hartford, CT 06103
(203) 728-5151

Interlaken Inn
Route 112
Lakeville, CT 06039
(203) 435-9878

Harrison Conference Center
Heritage Village, CT 06488
(203) 264-8255/(914) 332-0144

Stamford Marriott
Two Stamford Forum
Stamford, CT 06901
(203) 357-9555

DISTRICT OF COLUMBIA
The Shoreham
2500 Calvert St., NW
Washington, D.C. 20008
(202) 234-0700

Washington Hilton Hotel
1919 Connecticut Ave., NW
Washington, D.C. 20009
(202) 483-3000

Washington Hotel
15th & Penn Ave., NW
Washington, D.C. 20004
(202) 638-5900

FLORIDA
Boca Raton Hotel & Club
Camino Real
Boca Raton, FL 33432
(305) 395-3000

Plantation Inn & Golf Resort
W. Kings Bay Rd.
Crystal River, FL 32629
(904) 795-4211

Daytona Hilton
2637 S. Atlantic Ave.
Daytona Beach, FL 32018
(904) 767-7350

Sandestin Resort
Highway 98 E
Destin, FL 32541
(904) 837-2121

Hilton Inn and Conference Center
   at Inverrary
3501 Inverray Blvd.
Lauderhill, FL 33320
(305) 485-0500

Inter-Continental Miami Hotel
801 S. Bayshore Dr.
Miami, FL 33131
(305) 377-1966

Court of Flags Hotel
5715 Major Blvd.
Orlando, FL 32805
(305) 351-3340

Sheraton Inn Winter Park
736 Lee Rd.
Orlando, FL 32810
(305) 647-1112

Sheraton Twin Towers Hotel
5780 Major Blvd.
Orlando, FL 32805
(305) 351-1000

La Coquille Club
P.O. Box 2528
Palm Beach, FL 33480
(305) 582-7411

Palm Beach Ocean Hotel
2770-2830 S. Ocean Blvd.
Palm Beach, FL 33480
(305) 582-5381

The World of Palm-Aire
2501 Palm-Aire Dr. N.
Pompano Beach, FL 33060
(305) 971-6000

Don CeSar Beach Resort
3400 Gulf Blvd.
St. Petersburg Beach, FL 33706
(813) 360-1881

Saddlebrook Resort
Highway 54
Wesley Chapel, FL 33599
(813) 973-1111

GEORGIA
Atlanta Hilton Hotel
255 Courtland and Harris Sts., NE
Atlanta, GA 30043
(404) 659-2000

Atlanta Marriott Hotel
Courtland and
   International Blvd., NE
Atlanta, GA 30043
(404) 659-6500

Peachtree Plaza
Peachtree at International
Atlanta, GA 30343
(404) 659-1400

Augusta Hilton Hotel
640 Broad St.
Augusta, GA 30902
(404) 722-5541

Thunderbird Inn
919 15th St.
P.O. Box 10083
Augusta, GA 30903
(404) 724-9625

Big Canoe Conference Center
Big Canoe, GA 30143
(404) 579-3333

Callaway Gardens Inn
US Highway 27 S
Pine Mountain, GA 31822
(404) 663-2281

Sheraton Savannah Inn
   & Country Club
612 Wilmington Island Rd.
Savannah, GA 31410
(912) 897-1612

Holiday Inn of Thomasville
US Highway 19S
Box 1055
Thomasville, GA 31792
(912) 226-7111

HAWAII
Hyatt Regency-Maui
200 Nohea Kai Dr.
Lahaina-Maui, HI 96761
(808) 922-9292

IDAHO
North Shore Motor Hotel
Convention Center
North Shore Plaza
Coeure D'Alene, ID 83814
(208) 664-9241

University Inn-Best Western
1516 Pullman Rd.
Moscow, ID 83843
(208) 882-0550

Pocatello Hilton Inn
1555 Pocatello Creek Rd.
Pocatello, ID 83201
(208) 233-2200

Elkhorn Village Inn &
   Condominiums
Elkhorn Rd.
Box 1067
Sun Valley, ID 83353
(208) 622-4511

ILLINOIS
Ramada Inn-Convention Center
1501 S. Neil St.
Champaign, IL 61820
(217) 352-7891

Chicago Marriott Hotel
540 N. Michigan Ave.
Chicago, IL 60611
(312) 836-0100

McCormick Inn
23rd St. and Lake Shore Dr.
Chicago, IL 60616
(312) 791-1900

Holiday Inn-City Centre
300 E. Ohio St.
Chicago, IL 60611
(312) 787-6100

Radisson Chicago Hotel
505 N. Michigan
Chicago, IL 60611
(312) 944-4100

Holiday Inn
US 36 and Wyckles Rd.
Decatur, IL 62522
(217) 422-8800

Ramada The O'Hare Inn
Mannheim and Higgins Rd.
Des Plaines, IL 60018
(312) 827-5131

Chateau Louise Resort
Route 31
Dundee, IL 60118
(312) 426-8000

Keller's Ramada Inn
I-70 and 57 111
Routes 32-33
Box 747
Effingham, IL 62401
(217) 342-2131

Holiday Inn-Elk Grove
1000 Busse Rd.
Elk Grove Village, IL 60007
(312) 437-6010

Midway Motor Lodge
1600 Oakton St.
Elk Grove Village, IL 60007
(312) 981-0010

Eagle Ridge Inn & Resort
Galena Territory
Route 20
Galena, IL 61036
(815) 777-2444

La Quinta Motor Inn
U.S. Highways 150 and 92
Moline, IL 61265
(309) 762-9008

Sheraton North Shore Inn
933 Skokie Blvd.
Northbrook, IL 60062
(312) 498-6500

Drake OakBrook Hotel/Conference
  Center
York and Cermak Rds.
Oak Brook, IL 60521
(312) 654-2230

Holiday Inn O'Hare/Kennedy
5440 N. River Rd.
Rosemont, IL 60018
(312) 671-6350

Pheasant Run Lodge
North Ave Route 64
P.O. Box 64
St. Charles, IL 60174
(312) 584-6300

Holiday Inn-O'Hare Airport
3801 N. Mannheim Rd.
Schiller Park, IL 60176
(312) 678-0670

Howard Johnson's O'Hare
International Hotel/Conference
  Center
10249 W. Irving Park Rd.
Schiller Park, IL 60176
(312) 671-6000

Holiday Inn-East
3100 S. Dirksen Pkwy.
Springfield, IL 62703
(217) 529-7171

Springfield Hilton
700 E. Adams St.
Springfield, IL 62701
(217) 789-1530

Sheraton Waukegan Inn &
  Conference Center
200 N. Greenbay Rd.
Waukegan, IL 60085
(312) 244-2400

INDIANA
Evansville Executive Inn
600 Walnut St.
P.O. Box 3246
Evansville, IN 47731
(812) 424-8000

Howard Johnson's Motor Lodge East
2141 N. Post Rd.
Indianapolis, IN 46219
(317) 897-2000

Marten House
1801 W. 86th St.
Indianapolis, IN 46260
(317) 872-4111

Sheraton West Hotel &
  Conference Center.
2544 Executive Dr. at Airport
Indianapolis, IN 46241
(317) 248-2481

Holiday Inn/Holiday Plaza Hotel
  and Resort
800 E. 81st Ave.
Holiday Plaza
Merrillville, IN 46410
(219) 769-6311

IOWA
Gateway Center Motor Hotel
U.S. 30 and ISU Center Exit
Ames, IA 50010
(515) 292-8600

Blackhawk Hotel
3rd and Perry St.
Davenport, IA 52801
(319) 323-2816

New Savery Hotel
4th and Locust St.
Des Moines, IA 50309
(515) 244-2151

Best Western Regency Inn
Junction Highways 14 and 30
Marshalltown, IA 50158
(515) 752-6321

KANSAS
Glenwood Manor Motor Hotel
9200 S. Metcalf, Highway 69
Overland Park, KS 66212
(913) 649-7000

Ramada Inn & Tower-Downtown
420 East 6th St.
Box 1598
Topeka, KS 66614
(913) 233-8981

KENTUCKY
Cincinnati Drawbridge Inn
I-75 at Buttermilk Pike
Fort Mitchell, KY 41017
(606) 341-2800

LOUISIANA
The Oak Manor Motor Hotel
8181 Airline Highway
Baton Rouge, LA 70815
(800) 535-8486

Royale Rouge Hotel
1575 Riverside N
Baton Rouge, LA 70802
(504) 387-4444

International Hotel
300 Canal St.
New Orleans, LA 70140
(504) 581-1300

Sheraton Bossier Inn
2015 Old Minder Rd., Bossier
Shreveport, LA 71111
(318) 742-9700

MAINE
Holiday Inn-Downtown
88 Spring St.
Portland, ME 04111
(207) 775-2311

MARYLAND
Baltimore Hilton Inn
1726 Reisterstown Rd.
Pikesville, MD 21208
(301) 653-1100

Marriott's Hunt Valley Inn
I-83 at Shawan Rd.
Hunt Valley, MD 21031
(301) 666-7000

Sheraton Fountainebleau Inn/Spa
10100 Ocean Highway
Ocean City, MD 21842
(301) 524-3535

MASSACHUSETTS
Boston Park Plaza Hotel
Arlington St. at Park Sq.
Boston, MA 02117
(617) 426-2000

Sheraton Inn/Conference Center
242 Sheraton Rd.
I-495, Exit 28
Boxborough, MA 01719
(617) 263-8701

Wychmere Harbor Club/Hotel
23 Snow Inn Rd.
Harwichport, MA 02646
(617) 432-1000

Dunfey Hyannis Hotel
35 Scudder Ave., West End Circle
Hyannis, MA 02601
(617) 775-7775

Howard Johnson's Motor Lodge
320 Washington St.
Newton, MA 02158
(617) 969-3010

Oak N' Spruce Resort
  "In the Berkshires"
South Lee, MA 01260
(413) 243-3500

Sheraton Sturbridge Inn
U.S. Route 20
Sturbridge, MA 01566
(617) 347-7393

Hilton Inn Resort &
  Conference Center
Route 128 at Audubon Rd.
Wakefield, MA 01880
(617) 245-9300

Sheraton Inn-Springfield West
1080 Riverdale St. at I-91
West Springfield, MA 01089
(413) 781-8750

Sheraton Lincoln Inn &
  Conference Center
500 Lincoln St.
Worcester, MA 01606
(617) 852-4000

MICHIGAN
Grand Traverse Hilton
Conference Center and Resort
Grand Traverse Village

Acme, MI 49610
(616) 938-2100

Holiday Inn of Alpena
1000 US 23 N
Alpena, MI 49707
(517) 356-2151

Briarwood Hilton
610 Hilton Blvd. and State St.
Ann Arbor, MI 48104
(313) 761-7800

Marriott Inn
3600 Plymouth Rd.
Ann Arbor, MI 48105
(313) 769-9800

Boyne Mountain Lodge
Boyne Falls, MI 49713
(616) 549-2441

McGuire's Resort & Conference
  Center
7880 Mackinaw Trail
Cadillac, MI 49601
(616) 775-9947

Sugar Loaf Mountain Resort
  and Conference Center
Route 1
Cedar, MI 49621
(616) 228-5461

Northfield Hilton-Troy
5500 Crooks Rd. at I-75
Detroit, MI 48098
(313) 879-2100

Best Western Chalet
  Motor Lodge & Inn
1042 W. Main St.
Gaylord, MI 49735
(517) 732-9091

Grand Rapids Airport Hilton Inn
4747 28th St. SE
Grand Rapids, MI 49508
(616) 957-0100

Midway Motor Lodge
4101 28th St. SE
Grand Rapids, MI 49508
(616) 942-2550

Boyne Highlands Inn
Harbor Springs, MI 49740
(616) 549-2441

Holiday Inn
2000 Holiday Inn Dr.
Jackson, MI 49202
(517) 783-2681

Kalamazoo Center Hilton Inn
100 W. Michigan Ave.
Kalamazoo, MI 49007
(616) 381-2130

Grand Hotel
Mackinac Island, MI 49757
(906) 847-3331

Inn at the Bridge
I-94 at Hancock
Port Huron, MI 48060
(313) 984-2661

Hilton Airport Inn
31500 Wick Rd.
Detroit Metro Airport
Romulus, MI 48174
(313) 292-3400

Radisson Inn Saginaw
400 Johnson St.
Saginaw, MI 48607
(517) 755-1161

Holiday Inn on the Beach
615 E. Front St.
Traverse City, MI 49684
(616) 947-3700

Park Place-Best Western
300 E. State St.
Traverse City, MI 49684
(616) 946-5410

Hilton Inn
1455 Stephenson Highway
Troy, MI 48084
(313) 583-9000

Midway Motor Lodge
31800 Van Dyke
Warren, MI 48093
(313) 939-2860

MINNESOTA

Radisson Arrowwood Inn and Resort
P.O. Box 639
Alexandria, MN 56308
(612) 762-1124

Holiday Inn-Bloomington Central
1201 West 94th St.
Bloomington, MN 55431
(612) 884-8211

L'hotel de France Minneapolis
5601 West 78th St.
Bloomington, MN 55435
(612) 835-1900

Radisson South Hotel
7800 Normandale
Bloomington, MN 55435
(612) 835-7800

Grand View Lodge/Tennis Club
Route 6
P.O. Box 22
Brainerd, MN 56401
(218) 963-2234: Summer
(612) 332-1667: Winter

Nelson's Resort
Crane Lake, MN 55725
(218) 993-2295

Holiday Inn of Detroit Lakes
Highway 10 East
Detroit Lakes, MN 56501
(218) 847-2121

Best Western Normandy Inn
207 W. Superior St.
Duluth, MN 55802
(218) 722-1202

Golden Valley House-Best Western
4820 Olson Memorial Highway
Golden Valley, MN 55422
(612) 588-0511

Holiday Inn-Downtown Minneapolis
1313 Nicollet Mall
Minneapolis, MN 55403
(612) 332-0371

Marquette Hotel
710 Marquette Ave. at IDS Center
Minneapolis, MN 55402
(612) 332-2351

Sheraton Inn Northwest
I-94 and US 52, Brooklyn Park
Minneapolis, MN 55428
(612) 566-8855

The Thunderbird Motel
2201 E. 78th St. Bloomington
Minneapolis, MN 55420
(612) 854-3411

Best Western Midway Motor Lodge
1517 16th St., SW
Rochester, MN 55901
(507) 289-8866

Holiday Inn North Roseville
2540 N. Cleveland Ave.
St. Paul, MN 55113
(612) 636-4567

MISSOURI

Holiday Inn
US 61 S at Market
Hannibal, MO 63401
(314) 221-2508

Holiday Inn of Joplin
3615 Range Line Rd.
I-44 and US 71
Joplin, MO 64801
(417) 782-1000

Sheraton Royal Hotel
9103 E. 39th St.
Kansas City, MO 64133
(816) 737-0200

The Lodge of the Four Seasons
Lake Rd HH
P.O. Box 215
Lake Ozark, MO 65049
(314) 365-3001

Marriott's Tan-Tar-A Resort
State Rd KK
P.O. Box 188
Osage Beach, MO 65065
(314) 348-3131

Howard Johnson's Motor Lodge—
   Airport West
I-70 and 1425 S. 5th St.
St. Charles, MO 63301
(314) 946-6939

Bel Air Hilton
333 Washington Ave
St. Louis, MO 63102
(314) 621-7900

The Clayton Inn Hotel
7750 Carondelet
Clayton, MO 63105
(314) 726-5400

Harley Hotel
13440 Riverglen Dr.
St. Louis, MO 63045
(314) 291-6800

Holiday Inn—Clayton Plaza
7730 Bonhomme
Clayton, MO 63105
(314) 863-0400

Marriott's Pavilion Hotel
1 S. Broadway
St. Louis, MO 63102
(314) 421-1776

Midway Motor Lodge
   St. Louis Westport
2434 Old Dorsett Rd.
St. Louis, MO 63043
(314) 291-8700

Stouffer's Riverfront Towers
200 S. 4th St.
St. Louis, MO 63102
(314) 241-9500

MONTANA

Huntley Lodge
P.O. Box 1
Big Sky, MT 59716
(406) 995-4211

Best Western Ponderosa Inn
2511 First Ave. N
Billings, MT 59101
(406) 248-7701

Holiday Inn of Bozeman
5 Baxter Lane
Bozeman, MT 59715
(406) 587-4561

Sheraton Great Falls Inn
400 Tenth Ave. S.
Great Falls, MT 59405
(406) 727-7200

Best Western Colonial Inn
2301 Colonial Dr.
Helena, MT 59601
(406) 443-2100

Helena TraveLodge
22 N. Last Chance Gulch
Helena, MT 59601
(406) 443-2200

NEBRASKA

Holiday Inn
Highways 281 and I-80
Grand Island, NE 68801
(308) 384-7770

Ramada Inn-Central
7007 Grover St.
Omaha, NE 68106
(402) 397-7030

NEVADA

Caesars Palace Hotel
3570 Las Vegas Blvd. S
Las Vegas, NV 89109
(702) 731-7201

Las Vegas Hilton Hotel
3000 Paradise Rd.
Las Vegas, NV 89109
(702) 732-5111

Tropicana Hotel and Country Club
3801 Las Vegas Blvd. S
Las Vegas, NV 89109
(702) 739-2222

Harrah's Reno Hotel & Casino
219 N. Center St.
P.O. Box 10
Reno, NV 89504
(702) 788-3043

NEW HAMPSHIRE

Mount Washington Hotel
Route 302
Bretton Woods, NH 03575
(603) 278-1000

Christmas Farm Inn
Route 16-B
Jackson, NH 03846
(603) 383-4313

Margate Resort
76 Lake St.
Laconia, NH 03246
(603) 524-5210

Fox Ridge Resort Inn
Route 16
North Conway, NH 03860
(603) 356-3151

Red Jacket Mt. View Motor Inn
Routes 16 and 302
North Conway, NH 03860
(603) 356-5411

Sheraton North Country Inn
Airport Rd.
West Lebanon, NH 03784
(603) 298-5906

NEW JERSEY

Del Webb's Claridge
Indiana Ave and Boardwalk
Atlantic City, NJ 08404
(609) 340-3500

Resorts International Hotel Casino
North Carolina Ave. and Boardwalk
Atlantic City, NJ 08404
(609) 340-6030

Golden Eagle Inn
Oceanfront at Philadelphia Ave.
Cape May, NJ 08204
(609) 884-5611

Sheraton Heights
650 Terrace Ave.
Route 80 & 17
Hasbrouck Heights, NJ 07604
(201) 288-6100

Holiday Inn-Jersey City
Holland Tunnel Plaza
Jersey City, NJ 07302
(201) 653-0300

Playboy Resort and Country Club
Route 517 Great Gorge
Box 637
McAfee, NJ 07428
(201) 827-6000

Port-O-Call Hotel and Motor Inn
1510 Boardwalk
Ocean City, NJ 08226
(609) 399-8812

Somerset Marriott Hotel
110 Davidson Ave.
Somerset, NJ 08873
(201) 560-0500

Travelodge at Franklin Mall
1850 Easton Ave.
Somerset, NJ 08873
(201) 469-5050

Woodcliff Lake Hilton Inn
Chestnut Ridge Rd.
Woodcliff Lake, NJ 07675
(201) 391-3600

NEW MEXICO

Classic Hotel Best Western
6815 Menaul Blvd. NE
Albuquerque, NM 87110
(505) 881-9666

Holiday Inn
Exit 16 W Interchange I-40
Gallup, NM 87301
(505) 722-2201

Inn of the Mountain Gods
Mescalero Highway 70
Box 259
Mescalero, NM 88340
(505) 257-5141

Bishop's Lodge
Bishop's Lodge Rd.
Box 2367
Santa Fe, NM 87501
(505) 983-6377

Sagebrush Inn
South Santa Fe Rd.
P.O. Box 1566
Taos, NM 87571
(505) 758-2254

NEW YORK

Pine Tree Point Resort
P.O. Box 68
Alexandria Bay, NY 13607
(315) 482-9911

Buffalo Hilton at the Waterfront
Church and Terrace
Buffalo, NY 14202
(716) 845-5100

Sheraton Inn—Buffalo East
2040 Walden Ave.
Cheektowaga, NY 14225
(716) 681-2400

Sheraton Canandaigua Inn
   on the Lake
770 S. Main St.
Canandaigua, NY 14424
(716) 394-7800

Inn-At-The-Peak
Clymer, NY 14724
(716) 355-4141

East Norwich Inn
Route 25-A at 106
East Norwich, NY 11732
(516) 922-1500

Villaggio Resort Hotel
O'Hara Rd. just off Route 23-A
Haines Falls, NY 12436
(518) 589-5000

Concord Resort Hotel
Kiamesha Lake, NY 12751
(914) 794-4000

Holiday Inn
Route 9
P.O. Box 231
Lake George, NY 12845
(518) 668-5781

Roaring Brook Ranch
   and Tennis Resort
Route 9N South
Lake George, NY 12845
(518) 668-5767

Hidden Valley Ranch
Hidden Valley Rd.
Lake Lucerne, NY 12846
(518) 696-2431

Howard Johnson's Motor Lodge
551 Route 211 E, I-84 Exit 4-W
Middletown, NY 10940
(914) 342-5822

Gurney's Inn/Oceanfront Resort
   and Conference Center
Old Montauk Highway
Montauk, NY 11954
(516) 668-2345

Montauk Yacht Club and Inn
Star Island Rd.
P.O. Box W
Montauk, NY 11954
(516) 668-3100

Parker Meridien Hotel
118 West 57th St.
New York, NY 10019
(212) 245-5000

Vista International Hotel
3 World Trade Center
New York, NY 10048
(212) 938-9100

The Warwick Hotel
65 West 54th St.
New York, NY 10019
(212) 247-2700

Pickwick Motor Inn
Exit 48 Long Island Expressway
Plainview, NY 11803
(516) 694-6500

Rye Town Hilton
699 Westchester Ave.
Port Chester, NY 10573
(914) 939-6300

Schenectady Ramada Inn
450 Nott St.
Schenectady, NY 12308
(518) 370-7151

Syracuse Marriott Inn
Marriott Dr. at Carrier Circle
Syracuse, NY 13057
(315) 432-0200

Stouffer's Inn of Westchester
80 W. Red Oak Lane
White Plains, NY 10604
(914) 694-5400

NORTH CAROLINA
Great Smokies Hilton Resort/
   Conference Center
1 Hilton Inn Dr.
Asheville, NC 28806
(704) 254-3211

Grove Park Inn/Country Club
290 Macon Ave.
Asheville, NC 28804
(704) 252-2711

Registry Inn
321 W. Woodlawn Rd.
Charlotte, NC 28210
(704) 525-4441

Sheraton Center Hotel
555 S. McDowell St.
Charlotte, NC 28204
(704) 372-4100

Ramada Inn Downtown
600 Willard St.
Durham, NC 27707
(919) 683-1531

Holiday Inn—Holidome
702 Memorial Dr.
P.O. Box 585
Greenville, NC 27834
(919) 758-3401

Pinehurst Hotel and Country Club
P.O. Box 4000
Pinehurst, NC 28374
(919) 295-6811

Pine Needles Lodges and
   Country Club
Off US 1 on NC 2
P.O. Box 88
Southern Pines, NC 28337
(919) 692-7111

OHIO
Sheraton Aurora Inn
800 N. Aurora Rd.
Aurora, OH 44202
(216) 562-9151

Sheraton Belden Inn
4375 Metro Center
Canton, OH 44720
(216) 494-6494

Cincinnati Plaza
  at Fountain Square
Cincinnati, OH 45202
(513) 621-7700

Holiday Inn Coliseum
4742 Brecksville Rd., Richfield
Cleveland, OH 44286
(216) 659-6151

Holiday Inn—Wickliffe
28500 Euclid Ave., Wickliffe
Cleveland, OH 44092
(216) 585-2750

Sheraton Hopkins Airport Hotel
5300 Riverside Dr.
Cleveland, OH 44135
(216) 267-1500

Best Western Royal Motor Inn
3232 Olentangy River Rd.
Columbus, OH 43202
(614) 261-7141

Holiday Inn—Airport Holidome
750 Stelzer Rd.
I-70 James Rd. Exit
Columbus, OH 43219
(614) 237-6360

La Quinta Motor Inn North
3636 N. Dixie Dr.
Dayton, OH 45414
(513) 276-6151

La Quinta Motor Inn South
840 Nicholas Rd.
Dayton, OH 45408
(513) 223-0166

Atwood Lake Lodge Resort
Route 542

P.O. Box 96
Dellroy, OH 44620
(216) 735-2211

Quail Hollow Inn
I-90 and Route 44
Painsville, OH 44077
(216) 352-6201

Midway Motor Lodge
30 Tri County Parkway
Springdale, OH 45246
(513) 772-5440

Americana Inn
11 W. Leffel Lane
Springfield, OH 45506
(513) 322-4941

Harley Hotel
1800 Miami St.
Toledo, OH 43605
(419) 666-5120

OKLAHOMA
Sheraton Inn Skyline East
6333 E. Skelly Dr.
Tulsa, OK 74135
(918) 627-1000

OREGON
The Inn of the Seventh Mountain
Century Dr.
P.O. Box 1207
Bend, OR 97701
(503) 382-8711

The Inn at Spanish Head
4009 S Highway 101
Lincoln City, OR 97367
(503) 996-2161

Marriott Hotel
1401 SW Front Ave.
Portland, OR 97201
(503) 226-7600

PENNSYLVANIA
Sheraton Altoona
Route 220 RD #2
P.O. Box 520
Altoona, PA 16601

Magic Valley USA
Bushkill, PA 18324
(717) 588-6661

Seven Springs Mountain Resort
RD #1
Champion, PA 15622
(814) 352-7777

Hershey Lodge &
  Convention Center
W. Chocolate Ave. & University Dr.
Hershey, PA 17033
(717) 533-3311

Sheraton Valley Forge Hotel
Route 363
King of Prussia, PA 19406
(215) 337-2000

Host Farm & Corral
2300 Lincoln Highway E.
Lancaster, PA 17602
(717) 299-5500

Host Town Resort
30 Keller Ave.
Lancaster, PA 17601
(717) 299-5700

Lancaster Treadway Resort Inn
222 Eden Rd.
Routes 30 & 272N
Lancaster, PA 17602
(717) 569-6444

Sheraton Harrisburg Inn
I-83 and PA Turnpike Exit 18
New Cumberland, PA 17070
(717) 774-2721

Franklin Plaza Hotel
2 Franklin Plaza
Philadelphia, PA 19103
(215) 448-2000

Sheraton Airport Inn
Philadelphia International Airport
Philadelphia, PA 19153
(215) 365-4150

Sheraton Motor Inn—Northeast
9461 Roosevelt Blvd.
Philadelphia, PA 19114
(215) 671-9600

Hyatt Pittsburgh at Chatham Center
112 Washington Place
Pittsburgh, PA 15219
(412) 391-5000

Pittsburgh Marriott—Greentree
101 Marriott Dr.
Pittsburgh, PA 15205
(412) 922-8400

Sheraton Pocono Inn
I-80 at Exit 48
Stroudsburg, PA 18360
(717) 424-1930

Mount Summit Inn
Route 40 East
Uniontown, PA 15401
(412) 438-8594

Hilton Inn Meadowlands
340 Racetrack Rd.
Washington, PA 15301
(412) 222-6200

RHODE ISLAND
Sheraton-Islander Inn
Goat Island
Newport, RI 02840
(401) 849-2600

Sheraton Airport Inn
1850 Post Rd., US Route 1
Warwick, RI 02886
(401) 738-4000

SOUTH CAROLINA
Kiawah Island Inn and Resort
P.O. Box 12910
Charleston, SC 29412
(803) 768-2121

TENNESSEE
Downtowner Motor Inn
Highway 73
P.O. Box 749
Gatlinburg, TN 37738
(615) 436-5043

Glenstone Lodge
Airport Rd.
Box 149
Gatlinburg, TN 37738
(615) 436-9361

The Peabody Hotel
149 Union Ave.
Memphis, TN 38103
(901) 529-4000

Continental Inn Interstate
303 Interstate Dr. off I-65
Nashville, TN 37213
(615) 244-6690

Music City Rodeway Inn
797 Briley Parkway at I-40
Nashville, TN 37217
(615) 361-5900

TEXAS
Amarillo Hilton Inn
I-40 Lakeside
Amarillo, TX 79105
(806) 373-3071

Best Western Villa Capri Hotel
2400 N. Interregional Highway 35
Austin, TX 78705
(512) 476-6171

Lakeway Resort
101 Lakeway Dr.
Austin, TX 78734
(512) 261-6000

Sheraton Marina Inn
300 N. Shoreline Blvd.
Corpus Christi, TX 78401
(512) 883-5111

Amfac Hotel & Resort
Dallas/Fort Worth Airport
Box 61025
Dallas, TX 75261
(214) 453-8400

Doubletree Inn at Campbell Center
8250 N. Central Expressway
Dallas, TX 75206
(214) 691-8700

Loews Anatole Dallas Hotel
2201 Stemmons Freeway
Dallas, TX 75207
(214) 748-1200

The Summit Hotel
2645 LBJ Freeway at I-35
Dallas, TX 75234
(214) 243-3363

Americana Hotel/Tandy Center
200 Main St.
Fort Worth, TX 76102
(817) 870-1000

Holiday Inn of Galveston
600 Strand
Galveston, TX 77550
(713) 765-5544

The Houstonian
111 N. Post Oak Lane

Houston, TX 77024
(713) 680-2626

Inn on the Park
4 Riverway
Houston, TX 77055
(713) 871-8181

Quality Inn—Intercontinental Airport
6115 Jetero Blvd.
Houston, TX 77205
(713) 446-9131

Stouffer's Greenway Plaza Hotel
6 Greenway Plaza E
Houston, TX 77046
(713) 629-1200

Best Western Inn of the Hills
1001 Junction Highway
Kerrville, TX 78028
(512) 896-2300

Holiday Inn Casa Grande
6624 Ave. H
Lubbock, TX 79412
(806) 745-2208

Four Seasons Plaza Nacional
555 S. Alamo
San Antonio, TX 78205
(512) 229-1000

Inn at Turtle Creek, The
3830 Parkdale Dr.
San Antonio, TX 78229
(512) 696-5600

Marriott Hotel San Antonio
711 E. Riverwalk
San Antonio, TX 78205
(512) 224-4555

Hilton South Padre Resort
5000 Padre Blvd.
P.O. Box 2081
South Padre Island, TX 78597

Woodcreek "Hill Country" Resort
1 Woodcreek Dr.
Wimberley, TX 78676
(512) 847-2221

Woodlands Inn and Country Club
2301 N. Millbend Dr.
Woodlands, TX 77380
(713) 367-1100

UTAH
Salt Lake Hilton
150 West 5th S
Salt Lake City UT 84101
(801) 532-3344

VERMONT
Stowehof Inn
Edson Hill Rd.
P.O. Box 1108
Stowe, VT 05672
(802) 253-8508

VIRGINIA
Crystal City Marriott Hotel
1999 Jefferson Davis Highway
Arlington, VA 22202
(703) 521-5500

Key Bridge Marriott Hotel
1401 Lee Highway
P.O. Box 9191
Arlington, VA 22209
(703) 524-6400

Quality Inn—Pentagon City
300 Army-Navy Dr.
Arlington, VA 22202
(703) 892-4100

Stouffer's National Center Hotel
2399 Jefferson—Davis Highway
   Route 1
Arlington, VA 22202
(703) 979-6800

Twin Bridges Marriott Hotel
US 1 and I-395
Box 24240
Arlington, VA 20024
(703) 628-4200

Williamsburg Hilton/
   National Conference Center
50 Kingmill Rd.
Williamsburg, VA 23185
(804) 220-2500

WASHINGTON
Bellevue Hilton
100 112th Ave. NE
Bellevue, WA 98004
(206) 455-3330

Aggie's Port Angeles Motor Inn
602 E. Front
Port Angeles, WA 98362
(206) 457-0471

Lake Quinault Lodge
2 Miles E of 101 So. Shore Exit
Quinault, WA 98575
(206) 288-2571

Doubletree Inn/
   Doubletree Plaza Hotel
205 Strander Blvd.
Seattle, WA 98188
(206) 246-8220

Park Hilton Hotel
6th and Seneca
Seattle, WA 98101
(206) 464-1980

Vance Airport Inn
18220 Pacific Highway S
Seattle, WA 98188
(206) 246-5535

Cavanaugh's Motor Inn
North 700 Div St.
Spokane, WA 99202
(509) 326-5577

WEST VIRGINIA
Wilson Lodge at Oglebay
Route 88 N
Wheeling, WV 26003
(304) 242-3000

The Greenbrier
White Sulphur Springs, WV 24986
(304) 536-1110

WISCONSIN
Midway Motor Lodge
3033 W. College Ave.
Appleton, WI 54911
(414) 731-4141

Best Western Midway Motor Lodge
2851 Hendrickson Dr.
Eau Claire, WI 54701
(715) 835-2242

Best Western Midway Motor Lodge
3900 Milton Ave.
Janesville, WI 53545
(608) 756-4511

Midway Motor Lodge
1835 Rose St.
La Crosse, WI 54601
(608) 781-7000

Playboy Resort and Country Club
Highway 50
Lake Geneva, WI 53147
(414) 248-8811

Holiday Inn—South Airport
6331 South 13th St.
Milwaukee, WI 53221
(414) 764-1500

Midway Motor Lodge Hwy 100—
   Best Western
254 N. Mayfair Rd.
Milwaukee, WI 53226
(414) 774-3600

Midway Motor Lodge—
   Milwaukee Airport
5105 S. Howell Ave.
Milwaukee, WI 53207
(414) 769-2100

Red Carpet Hotel
4747 S. Howell Ave.
Milwaukee, WI 53207
(414) 481-8000

Olympia Resort & Spa
1350 Royale Mile Rd.
Oconomowoc, WI 53066
(414) 567-0311

Pioneer Inn and Marina
1000 Pioneer Dr.
Oshkosh, WI 54901
(414) 233-1980

Best Western Midway Motor Lodge
2901 Martin Ave.
Wausau, WI 54401
(715) 842-1616

Holiday Inn—West
201 N. Mayfair Rd.
Wauwatosa, WI 53226
(414) 771-4400

Mead Inn
451 E. Grand Ave.
Wisconsin Rapids, WI 54494
(715) 423-1500

WYOMING
Jackson Hole Racquet Club Resort
Star Route 362-A
Jackson, WY 83001
(307) 733-3990

CANADA
Calgary Inn
320 4th Ave. SW
Calgary, Alberta (T2P 2S6)
(403) 266-1611

Tradewinds Hotel
6606 MacLeod Trail
Calgary, Alberta (T2H OL2)
(403) 252-2211

The Edmonton Inn
11830 Kingsway Ave.
Edmonton, Alberta (T5G OX5)
(403) 454-9521

Capri Hotel
1171 Harvey Ave.
Kelowna, British Columbia (V1Y 6E8)
(604) 860-6060

International Plaza Hotel
1999 Marine Dr.
North Vancouver, British Columbia
   (V7P 3E9)
(604) 984-0611

Brandon Red Oak Inn
3130 Victoria Ave. W
Brandon, Manitoba (R7A 5Z7)
(204) 728-5775

Airliner Inn
1740 Ellice Ave.
Winnipeg, Manitoba (R3H OB3)
(204) 775-7131

Birchwood Inn
2520 Portage Ave.
Winnipeg, Manitoba (R3J 3T6)
(203) 885-4478

TraveLodge Niakwa East
20 Alpine Ave.
Winnipeg, Manitoba (R2M OY5)
(204) 253-1301

Chateau Halifax
Scotia Square
Halifax, Nova Scotia
(902) 425-6700

Ramada Inn—Airport West
5444 Dixie Rd.
Mississauga, Ontario (L4W 2L2)
(416) 624-1144

Skyline Hotel
101 Lyon St.
Ottawa, Ontario (K1R 5T9)
(613) 237-3600

Red Oak Inn—
    Canadian Pacific Hotel
555 W. Arthur St.
Thunder Bay, Ontario (P7E 5R5)
(807) 577-8481

Constellation Hotel
900 Dixon Rd., Rexdale
Toronto, Ontario (M9W 1J7)
(416) 675-1500

Four Seasons Toronto
21 Avenue Rd.
Toronto, Ontario (M5R 2G1)
(416) 964-0411

Inn on the Park
1100 Eglinton Ave. E
Toronto, Ontario (M3C 1H8)
(416) 444-2561

The Sheraton Centre
123 Queen St. W
Toronto, Ontario (M5H 2M9)
(416) 361-1000

The Skyline Toronto
655 Dixon Rd. Rexdale
Toronto, Ontario (M9W 1J4)
(416) 244-1711

Sutton Place Hotel
955 Bay St.
Toronto, Ontario (M5S 2A3)
(416) 924-9221

Valhalla Inn
1 Valhalla Inn Rd.
Toronto, Ontario (M9B 1S9)
(416) 239-2391

Richelieu Inn
430 Ouellette Ave.
Winsor, Ontario (N9A 1B2)
(519) 253-7281

Montreal Aeroport Hilton
   International
12505 Cote de Liesse Rd.
Doryal, Quebec (49P 1B7)
(514) 631-2411

Cantrakon Conference Centre
   at Mont Ste. Marie Resort
Lac Ste. Marie, Quebec (J0X 1Z0)
(819) 467-5200

CP Hotels—Le Chateau
   de l'Aeroport
Montreal International Airport
Box 60
Mirabel, Quebec (J7N 1A2)
(514) 476-1611

Le Chateau Montebello
109 Notre-Dame St.
Montebello, Quebec (J0V 1L0)
(819) 423-6431

Gray Rocks Inn and Le Chateau
Mt. Tremblant
P.O. Box 1000 St. Jovite
Mont-Tremblant, Quebec (J0T 2H0)
(819) 425-2771

Loews Le Concorde
1225 Place Montcalm
Quebec City, Quebec (G1R 4W6)
(418) 647-2222

THE JEWEL BOX GARDEN

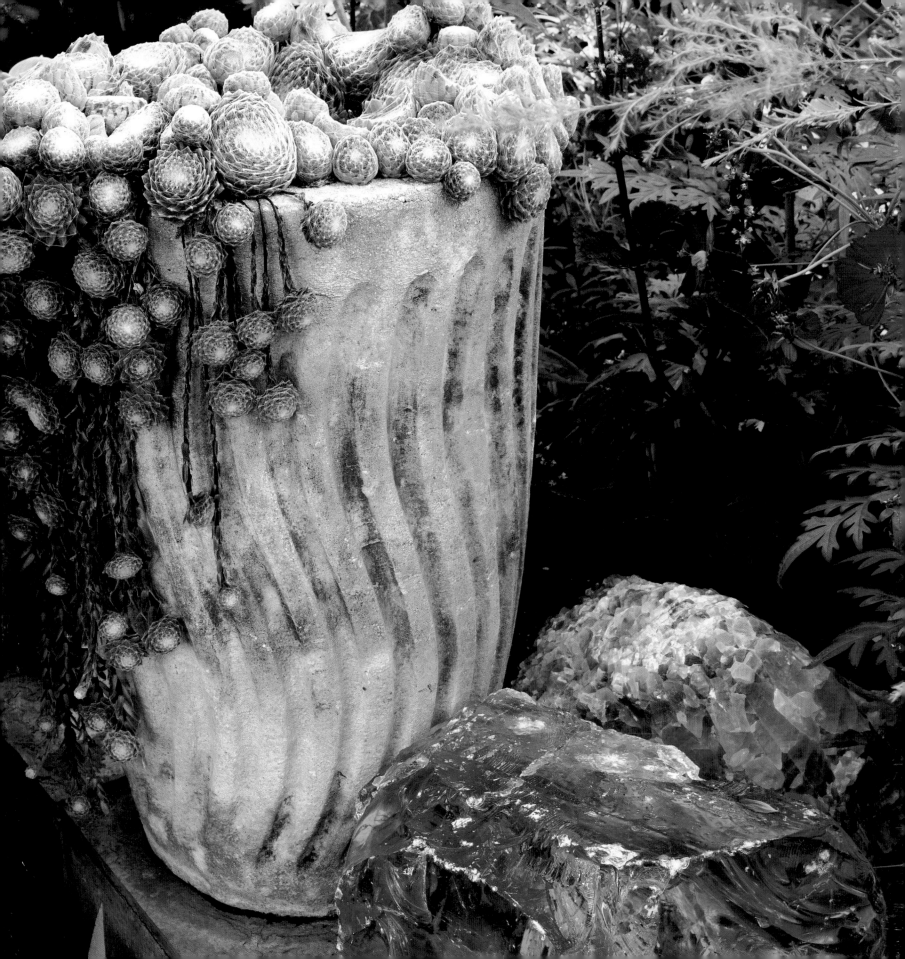

THE JEWEL BOX GARDEN

THOMAS HOBBS
PHOTOGRAPHS BY DAVID McDONALD

TIMBER PRESS

Portland • Cambridge

Published in the United States and the United Kingdom in 2004 by

Timber Press, Inc.
The Haseltine Building
133 S.W. Second Avenue, Suite 450
Portland, Oregon 97204-3527, U.S.A.

Timber Press
2 Station Road
Swavesey
Cambridge CB4 5QJ, U.K.

www.timberpress.com

This book was created and published in Canada by Raincoast Books
9050 Shaughnessy Street, Vancouver, British Columbia V6P 6E5
www.raincoast.com

Edited by Scott Steedman
Interior Design by Stacey Noyes

ISBN 0-88192-646-9

Catalog records are available from the Library of Congress and the British Library.

Printed & Bound in Hong Kong by Book Art Inc., Toronto

PREVIOUS PAGE *A **Sempervivum** tableau by* DAVIS DOLBAK, *see page 26.*

"At long last I saw the door in the wall. I hadn't gone through it, but at least I saw it."

ALAN HELMS

CHAPTER 1

Life, as we dream it could be

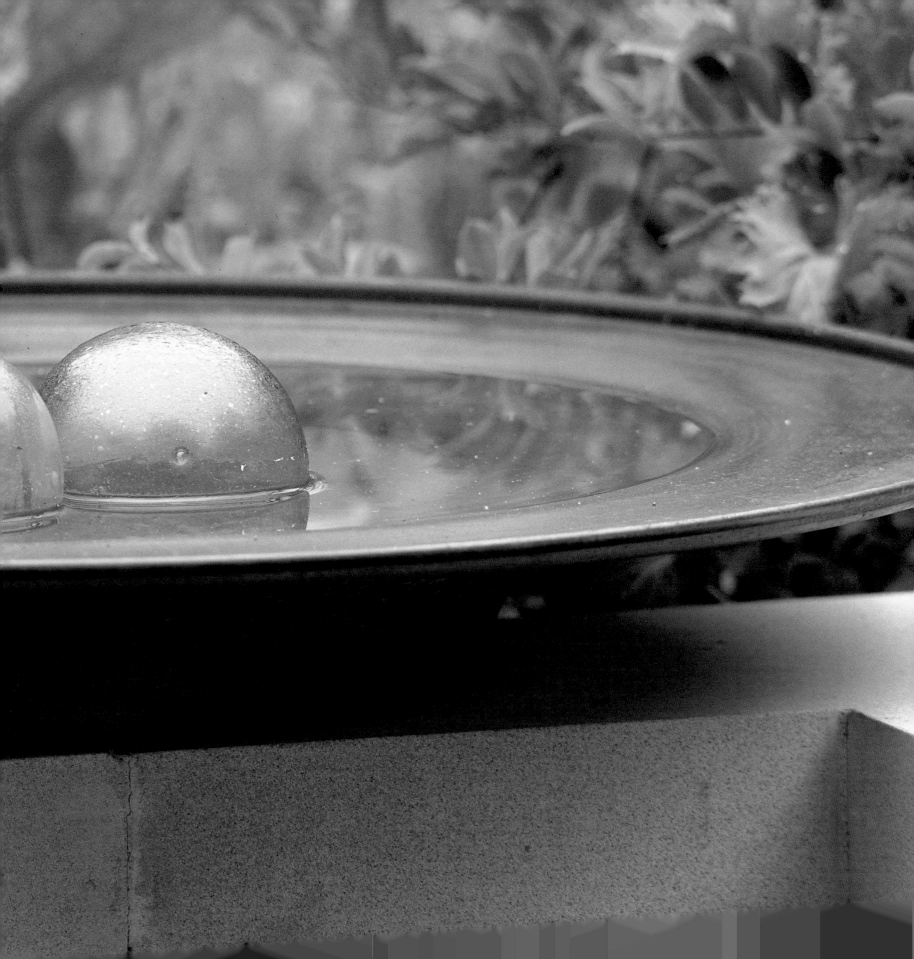

NOTICE I DIDN'T SAY, "LIFE, AS WE DREAM IT IS," BUT AS IT could be. One of the few aspects of life we do have some control over is our gardens. Whether it is an outdoor terrace or balcony or a city plot, we can turn dreams into visions and visions into reality. All you need are patience, money (sad, but true) and commitment.

I prefer the word "commitment" to the word "work," because gardening isn't work when it's for yourself. Most people use gardening as therapy, to unwind after a busy day or a hectic week. By letting yourself get in contact with the earth, by dealing with plants instead of people, you will feel refreshed, calmed — and gratified because you're accomplishing something. As I putter about in the garden, I like to envision one current going out of me and a different current coming in. I deliberately try to connect to *something*, and that is why my garden stops traffic.

Try to create an oasis of beauty. The smaller your space, the easier this is going to be. Larger gardens need divisions to break them up, but I cannot stand the phrase "garden rooms" — it sounds too *planned*. I would rather experience a series of surprise visions, without walls. This could happen on a small terrace, or between two houses. It could be a well-placed water feature, followed by a collection of treasured potted ferns or succulents on a charming antique plant stand, approached on a pebble mosaic sidewalk.

PREVIOUS PAGE *In the* SEATTLE *garden of* GLENN WITHEY *and* CHARLES PRICE, *a few glass fishing floats in a copper dish create a simple water feature. Endlessly rearranged by the wind, they remind us that not all containers must hold plants.*

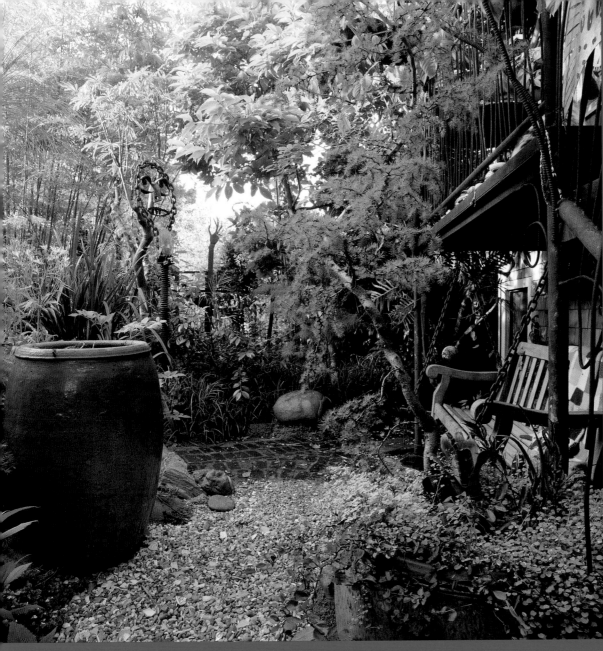

LEFT *In* MARCIA DONAHUE'S BERKELEY, CALIFORNIA, *garden, a pebble beach complete with colorful bits of sea glass also serves as a pathway. A swinging bench offers a perfect place to escape … and dream.*

BELOW *An open gate is irresistibly welcoming in* SUZANNE PORTER'S BERKELEY, CALIFORNIA, *garden. Choice potted foliage plants include the silvery spears of my favorite plant of the moment,* **Astelia chathamica.** *The plum-colored foliage of* **Loropetalum chinense** *'Razzleberry' and a potted pair of* **Lophomyrtus x ralphii** *'Sundae' reveal that plant sophistication dwells here! All these foliages benefit from the extra shelter they receive by being grown in the often-ignored space between neighboring houses.*

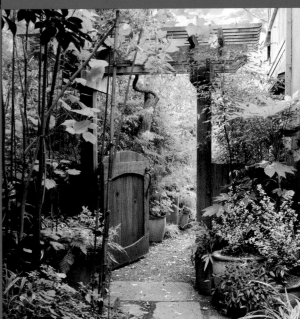

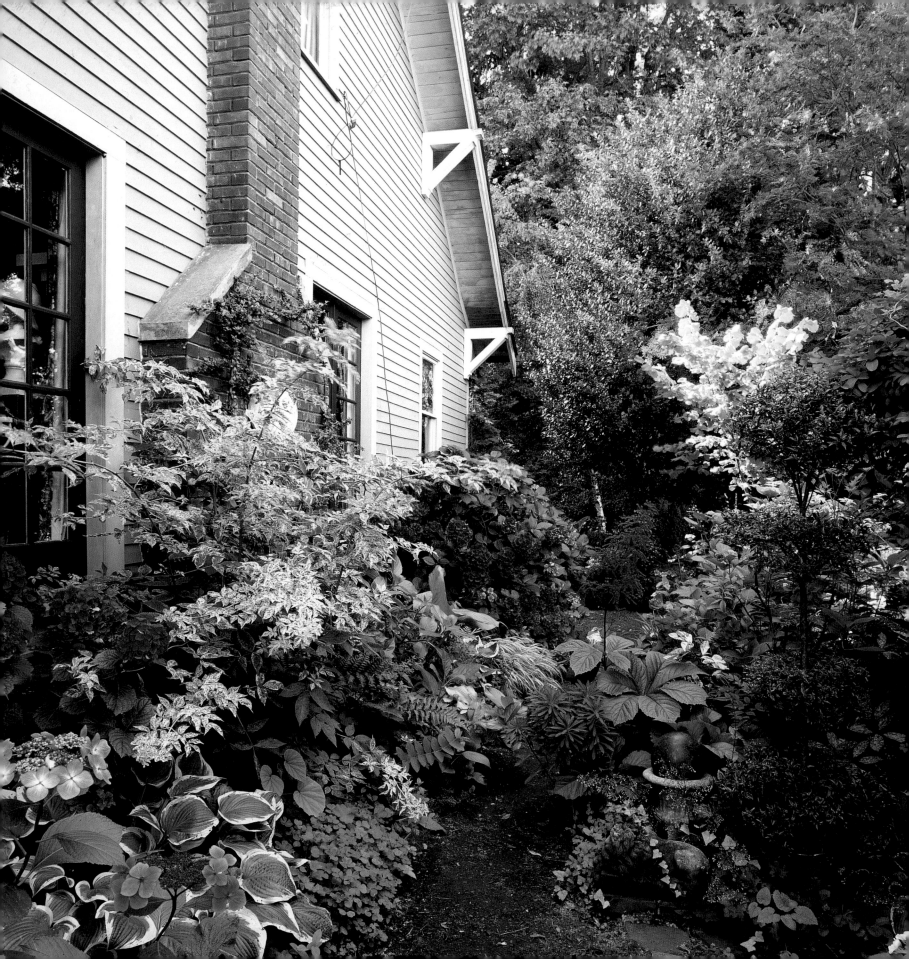

LEFT *Plants will take care of themselves when properly placed. Hydrangeas thrive in the cool, shaded sideyard of* MARK HENRY'S *garden in* SNOHOMISH, WASHINGTON. *A variegated elderberry,* **Sambucus nigra** *'Pulverulenta', adds spectacle and airy variation in height to this mixed planting of shade-loving perennials.*

RIGHT *The already subtle shades of* **Lilium** *'Peach Butterflies' is softened even further when combined with neighboring soft textures. The felted foliage of* **Phlomis fruticosa** *and the wispy grass* **Nassella tenuissima** *combine artfully with* **Hemerocallis** *'Pandora's Box' in the* SEATTLE *garden of the late* STEVE ANTONOW.

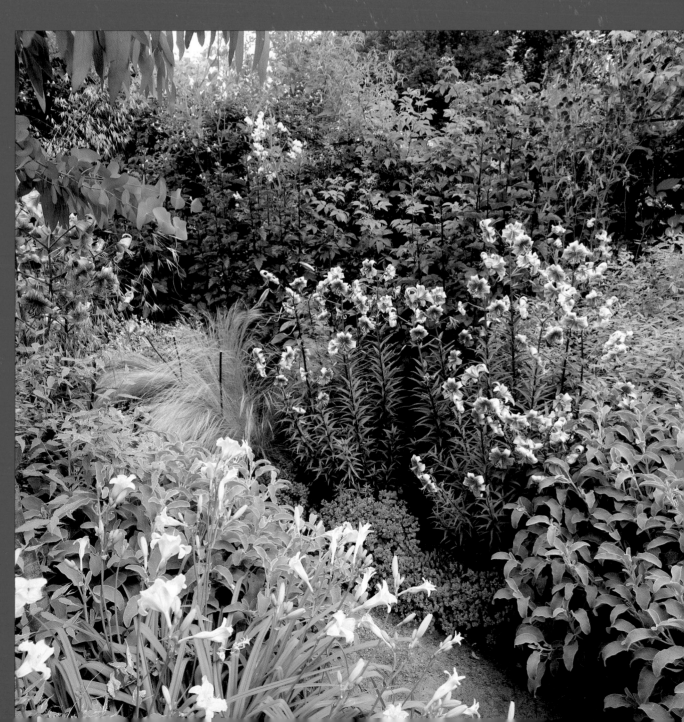

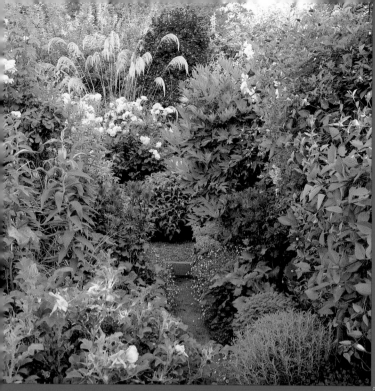

RIGHT *Wachendorfia thyrsi-flora's spikes of bright yellow echo the vertical foliage of phormiums and Japanese irises* (Iris ensata) *in* BOB CLARK'S OAKLAND, CALIFORNIA, *botanical wonderland. A softening tuft of the Japanese grass* **Hakonechloa macra** *'Aureola' clues visitors to choose the left path when given a choice.*

ABOVE *A New Zealand pampas grass,* **Cortaderia richardii,** *arches in a refined focal point in* STEVE ANTONOW'S SEATTLE *garden. It is important to lead the eye, and even more important not to disappoint. David Austin's rose 'Graham Thomas' doubles the beauty quotient without upstaging the star of this vignette.*

RIGHT *"The Elvis Bench" by* RAOUL ZUMBA *provides more than a place to sit in his and* BOB CLARK'S *spectacular* OAKLAND, CALIFORNIA, *garden. Mirror fragments reflect changing falling cherry petals and magnify the beauty all around as disco memories and the seasons go by.*

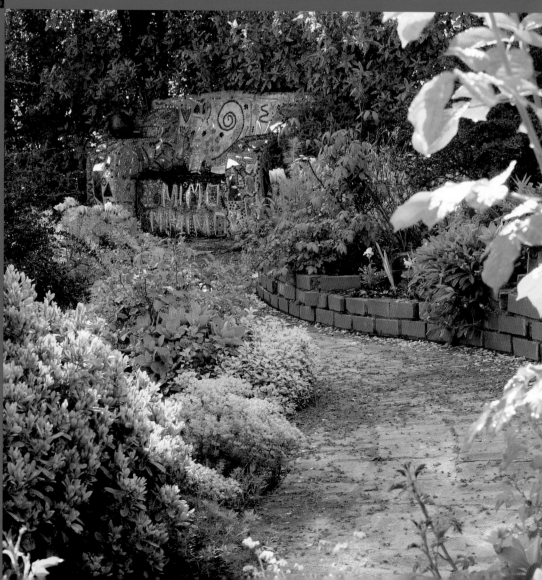

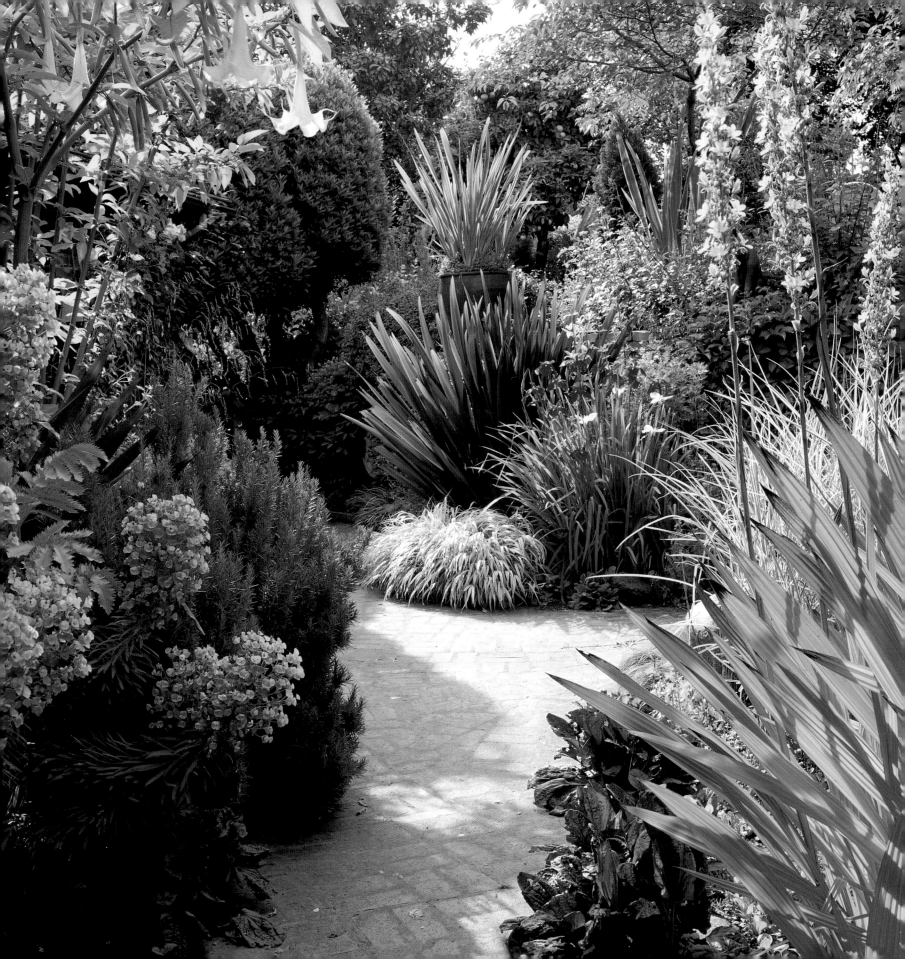

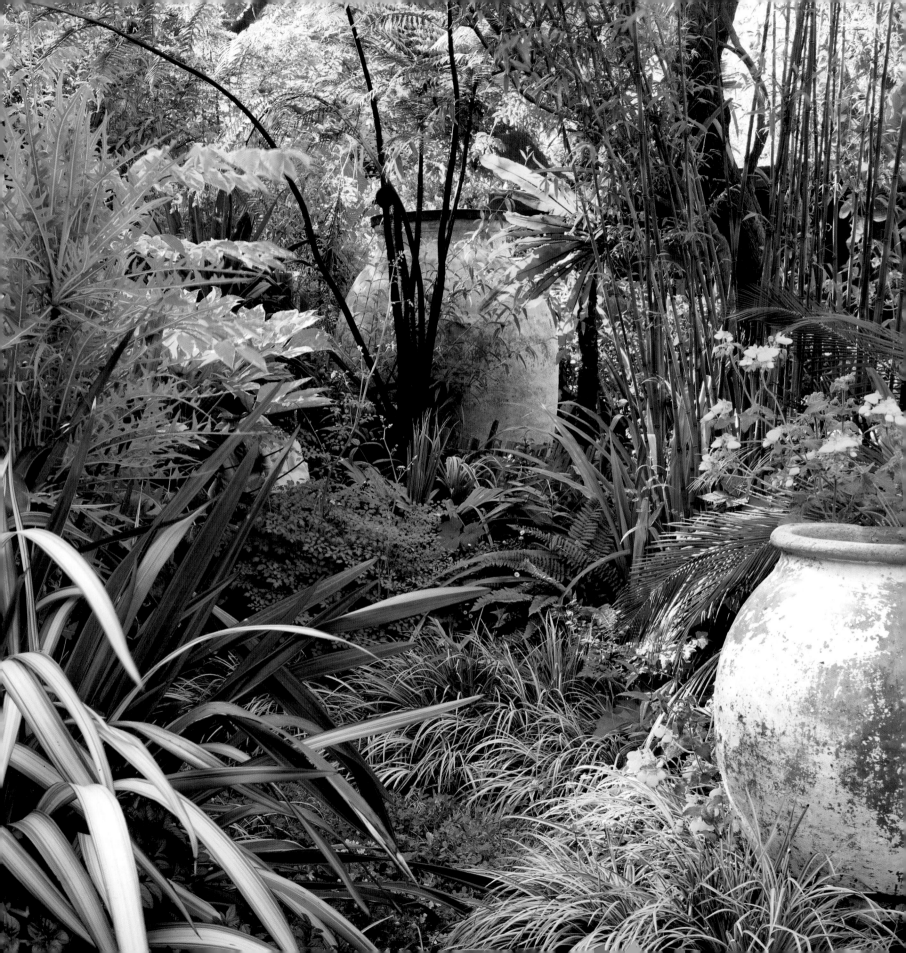

CONSIDER THE BEAUTY VALUE OF EVERY SURFACE AND DO something about it. A deck doesn't have to remain unadorned. Walls are blank canvases, waiting for a patina of age. I zero in on ancient villa walls in Italy and notice the beautiful staining, left for centuries by wise owners who could well afford to repaint. I have always loved the Italian phrase *bel'occhio,* which roughly translated means "beautiful eye." Plants look much better against a mellowed, knocked-back background.

Make sure your oasis-to-be is not sabotaged by a clinical white paint job. Apartment dwellers and townhouse gardeners may have to disguise rather than repaint. Clever use of trellises, matchstick blinds, bamboo fencing and strategically placed plants can transform a prison cell, let alone a balcony. A bit of "set-dec" is crucial to all forms of gardening.

FACING PAGE ROGER RAICHE *and* DAVID MᶜCRORY *have achieved a grotto effect in their* BERKELEY, CALIFORNIA, *garden by planting low-growing **Acorus gramineus** 'Ogon' in the center of an outstanding collection of foliage. The very beautiful black-stemmed tree fern (**Cyathea medullaris**) is cleverly showcased against an enormous urn. Creating refuges in or of our gardens should be a top priority.*

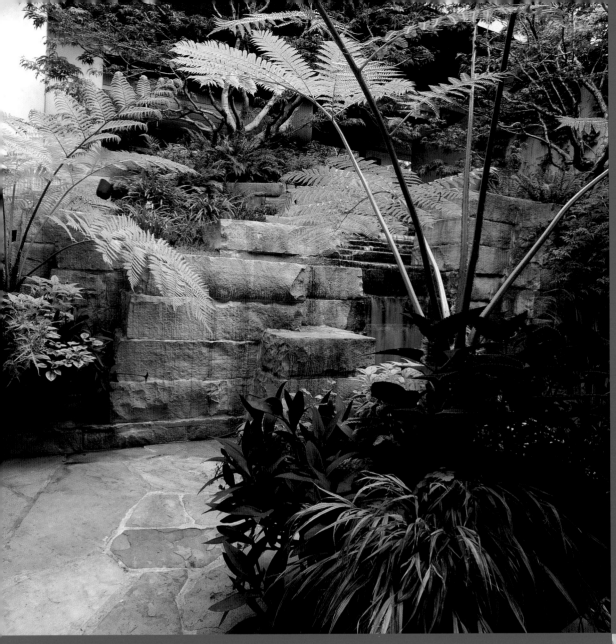

BELOW *The Canary Island ivy,* **Hedera canariensis** *'Variegata', cloaks an entire wall in* VALERIE MURRAY'S VICTORIA, B.C., *garden. Retro garden chairs are painted a matching creamy yellow, keeping the scene as neutral (and peaceful) as possible.*

ABOVE *The entrance court of the* LUNN *garden in* VANCOUVER, B.C., *features a cooling waterfall and unexpected potted tree ferns (**Alsophila australis**). Dramatic foliages spilling from the custom-made bronze containers include the bright purple* **Setcreasea purpurea** *and a burgundy-tinged splash of* **Hakonechloa macra** *'Aureola'. The golden variegated* **Plectranthus** *'Troy's Gold' is only happy in shady situations like this.*

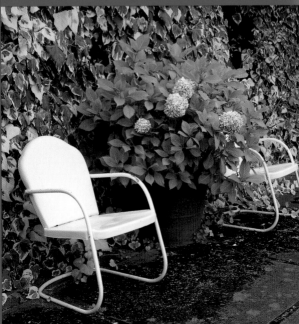

16

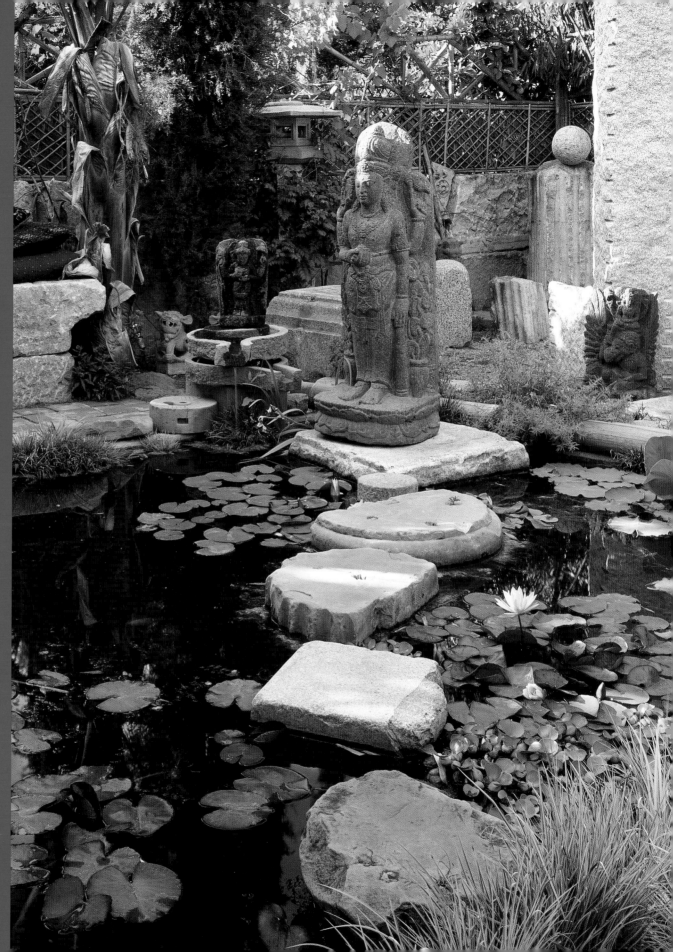

RIGHT *Stone, not plants, provides the landscape in this part of* CEVAN FORRISTT'S SAN JOSE, CALIFORNIA, *garden. This water garden has taken on spiritual importance. Make a wish, or bring an offering? Hmmm …*

ONE OF THE MYSTERIES OF MY LIFE IS REPEATED EVERY DAY. I drive to and from work and cannot help but notice block after block of very average-income homes that appear hopelessly un-gardeny. It is almost a case of one-upmanship to be the most unplanted, least cared for but absolutely occupied. To me, it is a drive through the Valley of Death. Expensive cars, new basketball hoops, satellite television receivers and white plastic patio furniture are everywhere. I ask myself, "What *do* these people care about, anyway?" Occasionally I'll spot a stranded tree peony, blooming its heart out, stoned on ugly. Or a maypole-type clothesline bedecked with absolutely fried plastic hanging baskets. The botanical equivalent of a car crash.

What I have surmised, with a little help from Joan Rivers, is that "God Divides!" Not everyone received the *bel'occhio* gene. Those of us who did are the lucky ones. We take things like sunsets for granted and get excited over the first snowdrop. We save wrapping paper because it is *so beautiful,* not just to save money and reuse it (well, maybe). Being blessed with what amounts to an extra gene is like having a limitless credit card to go out and treat yourself to a wonderful life. Don't let it expire.

FACING PAGE *A simple copper pipe drips into a pool of lotuses in* CEVAN FORRISTT'S *garden. The sound of water makes us look for its source, and is one way to establish a focal point in even the most interesting of gardens.*

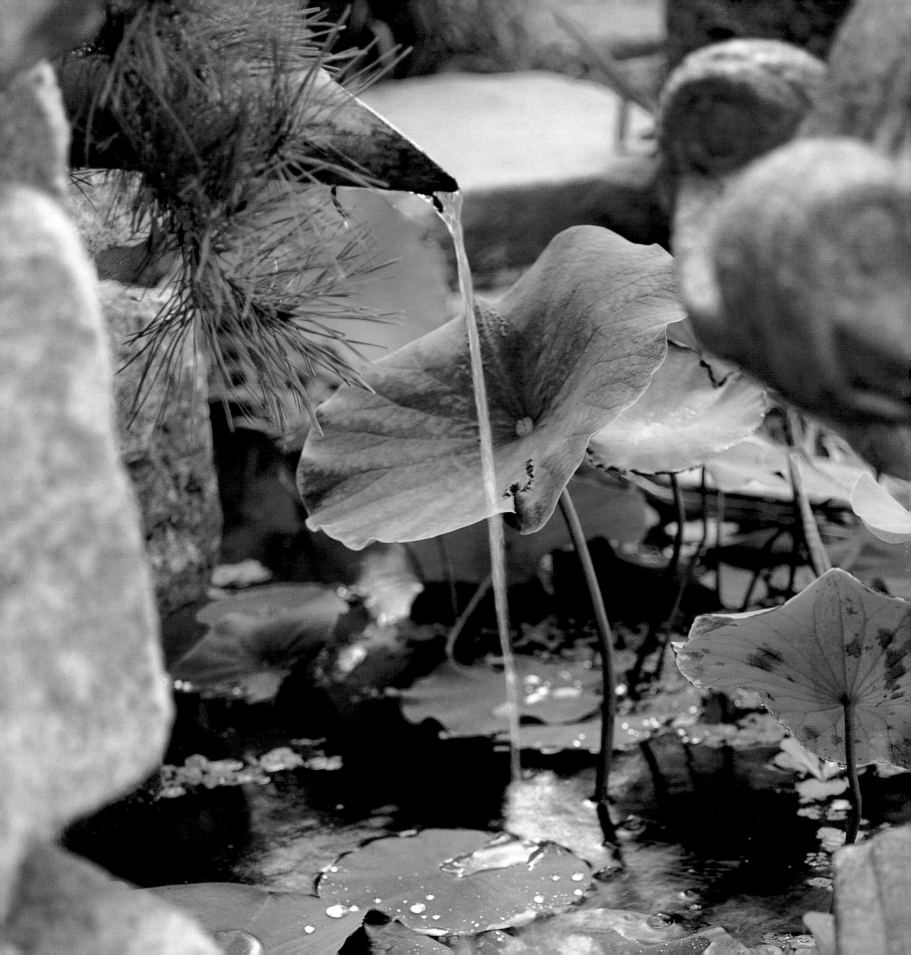

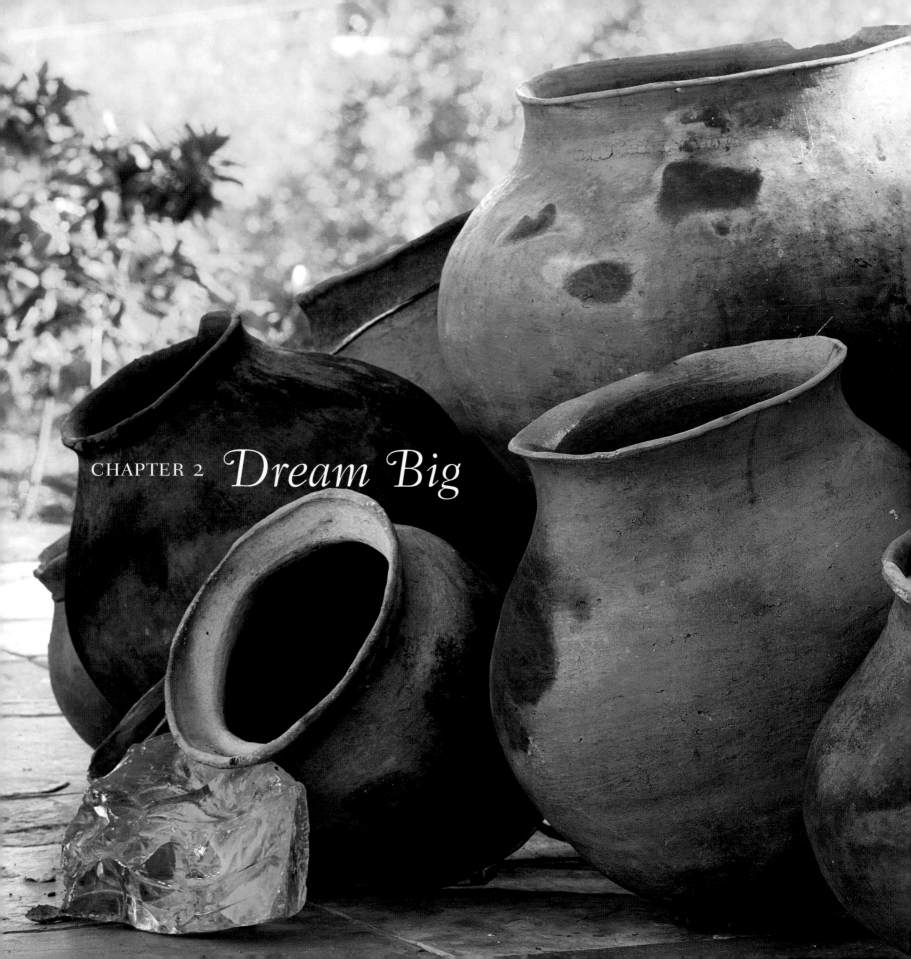

CHAPTER 2 *Dream Big*

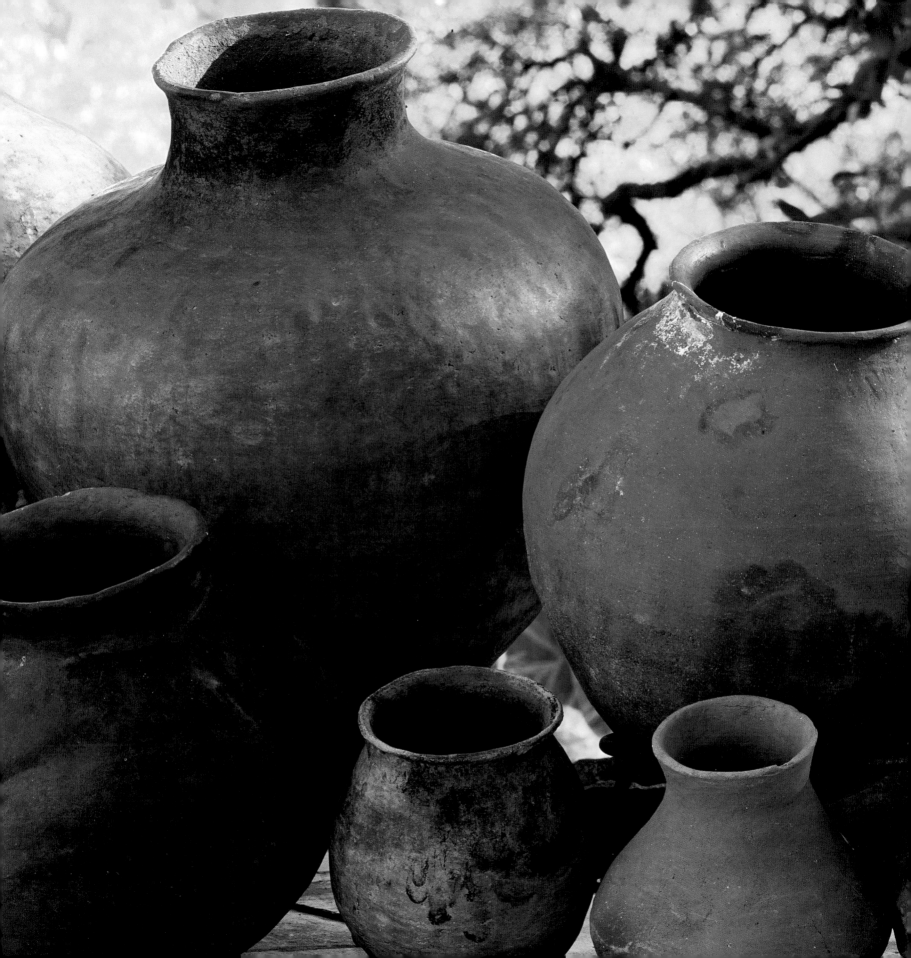

REALIZING A SPACE'S POTENTIAL HAS NOTHING TO DO WITH ITS actual size. So those who find themselves gardening in less space shouldn't feel short-changed. Envisioning what could be is actually easier when you're working with physical limitations.

When I garden, I am really setting up for what I hope will be, not what is presently visible. Although my body is working, my mind is months or even years down the road. It has to be. If I stayed in the present, I would never like what I saw. Dreaming while you work is one of gardening's big payoffs. I believe it must create chemical changes in the body. Stress levels disappear, voices become whispers and sore backs don't appear until the next day. The reward is worth any amount of effort.

I have discovered that gardening has no glass ceiling. You will not be held back by anything! The more you read, plant, listen and see, the more you will find available. Instead of going to university, I let the plants teach me. Observing their likes and dislikes gave me a career, a soulmate and a charmed life. Unknowingly, I allowed plants to enslave me as their spokesperson, caretaker and pimp.

PREVIOUS PAGE *The star in this composition of primitive pottery in* DAVIS DOLBAK'S *garden is the chunk of blue slag glass. In cooking, it is the addition of the unexpected that makes one chef better than another.*

FACING PAGE *Why be normal? By adding an architectural fragment of an exotic deity to a stone wall,* CEVAN FORRISTT *has magnified the wall's visual interest many times over. A little déjà vu never hurts.*

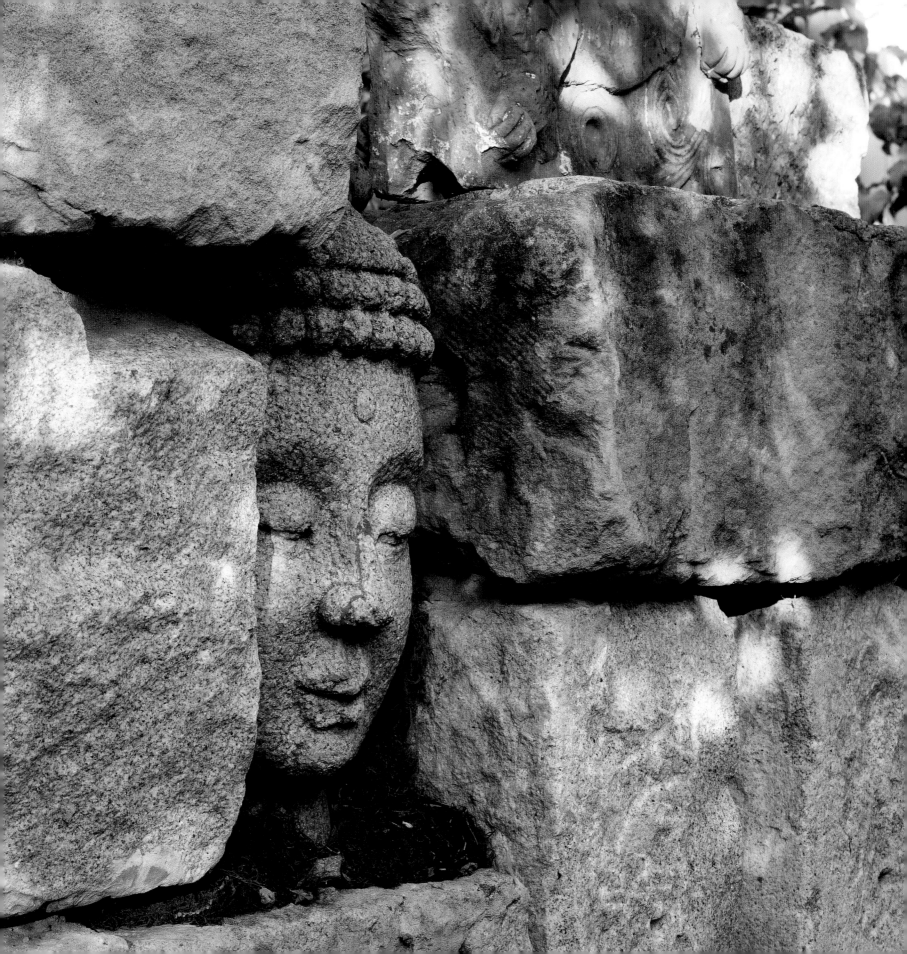

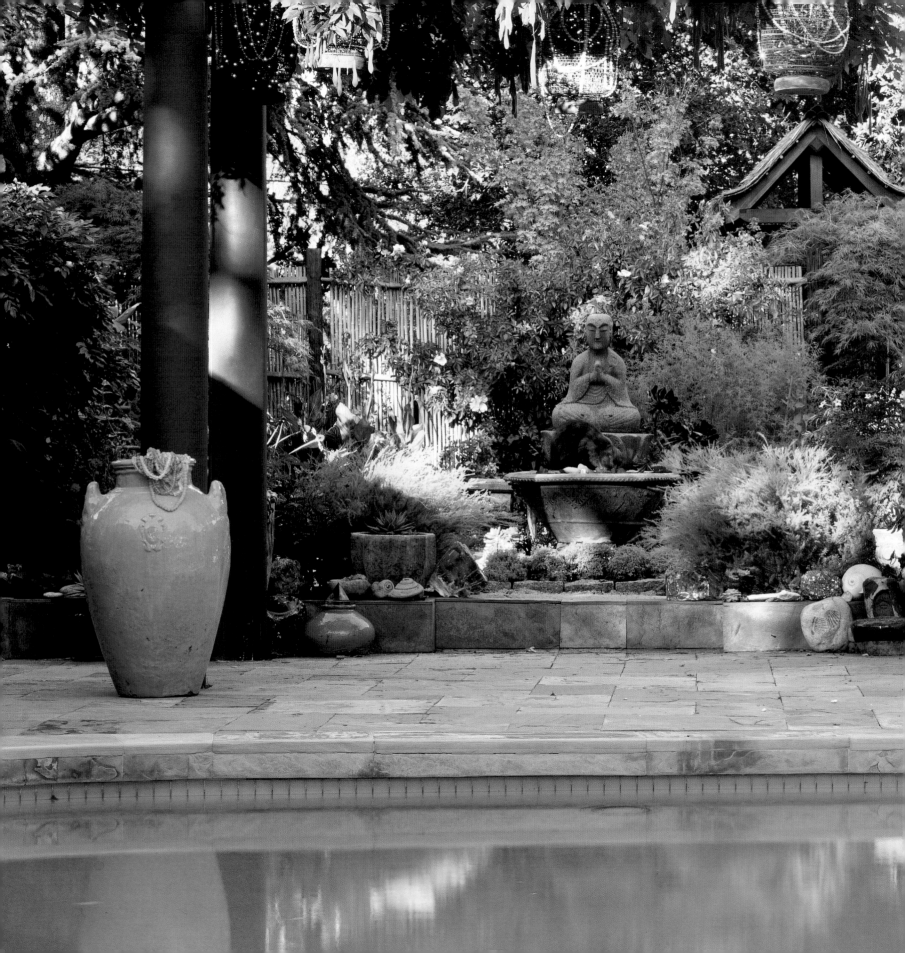

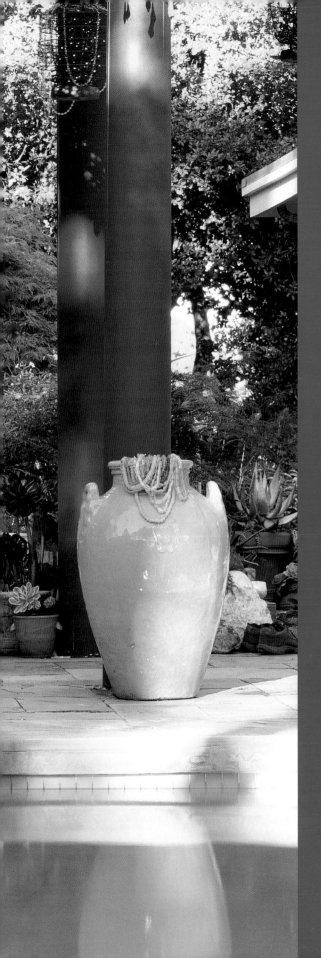

Magic — visual and mental — surrounds DAVIS DOLBAK'S *back-yard swimming pool in* SAN FRANCISCO. *A pair of glazed turquoise jars, a few pieces of slag glass, and all we see is turquoise!*

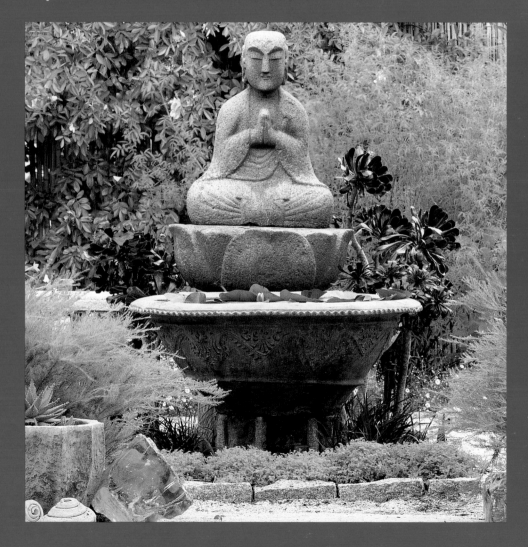

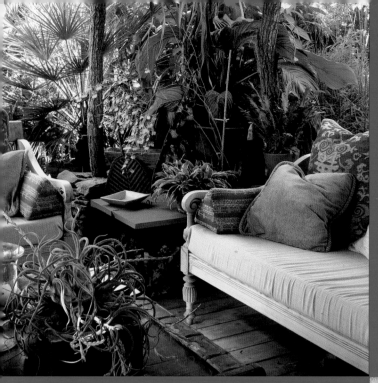

RIGHT *On his personal patio, San Francisco retail wizard* DAVIS DOLBAK *has installed a dramatic fire pit amid jungle-like greenery. A substitute for flowers, foliage adds texture and color. The red-tinged* **Ensete ventricosum** *'Maurelii' and the exotic tracery of an Australian tree fern (***Alsophila australis***) create privacy and act as a bold backdrop. Can you imagine white plastic patio chairs in this setting?*

ABOVE *An exotic outdoor living room in* DENNIS SCHRADER *and* BILL SMITH'S LONG ISLAND, NEW YORK, *garden. Tropical foliage, a yellow* **Oncidium** *orchid and a tussle of* **Tillandsia** *on the coffee table suggest faraway places. The Indonesian furniture reinforces the feeling of escape and adventure.*

RIGHT *It's all about texture.* DAVIS DOLBAK'S *grouping of seemingly ancient artifacts share a matte finish and a sense of history. There is time travel in this vignette; a nautical prism catches the light, but who left it there?*

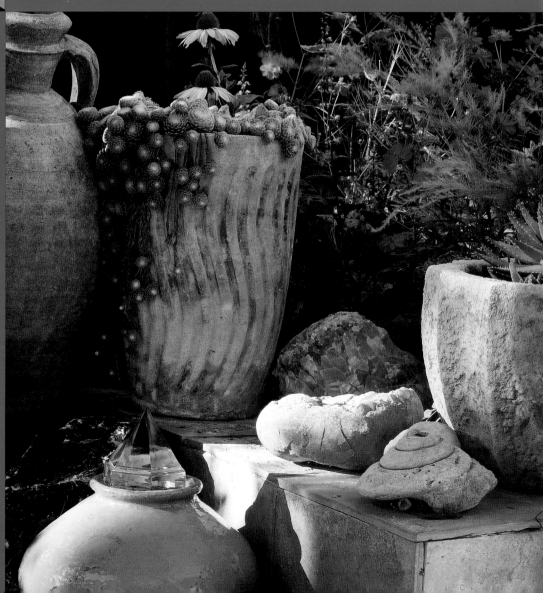

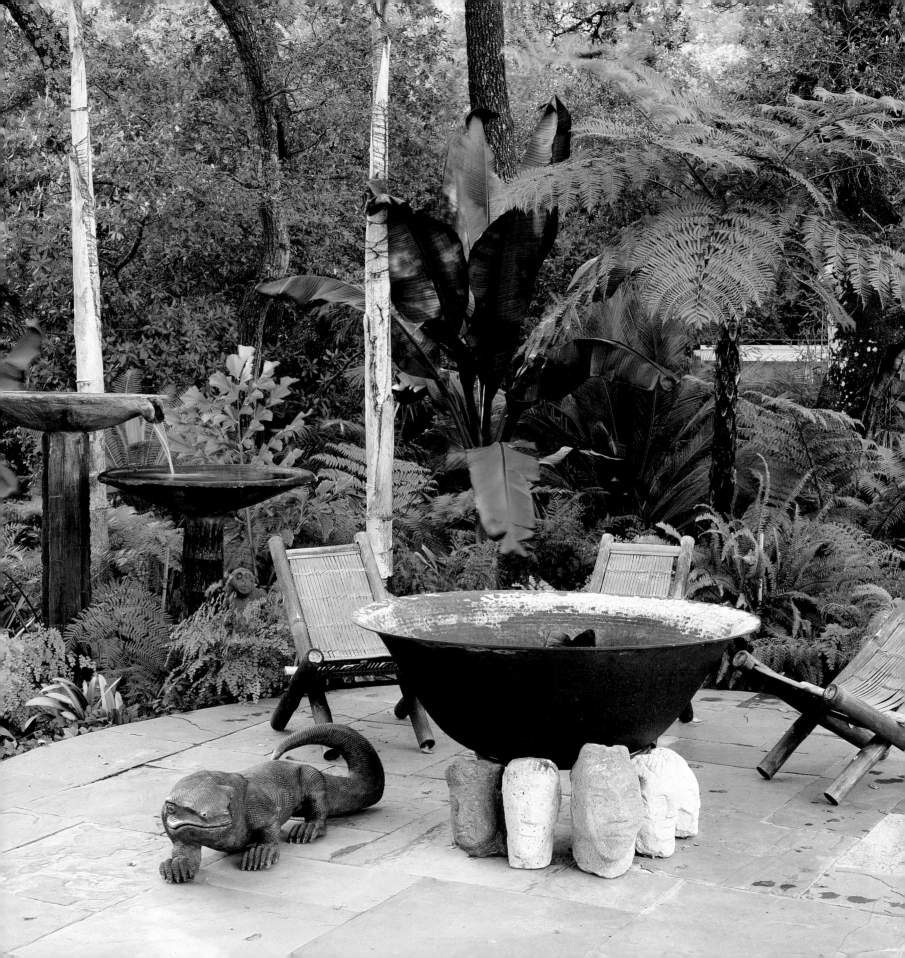

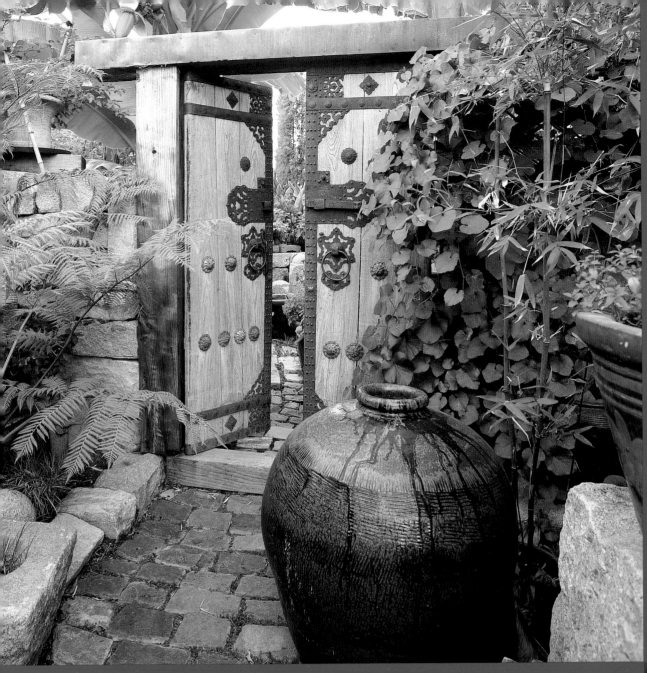

LEFT *Nothing says "come in" (or "stay out") better than a pair of tall gates. A sense of mystery is a very strong lure in* CEVAN FORRISTT'S SAN JOSE, CALIFORNIA, *garden. Plunking an oversize earthenware jar right in the pathway makes its boldness inescapable.*

BELOW *A simple offering or pure decoration, dried zinnias rest beautifully on the feet of a garden statue in* CEVAN FORRISTT'S *garden. Don't forget to say "thank you" every so often.*

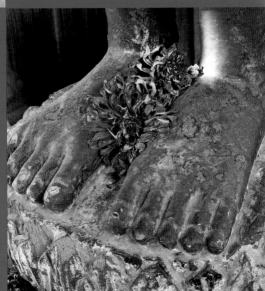

I WISH I KNEW WHO SAID, "IT IS NOT IRRITATING TO BE WHERE one is, it is only irritating to wish one was somewhere else." Oscar Wilde? Buddha? Jackie Collins? Regardless, I think this phrase applies perfectly to a lot of people and their gardens. Wishing your garden was better — i.e., less irritating — is a good sign. Now you must allow yourself to dream. Stay with the physical location but change everything else. Using your mind creatively is almost a lost art in the age of digital photos, camera-phones and wireless transmission, but conjuring is unavailable any other way (so far).

"Free your mind, the rest will follow" is a bit of pop radio that shouldn't be forgotten. I use this key phrase when a garden situation has me perplexed. What will look good and grow well together? The answer is not always apparent. Plant labels are not enough, and will not spark any creativity. You've got to let *artistry* do your plant shopping! Artistry is a channel, and you're either tuned in or you aren't. Sometimes you actually see people stumble onto this channel by accident. Watching people shop at a nursery is fascinating — you quickly see who is tuned in!

Dreaming big should be taught in schools. It applies to everything, not just gardening. Stifling potential in people is not only taught, it is sold. Most nurseries sell only common "popular" plants, which immediately limits the gardens in the surrounding neighborhood. Plantaholics will venture further afield, but the majority of homeowners settle for what they can get. I view this as tragic. Who wants to be limited to driving a Chrysler K-Car? I flee from them in traffic, especially if the driver is wearing a white Tilley hat, the dunce cap of the new millennium! The experience is powerful proof that someone forgot to dream.

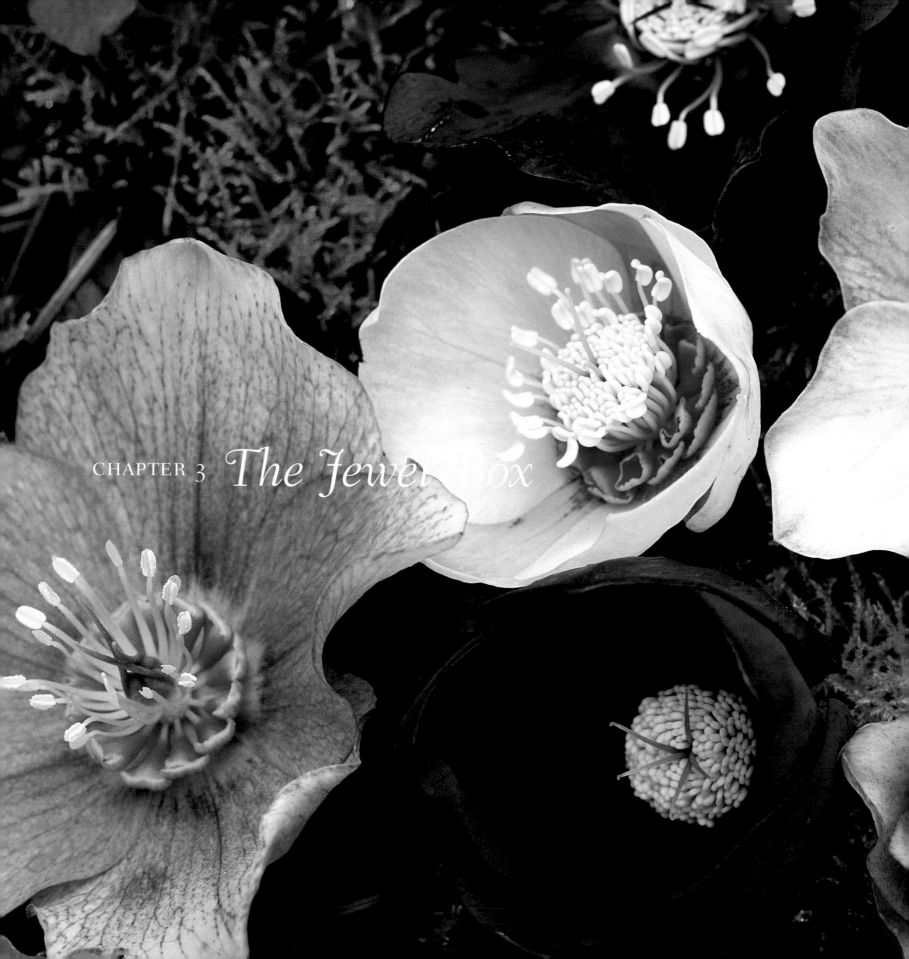

CHAPTER 3 *The Jewel Box*

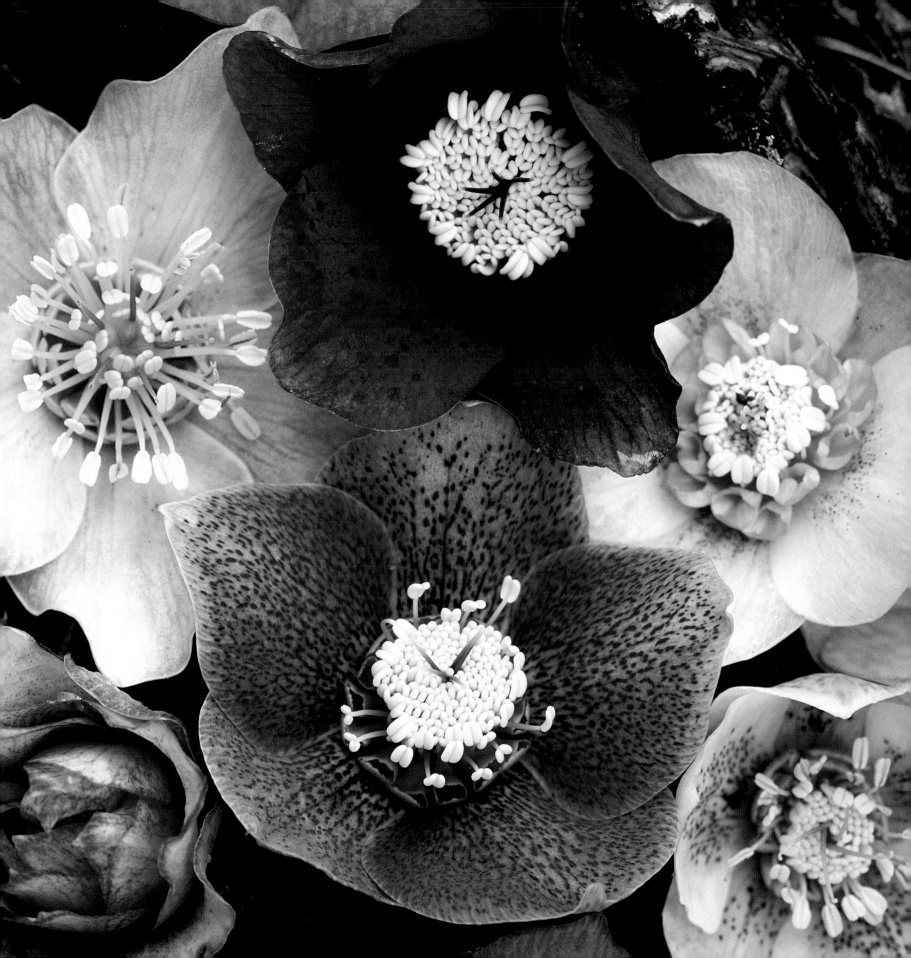

Wouldn't it be wonderful if you could describe your garden as a "jewel box full of beautiful plant treasures?" It is entirely possible, and the smaller your outdoor space, the easier it is going to be.

First of all, stop envisioning horizontally. It is much easier to plan from above. Imagine yourself in an art gallery. Instead of staring blankly at one canvas, you are free to float around the room and drink in the entire exhibition. Think of your garden, no matter how small, as an *exhibition space*. This will allow you to see the whole picture as a composite of all your gardening efforts. You still see and enjoy individual details, but rearranging becomes much easier. Is this astral gardening? I hope so.

Once you realize how valuable every square inch is, mediocrity becomes intolerable. Really small-space gardeners can use their eye, but larger-space gardeners will need their feet to make purging rounds, looking for weak spots. There are always plenty, which prompts us to keep tweaking and being creative. It also allows us to keep adding more plants to impossibly full gardens.

PREVIOUS PAGE *Modern hellebores are of such complex breeding they are now referred to as* **Helleborus x orientalis** *group. The strains keep improving: keep your eyes open for superior flower forms and clear colors. Picoteed petals, double flowers and more upward-facing blooms are waiting for you.*

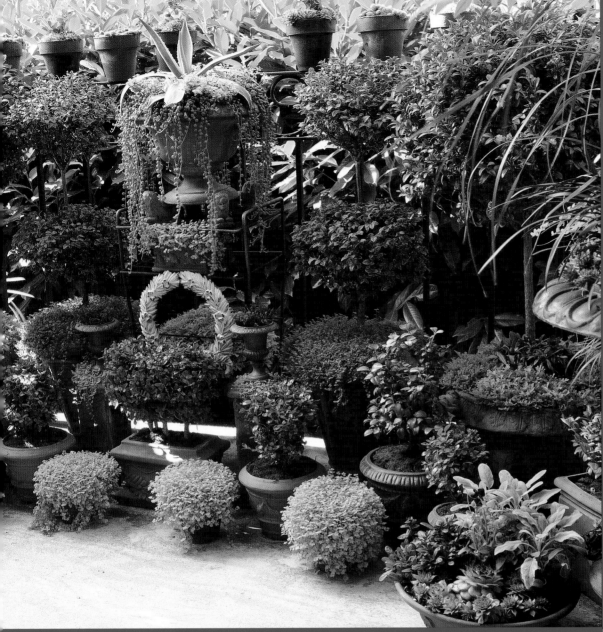

LEFT *On a tiny balcony in* VANCOUVER, B.C., DAMEN DJOS *creates a fantasy Versailles for himself. True dwarf boxwoods (**Buxus sempervirens** 'Suffruticosa') trained as tiny topiaries, pots of baby's tears (**Soleirolia soleirolii**) and an urn of trailing string of pearls (**Senecio rowleyanus**) all somehow conspire to make the* **Agave americana** *'Variegata' the star.*

BELOW *Tiny spaces are still ruled by scale and proportion. A touch of golden baby's tears (**Soleirolia soleirolii** 'Aurea') softens and marries a miniature cast-iron urn to its terra cotta base on* DAMEN DJOS'S *shady balcony.*

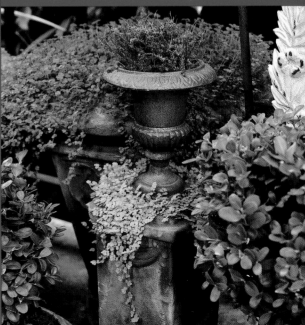

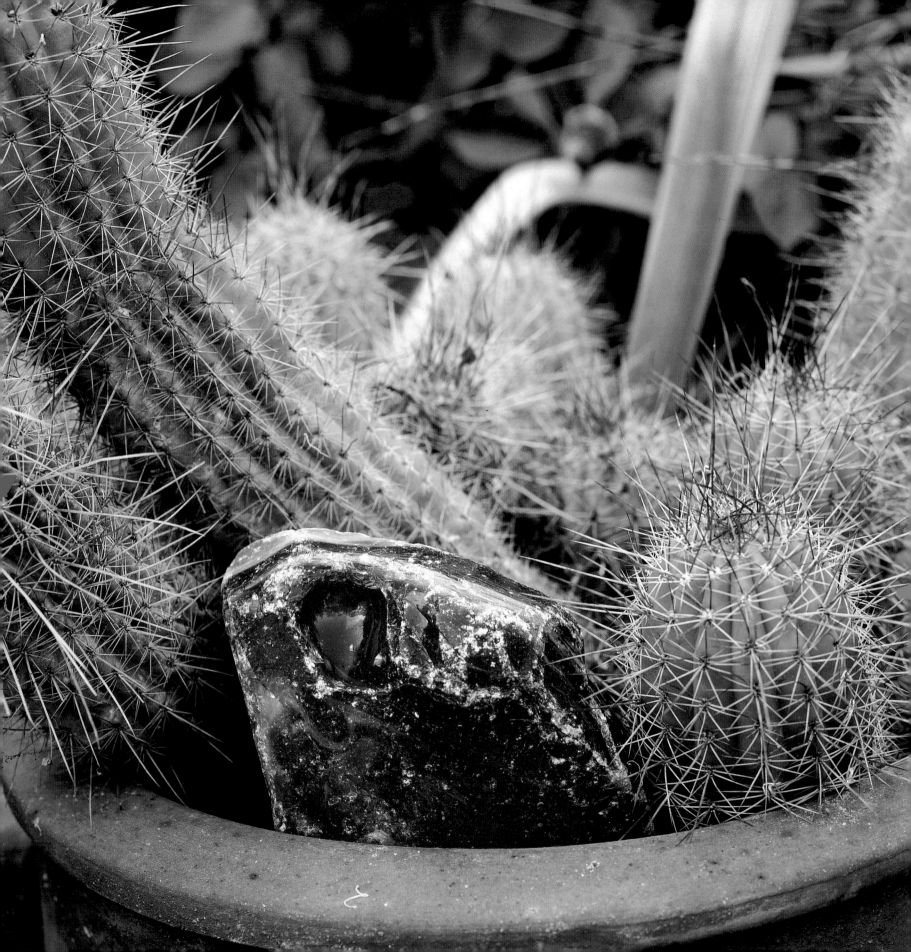

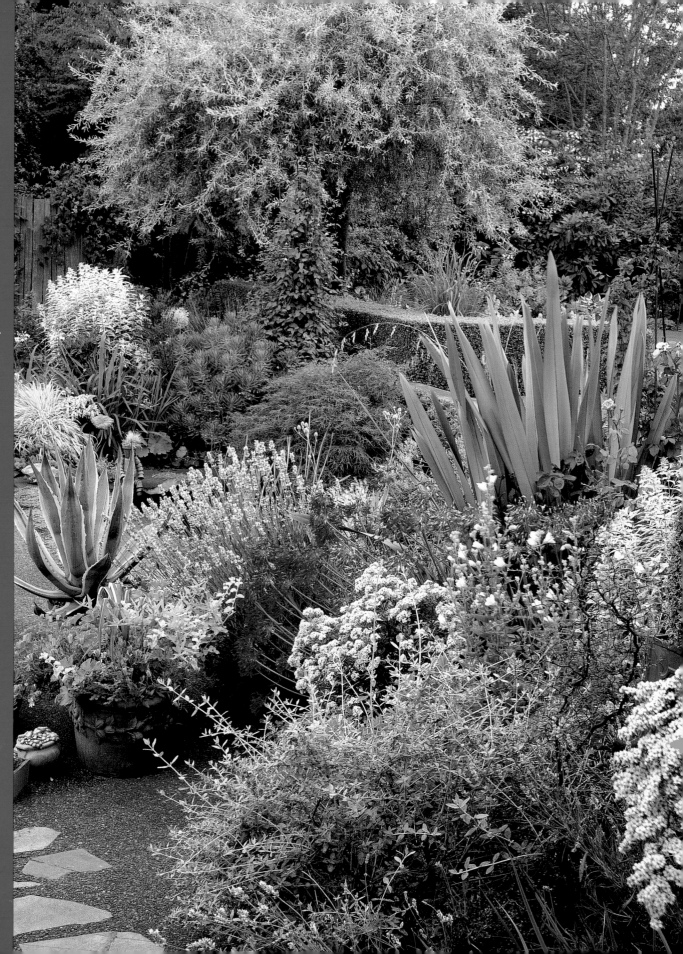

LEFT *A big chunk of cobalt blue glass makes a terrific substitute for flowers for this potted cactus in* ROGER RAICHE *and* DAVID McRORY'S *garden. Unexpected and unexplained, the mysterious deposit is guarded by fierce spines.*

RIGHT *Pyrus salicifolia 'Pendula' still manages to star in this complex planting in* SUSAN RYLEY'S VICTORIA, B.C., *garden. Her trademarked use of mellow yellows and silvery shades receives a well-placed punch from an unnamed dark blue* **Agapanthus** *and the bold spikes of* **Phormium tenax** *foliage.*

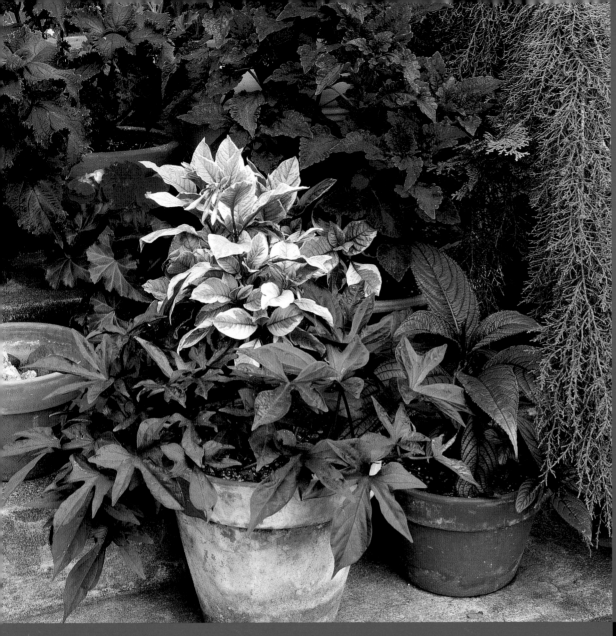

RIGHT *A spectacular staging of container plants in* DENNIS SCHRADER *and* BILL SMITH'S LONG ISLAND, NEW YORK, *garden. What appears to be black and white is really lots of green, silver and dark purple.* **Colocasia esculenta** *'Jet Black Wonder' contrasts with the cut-silver foliage of* **Centaurea gymnocarpa**. *The bold white rosettes of a potted pair of* **Furcraea gigantea** *'Striata' guard the entrance to this raised patio area.*

BELOW *At Southlands Nursery in* VANCOUVER, B.C., DAMEN DJOS *created this stunning "chandelier" of* **Rhodochiton atrosanguineum**. *String of pearls (***Senecio rowleyanus***) dangles out the bottom and* **Carex flagellifera** *tosses out the top. Planted and cared for much like a hanging basket, this eye-catching display continued to grow right through our mild winter.*

ABOVE *A collection of jewel-toned foliage softens a step in* SUSAN MACDONALD'S *garden in* SEATTLE. **Coleus, Fuchsia** *'Firecracker',* **Ipomoea batatus** *'Blackie' and the metallic magenta* **Strobilanthes dyerianus** *are now widely available. Sold as bedding plants, all are worth saving indoors over winter in cold climates.*

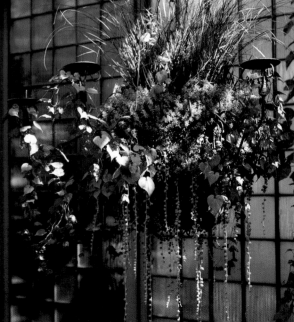

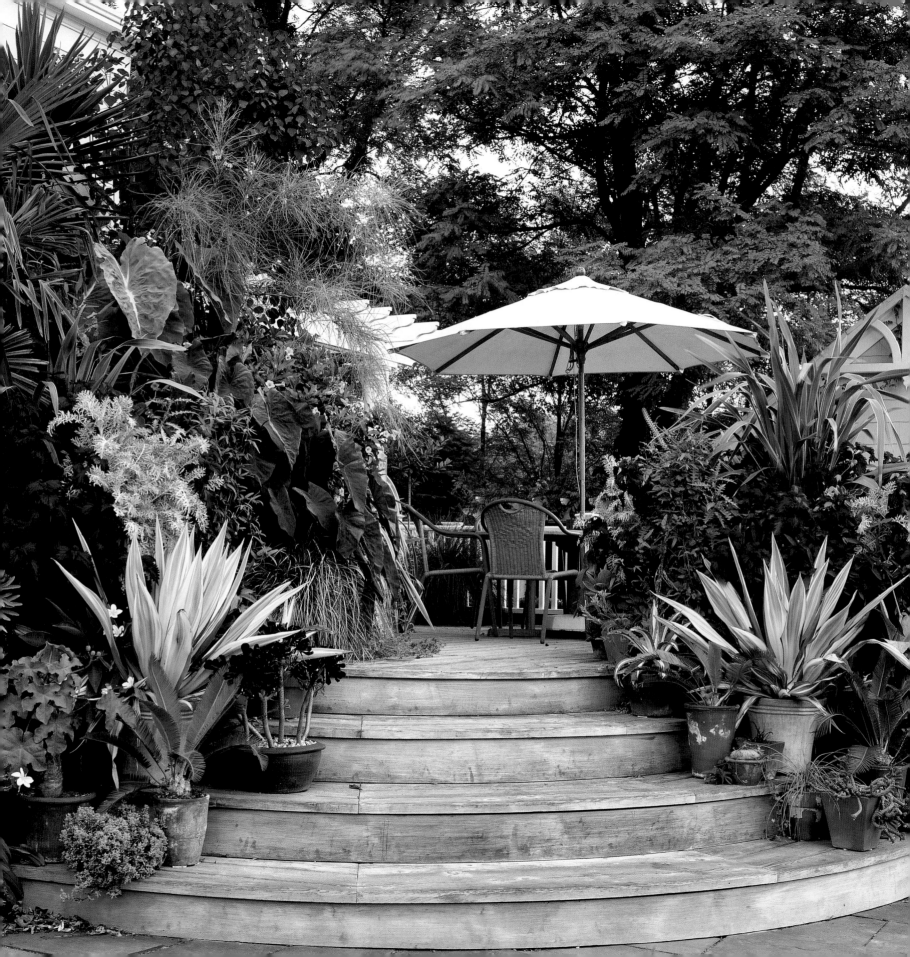

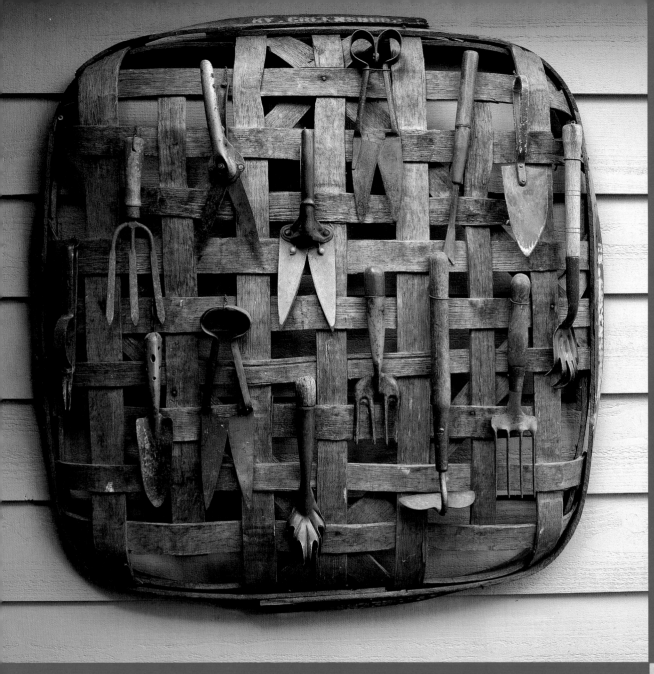

LEFT *A collection of old garden tools makes a beautiful wall display in* FREELAND TANNER'S CALIFORNIA, *garden. Such displays show personal talent that store-bought decor lacks.*

BELOW *An old bird cage makes an interesting garden accent. I like to change what's in it periodically. This time it houses an octopus-like* **Tillandsia xerographica** *for the summer. My favorite agave,* **Agave americana** *'Mediopicta', gets more appreciation up on a table.*

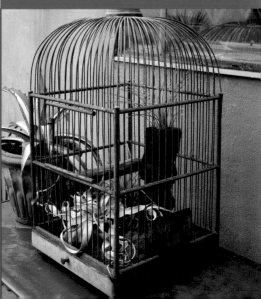

HAVE YOU NOTICED THAT SMART RETAILERS KNOW THAT WE need a "decompression space" upon entering a store? A bit of space to neutralize, form an instant opinion and be enticed further in. I think they stole this concept from gardening. Whether with a sweeping terrace, a groomed lawn area or an entry court, great gardens begin with some open space, which also keeps the vision changing. Japanese gardens use water this way. An artistic tableau always includes a platform. Those who garden in small spaces need to leave room to breathe, to prevent the Jewel Box from becoming a junk drawer!

The "hardscape" of a garden is often considered less important than the living portion. Good garden designers know that *the two are equals*. This is what separates amateurs from the pros. Patios, pathways, fences and walls should be given first priority, as they contain your dreams. But don't fret — there is a big difference between first and *top* priority, which is reserved for plants. It is for them that you are setting the stage.

Very ordinary surfaces are often inherited with the property, but that doesn't mean you are stuck with them *as is*. Plain concrete patios are the lowest common denominator, and a fact of life for apartment-dwellers. Happily, concrete stains beautifully! What a difference a wash of coppery-green makes. Concrete is also easily scored with a wet saw. Use a chalk snap-line to design a diagonal diamond grid pattern and make shallow cuts in boring concrete to add pattern. It is important to set the stage early in your garden plans. Don't sabotage your garden dreams by ignoring the hardscape.

I T IS TRAGIC THAT MONEY WORRIES CAN STOP PEOPLE FROM achieving anything attractive in their gardens. Lack of funds may excuse you from almost everything else, but it doesn't work this time. So much is free! A collection of stumps can be beautiful, so can rusty barbed wire. "Found objects" and piles of stones blend beautifully with plants. Skeletons of leaves, dried stalks and twigs, old windows and birdcages are all potential scene-stealers *once you realize it*. If necessity is the mother of invention, poverty just might have something to do with creativity. Start looking around and stop coming home empty-handed!

People with limited amounts of outdoor space should consider using plants with extra-value characteristics. Some plants have flashy new spring growth, often tinged in red or peach. The otherwise dreary **Pieris japonica** does this, as does **Euphorbia griffithii**. Herbaceous peonies emerge looking like red licorice, and tree peonies (**Paeonia suffruticosa** hybrids) have new foliage tinged in bronze. This is a very special family of plants that I would never be without. Their floral display in May is so short, it's as if they don't really want us to see it. The message I get from them is, "I'll be gone, so appreciate me now."

Concentrate on plants *that actually give you a thrill* instead of just filling up space or providing "color." For example, I have discovered the modern daylily. Hybridizers have completely transformed the frumpy old **Hemerocallis** into incredible works of art for the garden. They look like the ruffled glass sculptures of Dale Chihuly — imagine an orchid crossed with an Amaryllis that is completely hardy!

Being able to enjoy your Jewel Box from within means creating a place to sit, or even entertain others. The more multifunctional, the better. A barbecue or hot tub has to be attractive as well as functional. Tattoo that on your forehead.

RIGHT *The choice **Aralia elata** 'Aureavariegata' is allowed to star, without competition, in this corner of* TERRY LEBLANC'S VICTORIA, B.C., *garden. Such visually powerful plants need isolation to strut their stuff.*

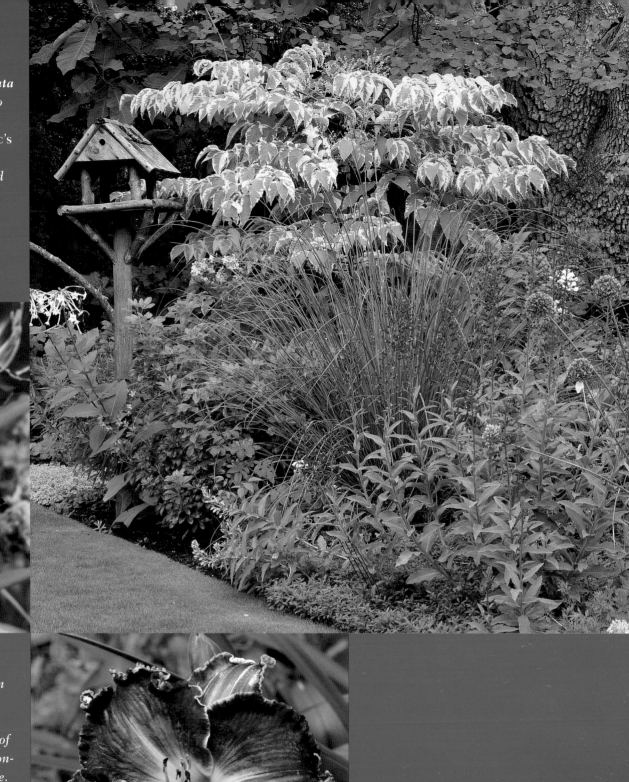

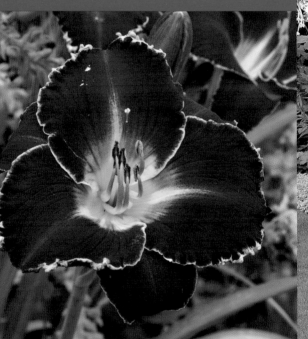

ABOVE *I employ modern daylilies as secret weapons in my garden. All of a sudden, amazing blooms such as this one —* **Hemerocallis** *'Lord of Lightning' — appear from non-descript tufts of green foliage.*

RIGHT **Hemerocallis** *'Forbidden Desires', one of the finest creations of my daylily guru Ted Petit.*

41

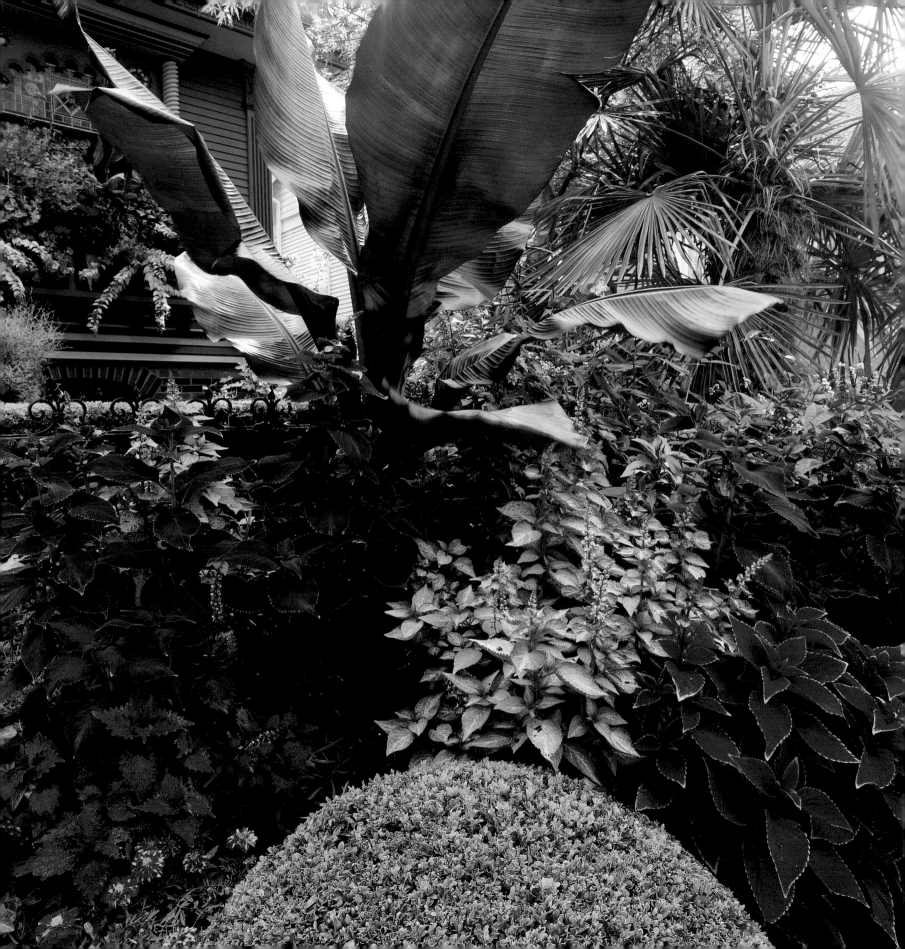

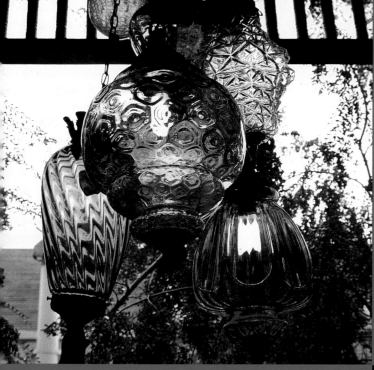

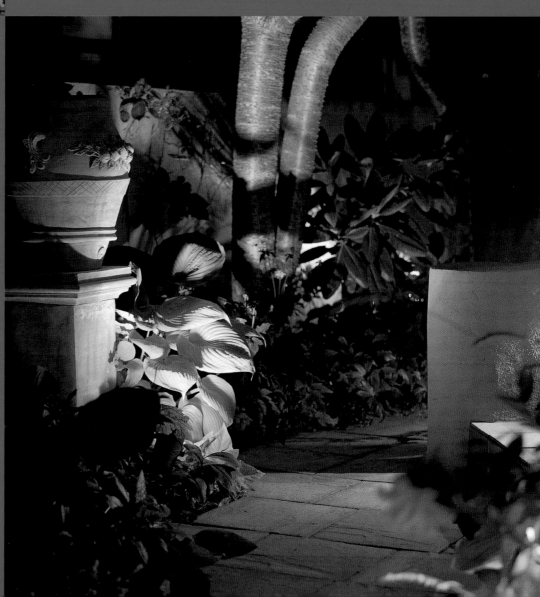

BELOW *Invest in garden lighting! Fixtures must not show. In my own garden, the bark of flowering cherries shows to best advantage at night. A large terra cotta oil jar from Impruneta, Italy, is lit as sculpture. This shady walkway between two houses would be scary if it wasn't nicely lit.*

ABOVE *Search and ye shall find wonder. In the whole world, only* MARCIA DONAHUE *could, and does, have a porch light made from 1960s' swag lamps!*

LEFT *An exotic tapestry planting by* GLENN WITHEY *and* CHARLES PRICE *balances form with color in the* SEATTLE *garden of* BRIAN COLEMAN. *The enormous red leaves of* **Ensete ventricosum** *'Maurelii' are able to compete with the mesmerizing foliage of coleus. Few plants can.*

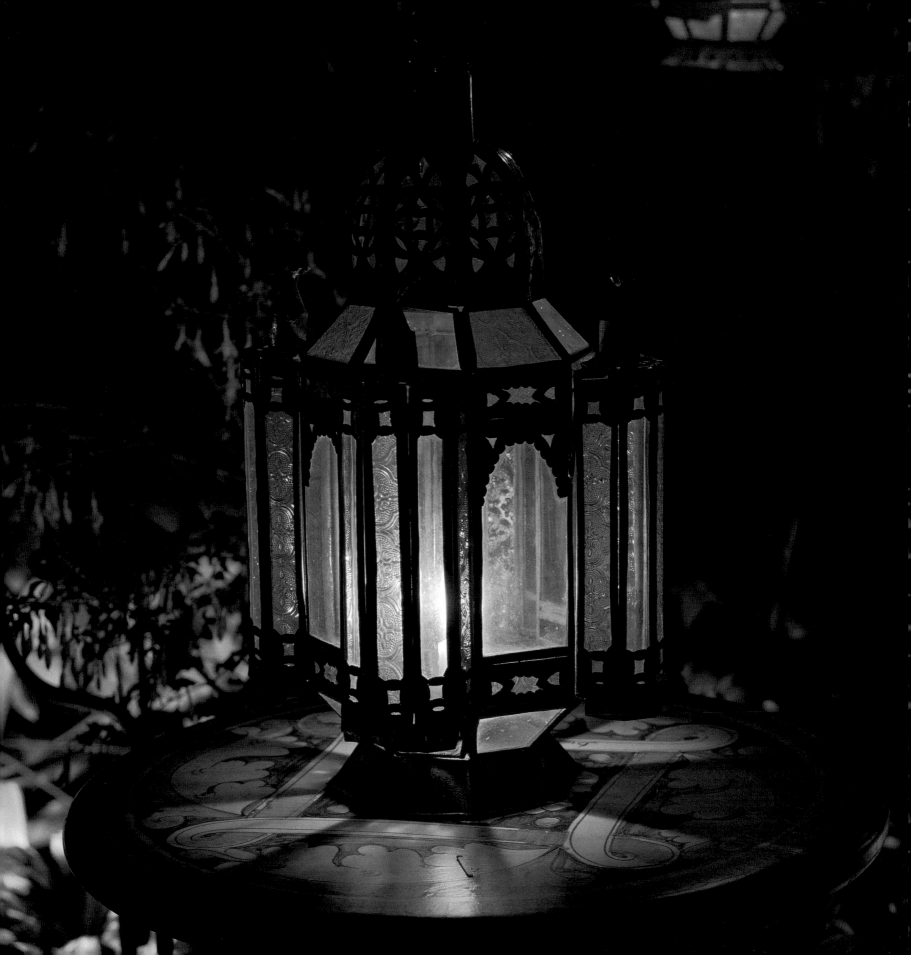

BRIGHT DAYLIGHT IS THE WORST TIME TO ENJOY YOUR PLANTS or your garden. Colors are bleached out and shadows disappear. Photographers know this. To see what you have achieved, make your rounds earlier or later. After dusk is the most dramatic time of all.

Patterns are exaggerated by adding night lighting. Tiny details can be projected as huge shadows against bare walls. I do this with my wrought-iron gates as well as foliage, projecting squirmy shapes and dramatic, gigantic leaves onto my house at night. I want it to look as weird as possible! For me, *gardening has become theater*. Don't waste space on dull, blobby-shaped plants. I cannot stand heathers or dwarf conifers. The spikes and spears of kniphofias, phormiums, cortaderias and yuccas exude drama. Garden lighting penetrates their open-leaf fountains and travels like neon up to their spiky tips. Roundy-moundy shapes just look like blackened footstools. Leave them for the gas stations.

Creating your own Jewel Box Garden should involve all of your senses. Sight and sound are always there, but taste, touch and scent are optional. Scent adds another dimension to our enjoyment of plants. I get lost there: even fragrance strips in magazines send me. At home, I try to include as many fragrant plants as possible. ***Helichrysum angustifolium***, the curry plant, grows right beside ***Daphne x burkwoodii*** for a wacky olfactory combo. A young ***Daphne bholua*** grows by my front door. I look forward to an immediate hit on winter mornings every time I leave the house. Every year I promise myself I'll grow pots of heliotrope, tubs of tuberoses and bushels of hyacinths (but I haven't yet: so many plants, so little space …). Intoxicating fragrance is something spiritually nutritious and these flowers are giving it away …

FACING PAGE *In my own garden, a Moroccan lantern creates magic! Remember how candles flicker and cast shadows in ways electric lights cannot. Try burning scented candles as well, for an extra scent in the night air.*

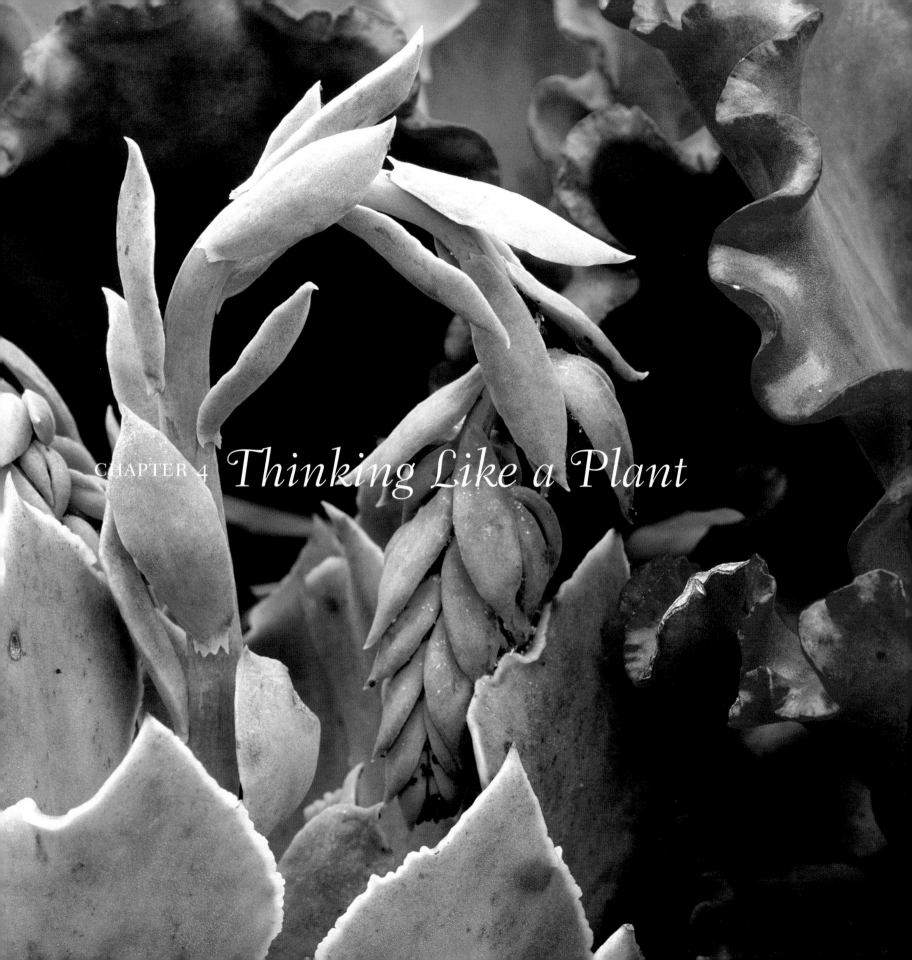

CHAPTER 4 *Thinking Like a Plant*

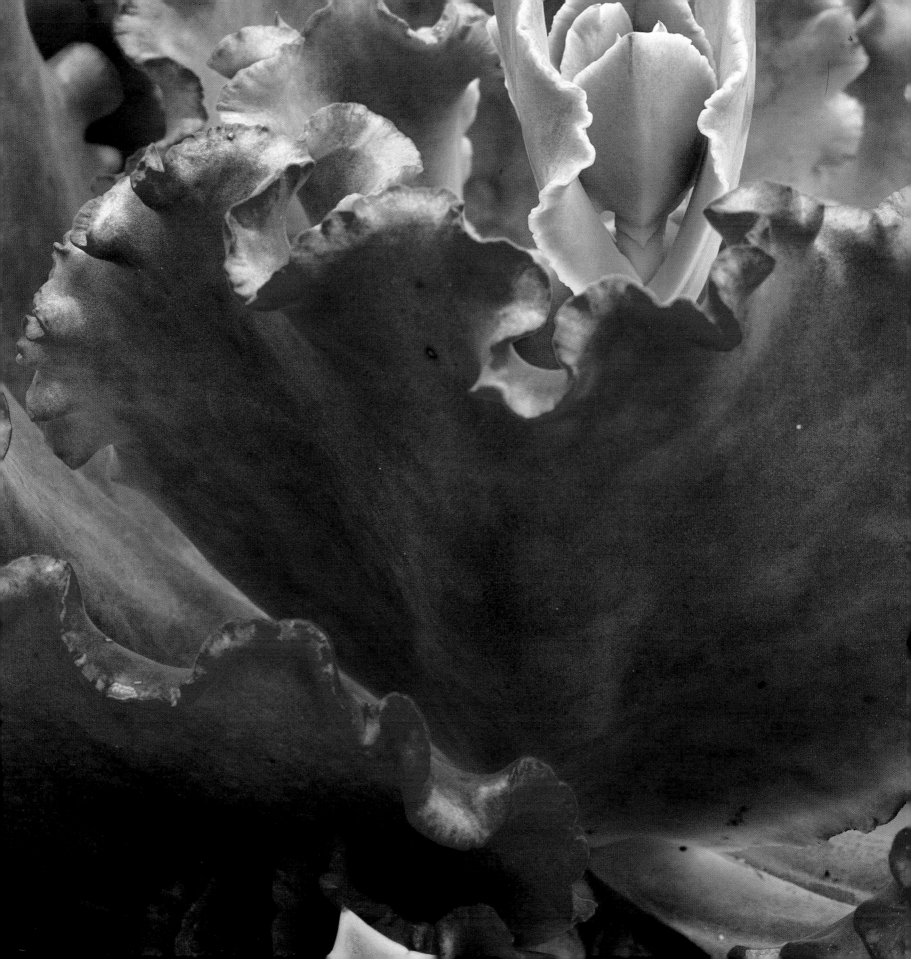

THERE IS MORE TO GARDENING THAN PROVIDING WATER, FERTILIZER and a spot to grow. To get maximum beauty out of your plants, you need to *bond* with them. Like puppies, they are really very easy to please and will show remarkable gratitude for your thoughtful efforts.

Realize that your plants really do depend on you. By thinking like a plant, you will site plants according to *their* wishes, *their* cultural needs, not yours. You will notice signs of stress, such as yellowing leaves, and learn to read them as cries for help, signals to attract your attention. Stop thinking of yourself as a gardener and become an artistic, psychic liaison between plant and animal.

All plants have a common goal — to flower, make seed and ensure their own continuation. To do so, they need help from insects, wind or animals to transfer their pollen. So they make themselves pretty, which happens to appeal to people as well. Realize that they are not putting on this show for *you*, but enjoy it anyway.

One of the last things a dying plant tries to do is flower. This seems very valiant to me, like a sappy movie. The final stages of its life are irreversible. Plants that complete their life cycle in one year are called annuals for a reason, and you must accept this. There is no point whining to hapless nursery employees that your alyssum/stocks/lobelia/marigolds are all done blooming by September, as it is their genetic time clock shutting them down. You can't fight Mother Nature!

PREVIOUS PAGE *Remember "Birds of a feather flock together" when planting. Group plants with the same needs, not the same looks. This allows for creative groupings and healthy plants. These* **Echeverias** *enjoy each other's company!*

FACING PAGE *The spiral aloe,* **Aloe polyphylla**, *wants to appear fierce and unmunchable to grazing animals in its native South Africa. Have your face shredded or eat something else — you decide!*

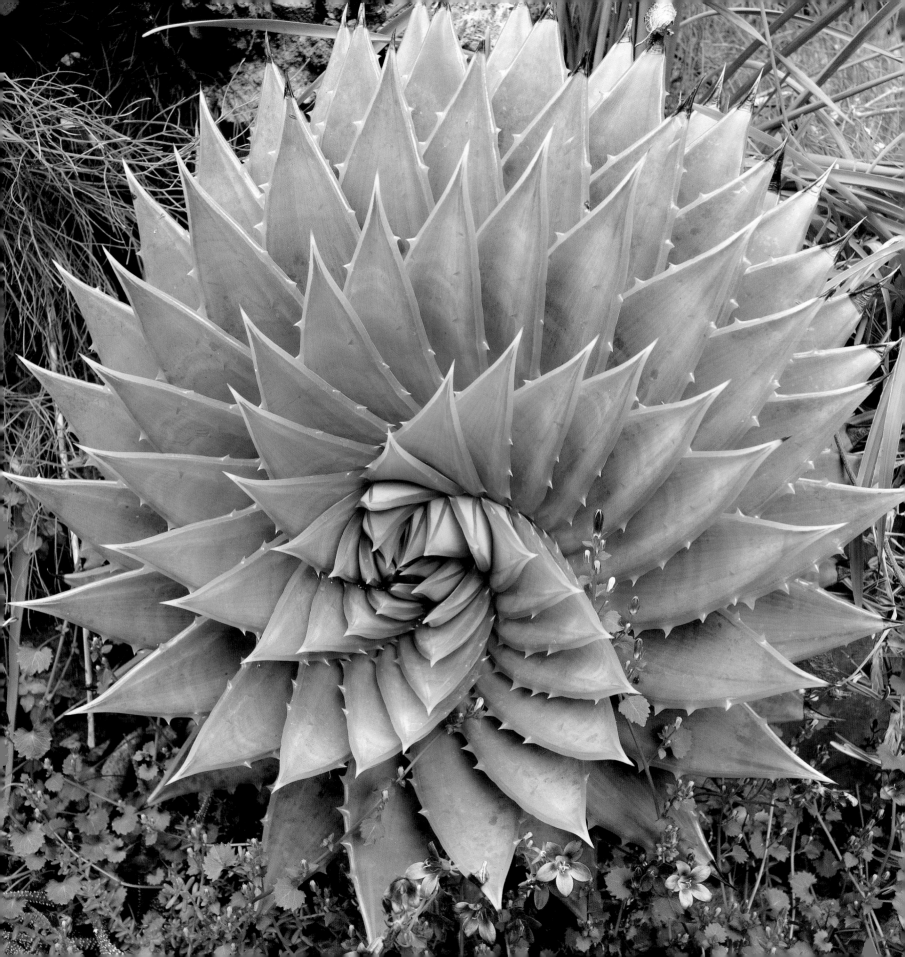

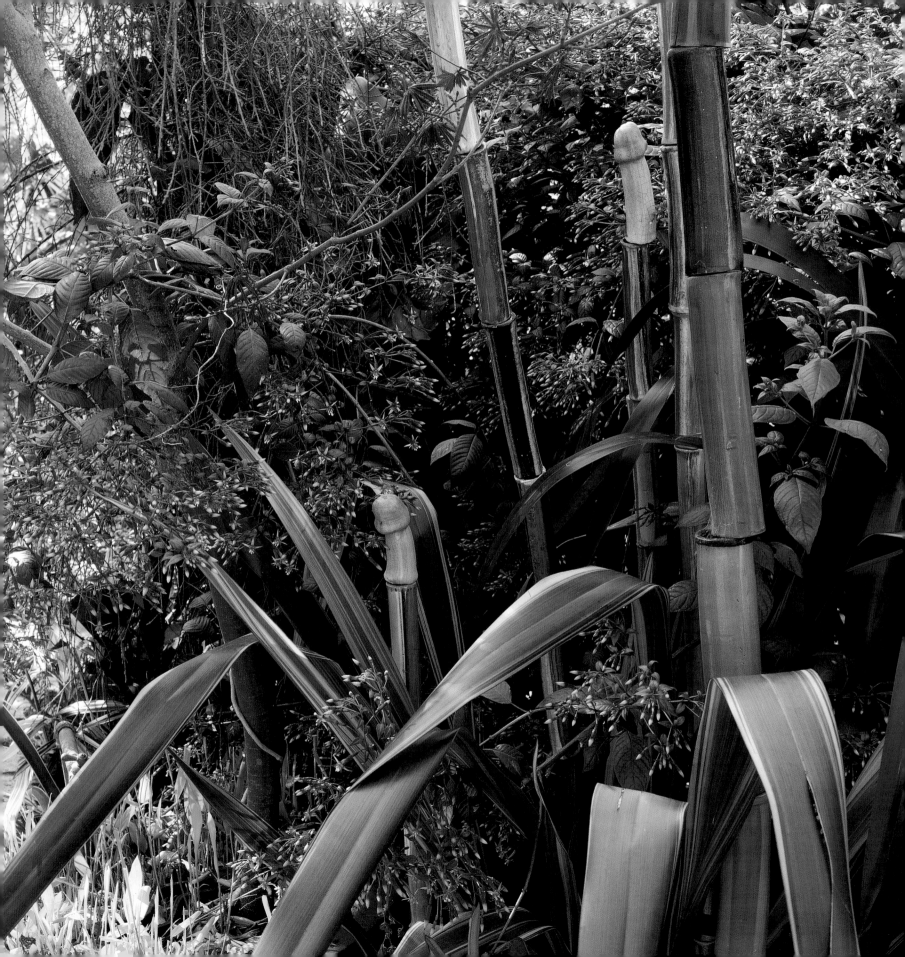

LEFT **Phormium** *'Sundowner' is very happy to see all visitors to the* RAICHE/McCRORY *garden in* BERKELEY, CALIFORNIA. *Marcia Donohue's ceramic "additions" help express an already sexy plant's true feelings!*

RIGHT **Hemerocallis** *'Bela Lugosi' beckons pollinators with its finest offerings. Daylilies really do only have one day to accomplish what most flowers do all summer: get laid! A remarkable, contrasting lime-green throat ensures this daylily will be noticed.*

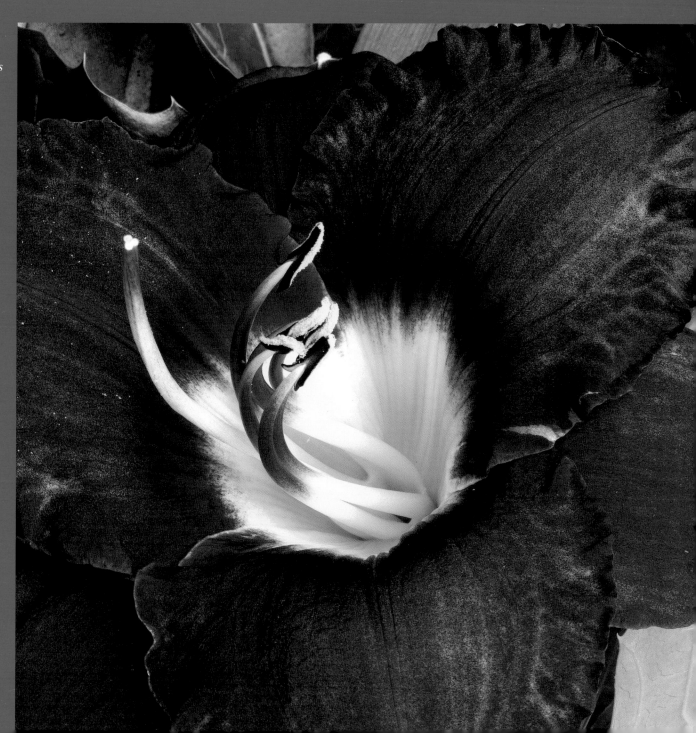

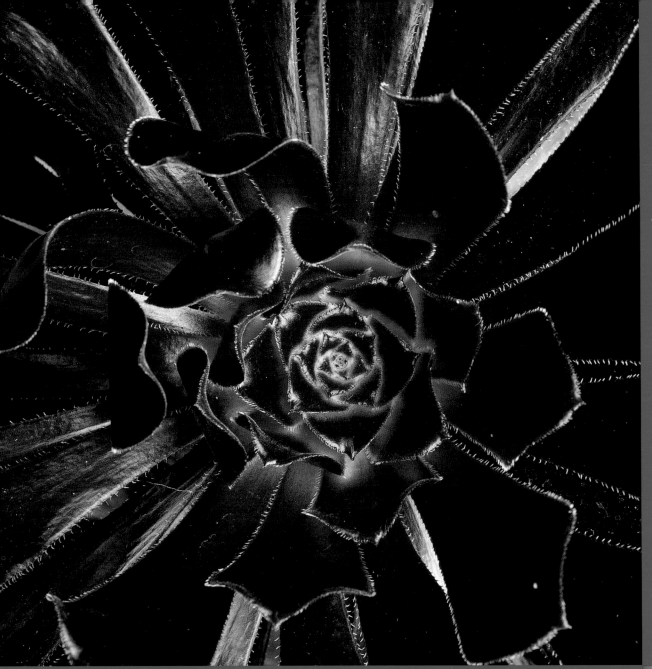

LEFT *Aeonium arboreum* 'Schwarzkopf' turns darker purple the more sun it gets. Cold-climate gardeners use this plant outside in summer pots and rarely get to see its blinding display of acid-yellow flowers. Other flower colors would disappear in its whorls of darkness.

BELOW *Hemerocallis* 'Sedona', bred by Pat Stamile, is one of my favorite daylilies. It is a perfect color match for my house, but I also love its ruffled gold edge and wide petals. Modern hybridizers have transformed those scraggy, orange things beside the ditch into breathtaking workhorses with names like 'Forbidden Desires' and 'Elusive Dream'.

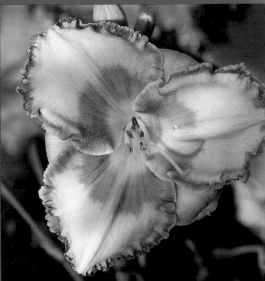

G REAT-LOOKING, HAPPY PLANTS ARE ALSO HAPPY UNDERGROUND. The part you can't see must be having a good time. To do so, it must have access to air, nutrition and, to varying degrees, moisture. Soil is really a vague term for a whole terrestrial universe. It provides an anchor for plants and a buffet meal they are stuck at for life. Roots will find and absorb nutrients *if they are there.* Soil is dirty hydroponics, using a variety of particles as support for roots as they search for something to eat and drink. This is hard to do without adequate moisture. Ever tried swallowing a pill without a glass of water?

Home gardeners can improve the "meal" in their soil just like organic farmers do. Natural materials such as composted leaves, mushrooms and steer manure add important texture and nutrition to the soil, and encourage an active bacterial component. This makes soil *alive*, which for your plants is like winning the lottery.

It should take years to create a happy soil system. Buying and plunking down "good" soil is not going to help unless it is dug in with what was already there. The earth wants to accept its new layer, but won't do so unless it is married! Many new homeowners find themselves dealing with pancakes of death installed by profit-obsessed contractors. With no attempt to create a *living soil,* plants never really thrive. They are letting you know the cupboard is bare by mysteriously refusing to grow.

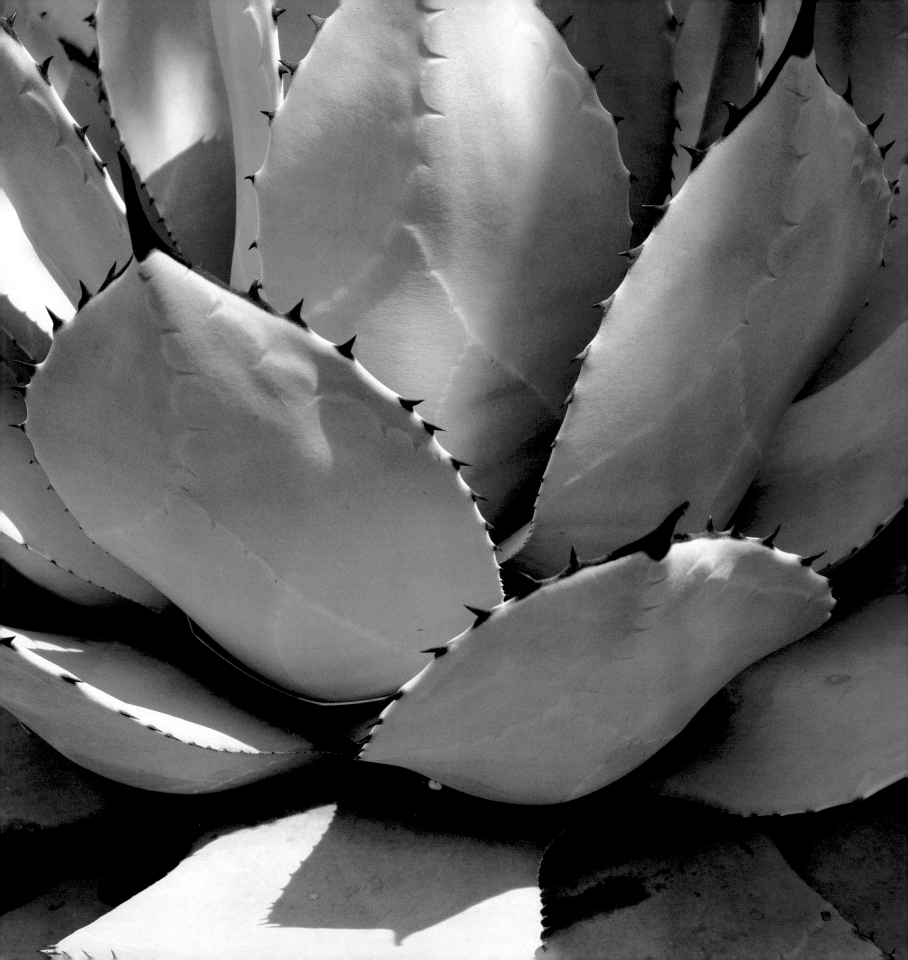

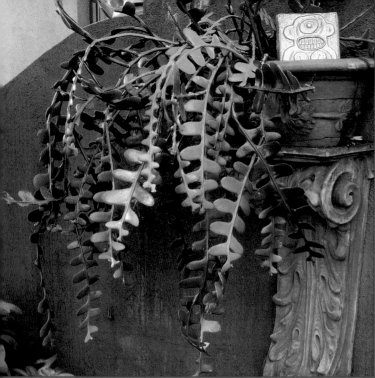

BELOW *The icy-blue sprawl of* **Mertensia simplicissima** *and tufts of* **Agropyron magellanicum** *grass create a feeling of dry heat in* LINDA COCHRAN'S *garden on* BAINBRIDGE ISLAND, *near* SEATTLE. *Flat rocks and a faded terra cotta painted wall set a scene far removed from the Pacific Northwest.*

ABOVE *It was the terra cotta wall bracket I wanted, to adorn a plain wall in my garden. Then it made a perfect home for a piece of living sculpture, a very kooky* **Cryptocereus** *I paired with a small sculpted tile by Bay area artist Mark Bullwinkle.*

LEFT *You know this* **Agave parryi** *wants sun, just by its appearance. Silvery colors and spines are clues, but its wide-open leaf arrangement is really a solar panel designed to catch as much light as possible and create little shadow. Notice the subtle tattoos created by the sun as leaves unfurl, one on top of another.*

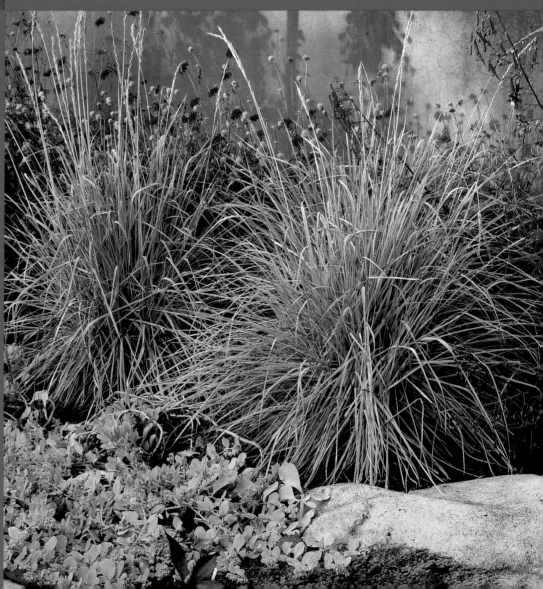

THIS SIGN OF UNHAPPINESS WILL LAST FOREVER UNLESS YOU take action. You need to improve the soil down where the plants are grazing. Stopping plant suicide is nearly impossible. It can be done, but it takes a long time to nurse a sentimental favorite back to health. A spa treatment, severe amputation or shock treatments may be necessary. I have tried massive doses of fertilizer, but soon learned that it was the weakest plants that overdosed. Plants on their last legs seem most willing to offer a cutting, a small part of themselves as a legacy of hope for the future. Withered orchids, dessicated jade plants and tortured pelargoniums can often be rescued and regrown from last-gasp tips.

Thinking like a plant means putting yourself in the plant's place for a while. How would you like to sit in front of your hot air duct in the living room all winter? Envision those *Ficus benjamina* leaves as skin flakes falling off. Then you die.

Television commercials have finally taught us about SP factor and tanning. Sun protection is now common sense, except when it comes to placing newly bought, greenhouse-grown plants outside. Many leaves are permanently scalded by this transfer to reality. Avoid this by first resting them under a shade tree for a day or two. Give the plants time to adjust their leaf surfaces after the cushy world of the greenhouse.

Make yourself more aware of how similar we are to plants. You should thrill them as much as they thrill you. The best gardeners have balanced relationships going with their gardens. A happy marriage. Any reward is incidental, but not unnoticed. In good times and bad ... sickness and health ... I do.

FACING PAGE *Cascading or trailing plants need to be displayed to best advantage. This means off the ground. I grow the hybrid oregano* **Origanum** *'Barbara Tingey' in an Italian terra cotta pot atop a garden wall, where its waterfall of ornamental "hops" delights me — and countless bees — all summer long.*

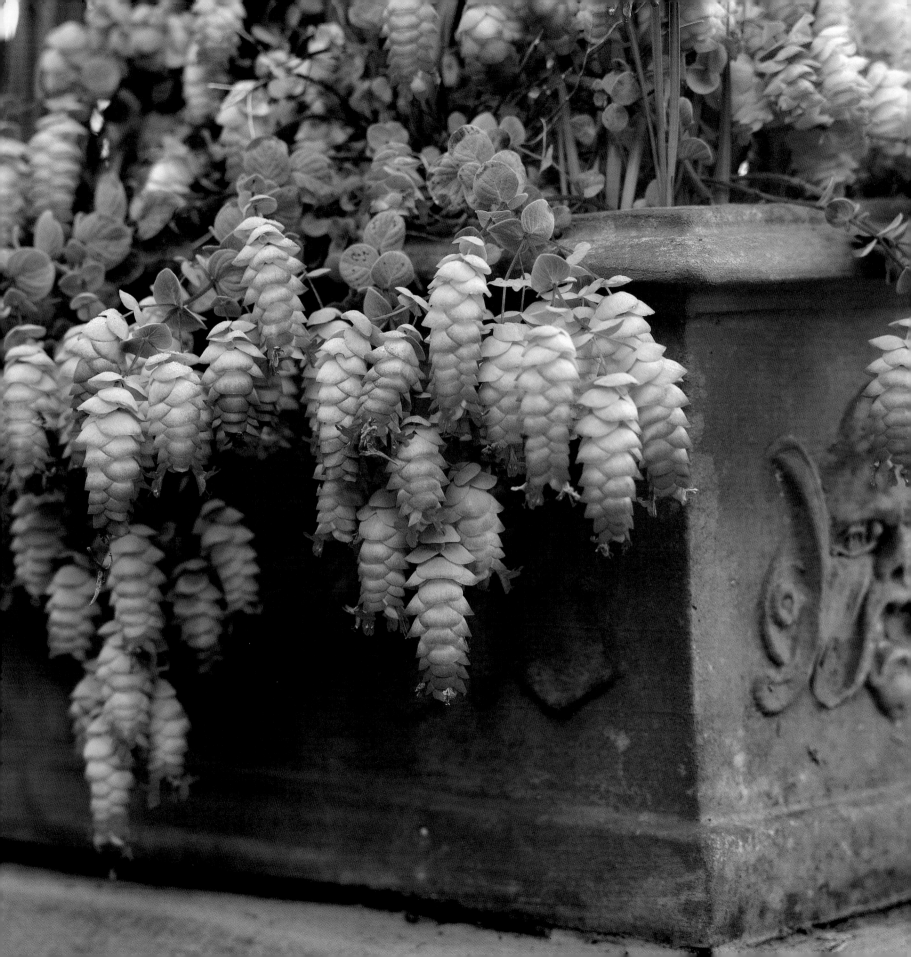

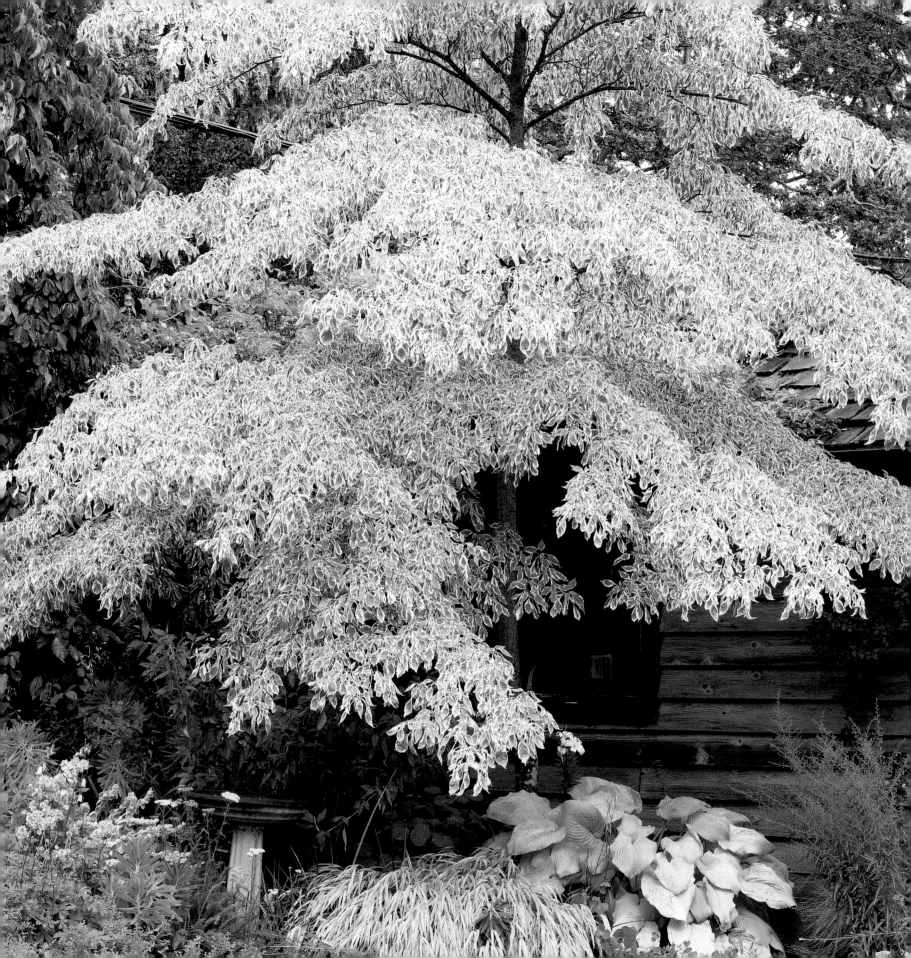

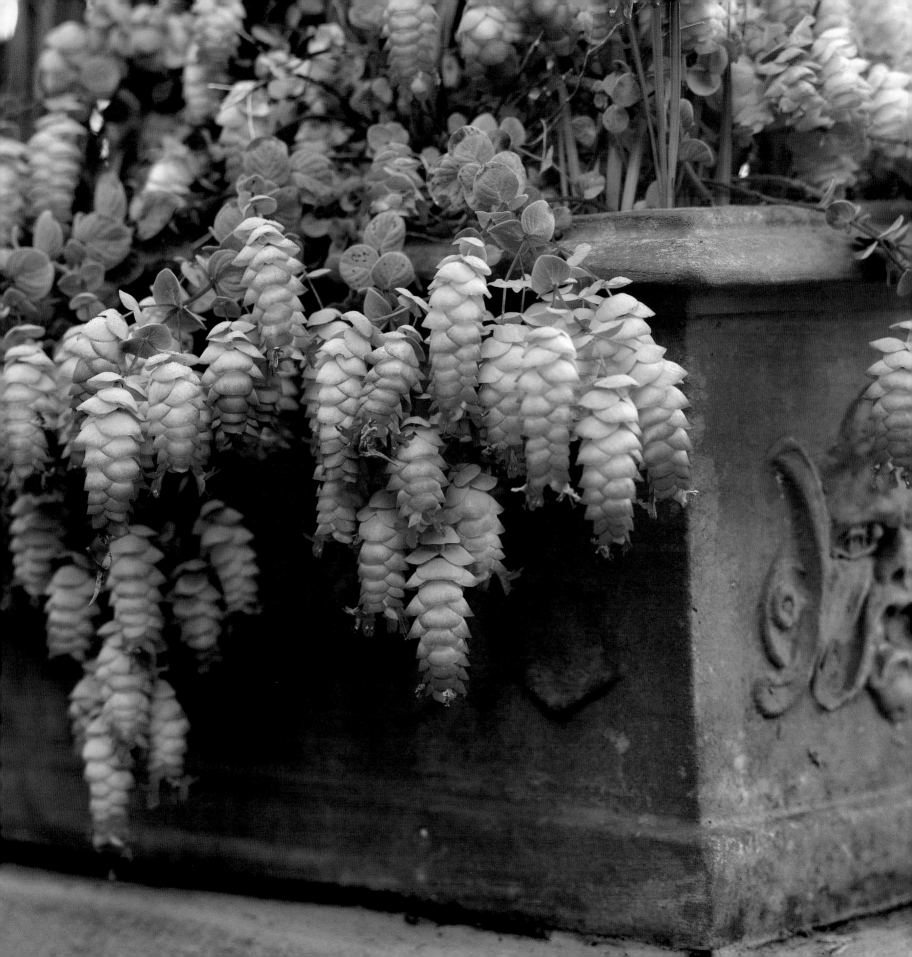

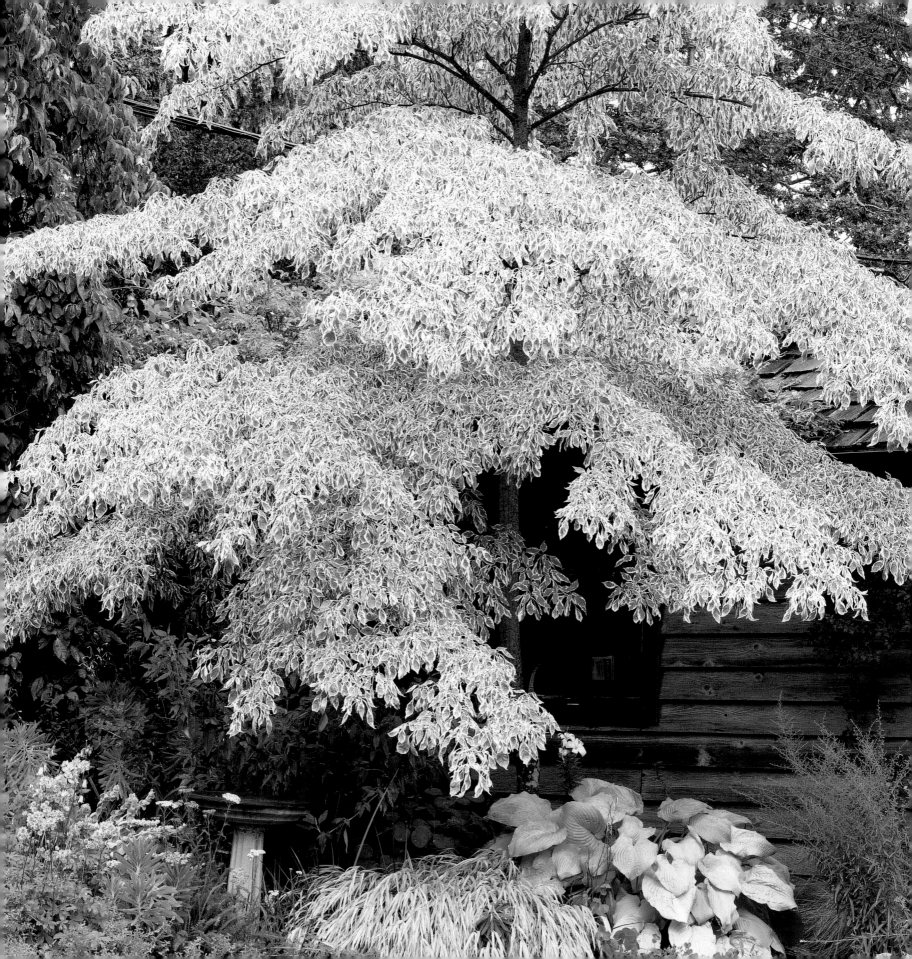

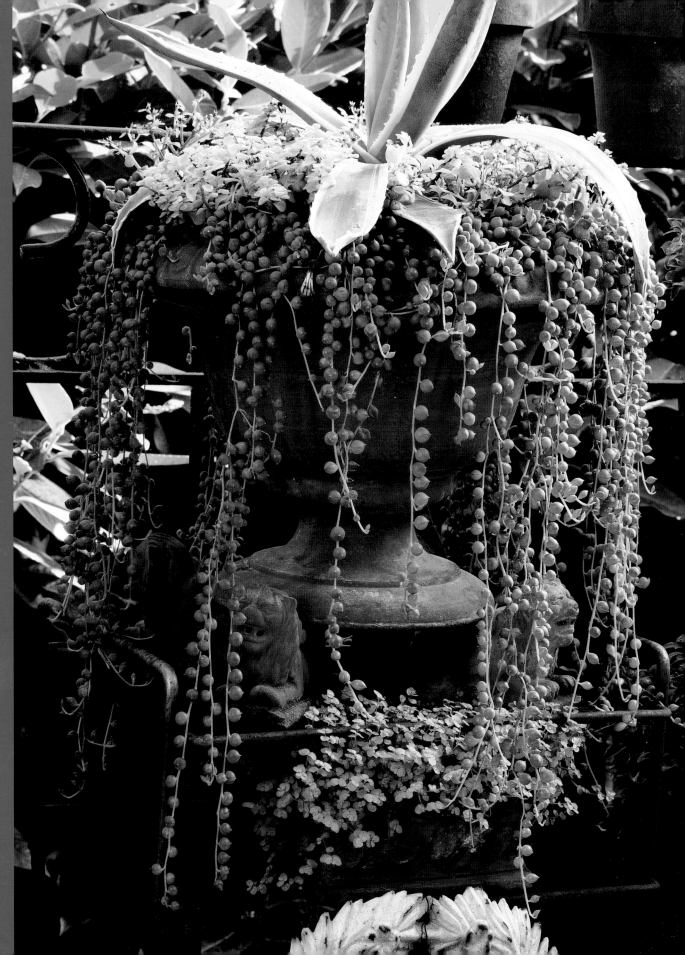

LEFT *If you've got it, flaunt it.* **Cornus controversa** *'Variegata' must always be treated like a star. In* SUSAN RYLEY'S VICTORIA, B.C., *garden, it reigns supreme in the back corner of what is really a bank vault, not a jewel box of a garden.*

RIGHT *String of pearls (***Senecio rowleyanus***) adds a fabulous fringe to* DAMEN DJOS'S *potted agave on his* VANCOUVER, B.C., *balcony.*

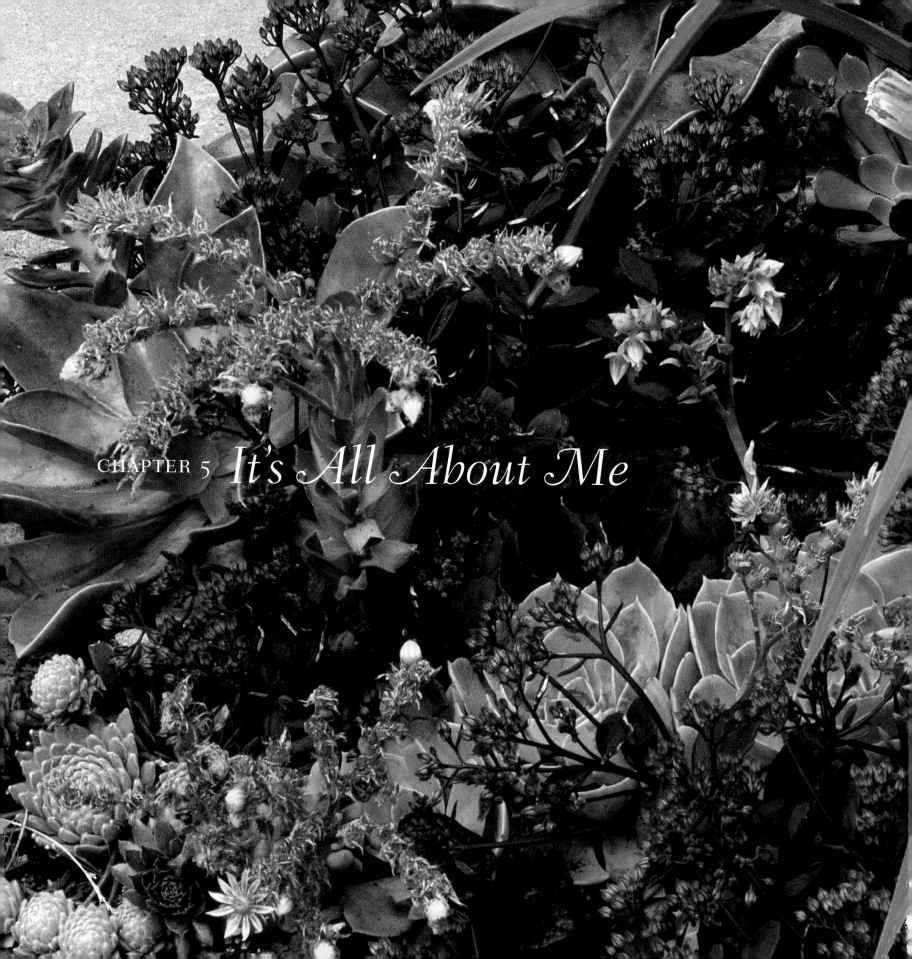

CHAPTER 5 *It's All About Me*

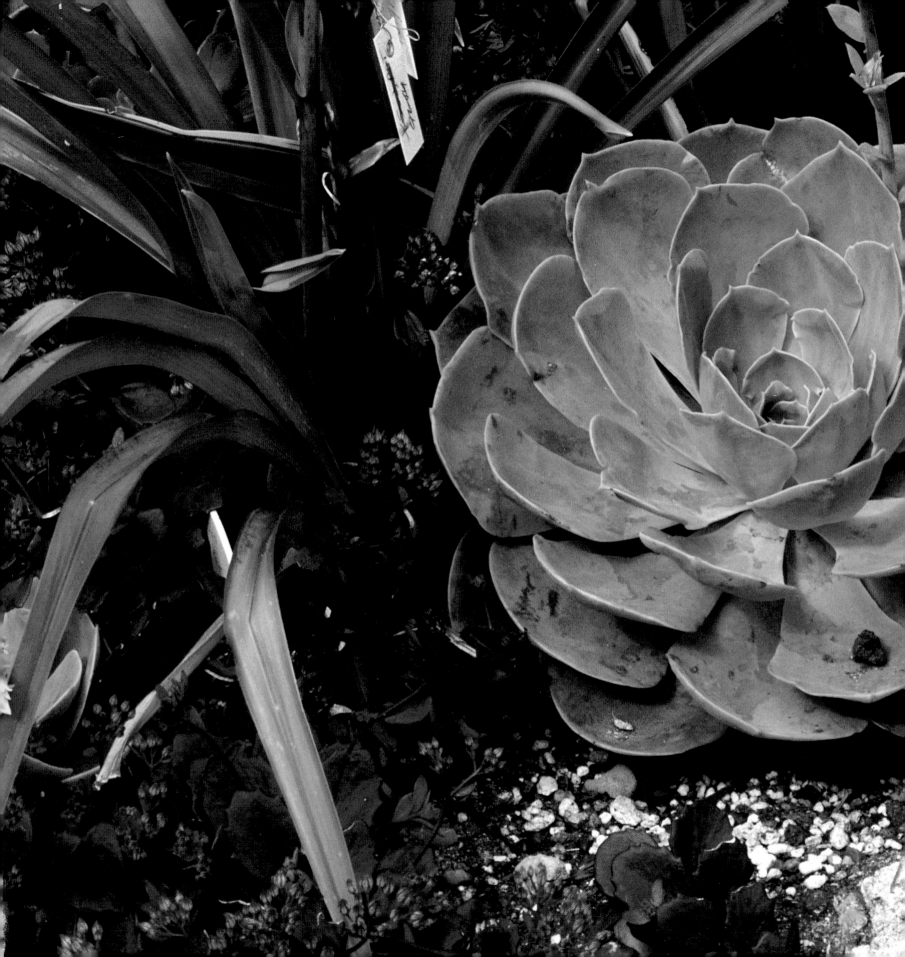

THE PLANTS YOU CHOOSE TO "PLAY WITH" END UP SAYING A LOT about you. "Saying it with flowers" is a valid form of expression. Try to adopt this slogan as your gardening mantra. Keep it in mind while plant shopping as well as when actually planting. How much are you willing to reveal?

Really good gardeners don't hold back. Mesmerizing, memorable plant pictures are created by the brave. Spines, teeth, spikes, thorns and even seed capsules add an edginess to plant compositions. "Safe" gardeners rely on flowers alone and leave theatricality out of it. Gardening is a chance to spread your wings — why do so many people never fly?

Beware of the botanical quicksand sold as "annuals." This huge industry dispenses humdrum goop like "supertunias" and the insanely popular bacopa (**Suteria cordata**). This trailing, white-flowered annual is the botanical equivalent of icicle lights — so overused and trite it has lost any attractiveness through overexposure. The discerning eye learns to avoid most popular plants. Why be like everyone else?

PREVIOUS PAGE *Cerinthe major* '*Purpurescens*' *froths about like a neon purple eucalyptus, while succulent* **Echeverias** *and the very dark purple* **Sedum x** '*Bertrum Anderson*' *bake in the sun in my small patio pocket garden.* **Phormium** '*Sundowner*' *adds another foliage texture to an already busy mixture.*

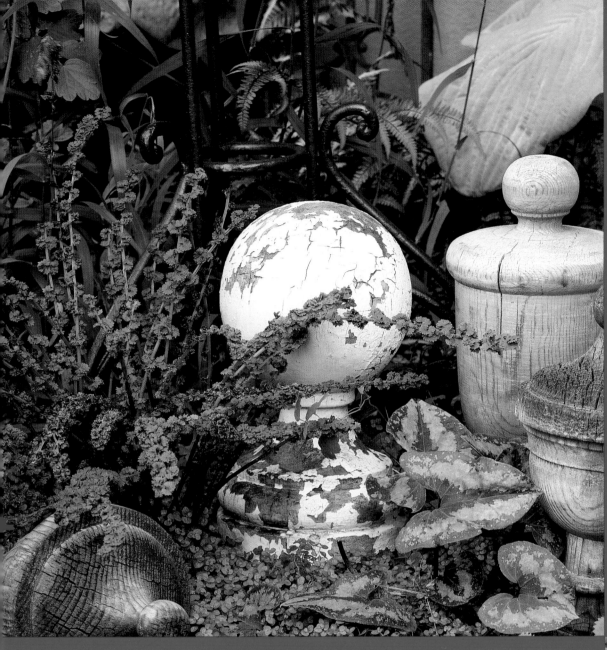

LEFT *In a small, shady corner of my garden, baby's tears (***Soleirolia soleirolii***) carpet the moist soil. A collection of old wooden fence finials forms a sculptural grouping in a "foliage only" composition. The silver-splashed, evergreen leaves of ***Asarum splendens*** are allowed to star, while the bizarre "tatting fern," ***Athyrium filix-femina*** 'Frizelliae', looks on. A self-sown ***Alchemilla mollis*** and ***Hosta*** 'Gold Standard' frame this tableau of less than one square yard.*

BELOW *The incredibly beautiful ***Saxifraga fortunei*** 'Miyuki's Purple' at Heronswood Nursery in Kingston, Washington.*

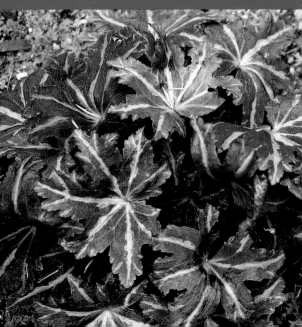

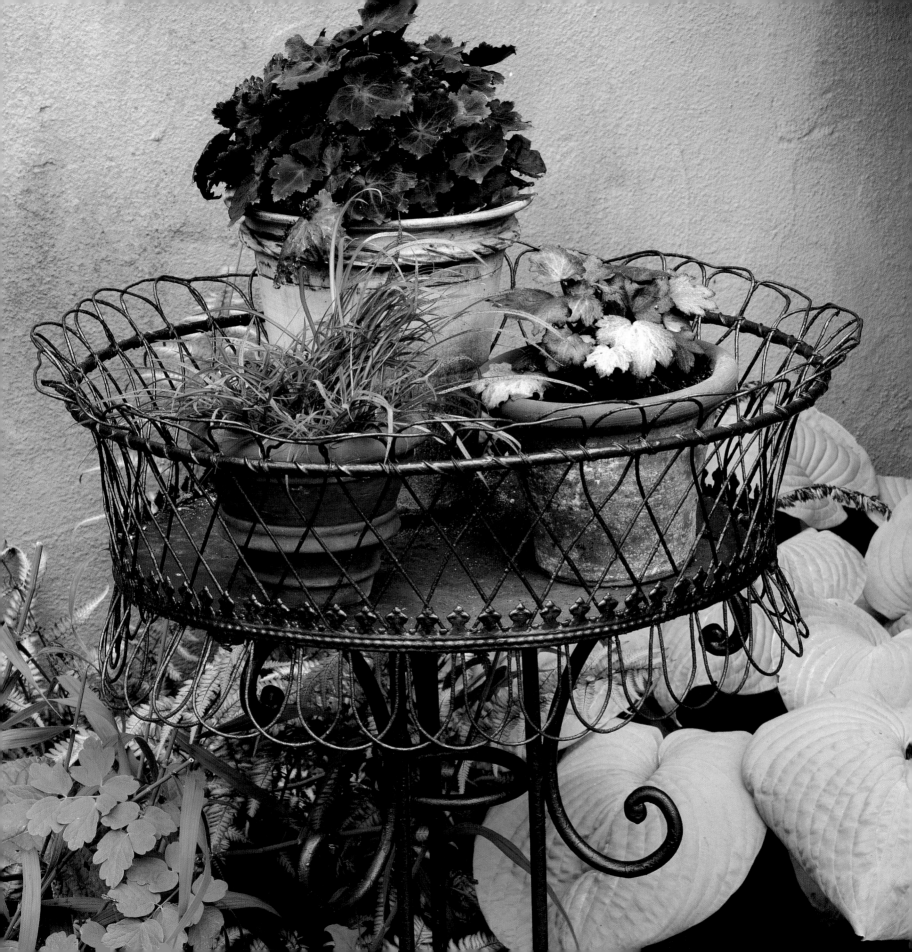

As you spend more time gardening, you develop a need for higher highs, a botanical fix that never satisfies. Walking around a nursery becomes more of a mission than an excursion. Avid gardeners become plant sharks, circling plant sales, hoping to score. This is what happens as you become a plant *addict*. Some become obsessed collectors who stash their hoard artlessly. Thankfully, most are changed into superb, artistic gardeners. They join a universal plant community whose members recognize each other instantly. Mutual respect is granted or withheld in direct proportion to botanical knowledge. Plant savvy has often led to friendship, even marriage. The mutual love of plants has an instant bonding effect, even amongst strangers.

Certain plants are practically an entree in themselves. Hellebores worked for several years, but are now losing their power; there are too many around. Double-flowered hellebores (the **Helleborus x orientalis** group) still enchant me, as do green-flowered species such as **Helleborus viridis**. The very dark-flowered, near-black hybrids are still in my garden, but no longer in my heart. It took five or six years, but the thrill of their funereal spring show is gone. A double-flowered black one is the hit I need now!

FACING PAGE *An antique plant stand from France holds personal favorites up where I can appreciate them. Pots of **Saxifraga fortunei** (the brown cultivar 'Velvet' and the multi-hued 'Five Color') would get lost in the garden. **Arthropodium candidum** is just the right brownish color to complement this grouping. This New Zealand native appears grass-like but is actually in the lily family.*

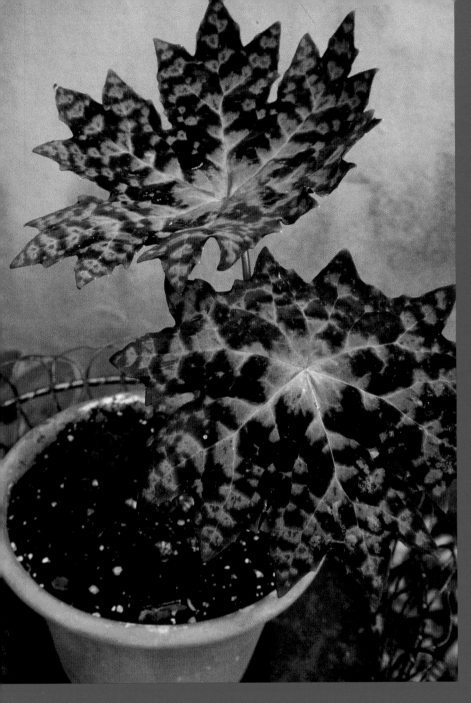

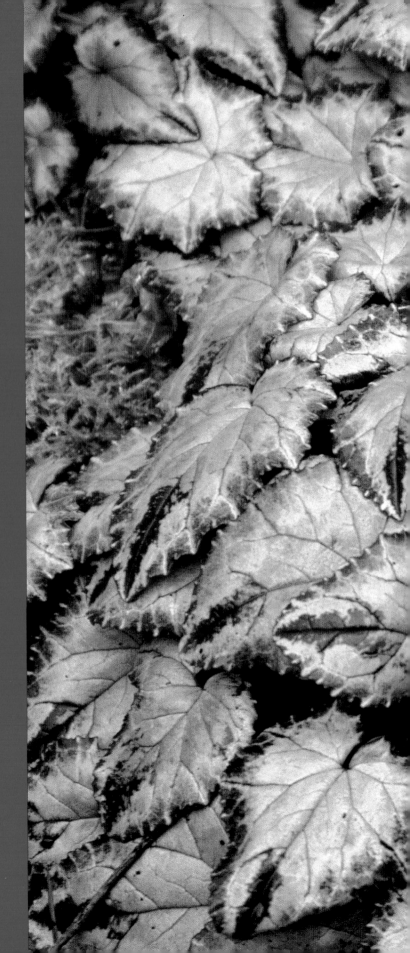

ABOVE *The first time I saw* **Podophyllum delavayi***, I screamed. This spectacular "Mayapple" from China is my most prized plant. I have grown it in a pot for years, and will now plant it out in moist, dappled shade.*

RIGHT *The hardy cyclamen are true jewels for almost anyone's garden. Patiently grown from seed, many spectacular forms are to be seen at Heronswood Nursery. This spectacular clump is from* **Cyclamen hederifolium** *'Bowle's Apollo group' seed. Needless to say, I am now growing some tiny seedlings myself.*

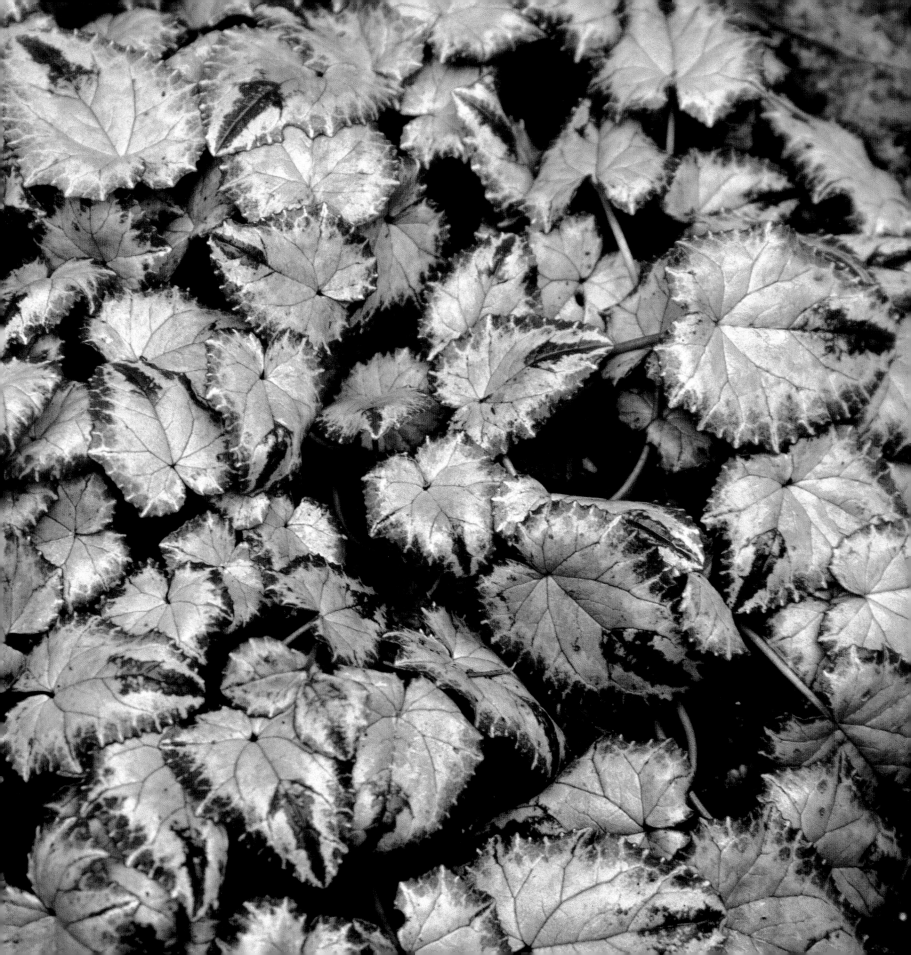

THERE IS SOMETHING EXTRA CHARMING ABOUT "SHY" PLANTS. I will stop what I am doing to admire the nodding flowers of *Deinanthe caerulea*. This herbaceous hydrangea relative from China produces clusters of nodding, waxy flowers in mid-summer. With particularly refined, cupped petals arranged very formally around a central "button," individual flowers appear as fine porcelain treasures.

I am also enchanted with the charm of many *Ranunculus ficaria* cultivars. These early bloomers, which come in bronzy-foliaged forms like 'Brazen Hussy' and 'Brambling', fill cracks between my steps. The small bright-gold flowers look like tiny calendulas atop miniature water lily foliage. Their show is completely over by late May, forcing me to really admire them while I can. One of my most treasured small perennials is the variegated *Hacquetia epipactis* 'Thor'. This subtle charmer produces celadon green- and white-striped flowers and foliage! Most people walk right past its discreet beauty. But I bought my car because it was the same shade of green as 'Thor'!

Being a left-handed, Gemini breach-birth *allows* me to love tetraploid daylilies. It is *who I am botanically*. Being able to appreciate the smaller, charming plants as well as the bold and dramatic makes me feel well rounded as a gardener. It also makes me believe in astrology. I am such a Gemini!

FACING PAGE *Deinanthe caerulea is a seldom-encountered, herbaceous relative of the hydrangea. I am smitten with its porcelain-like, soft lavender flowers*

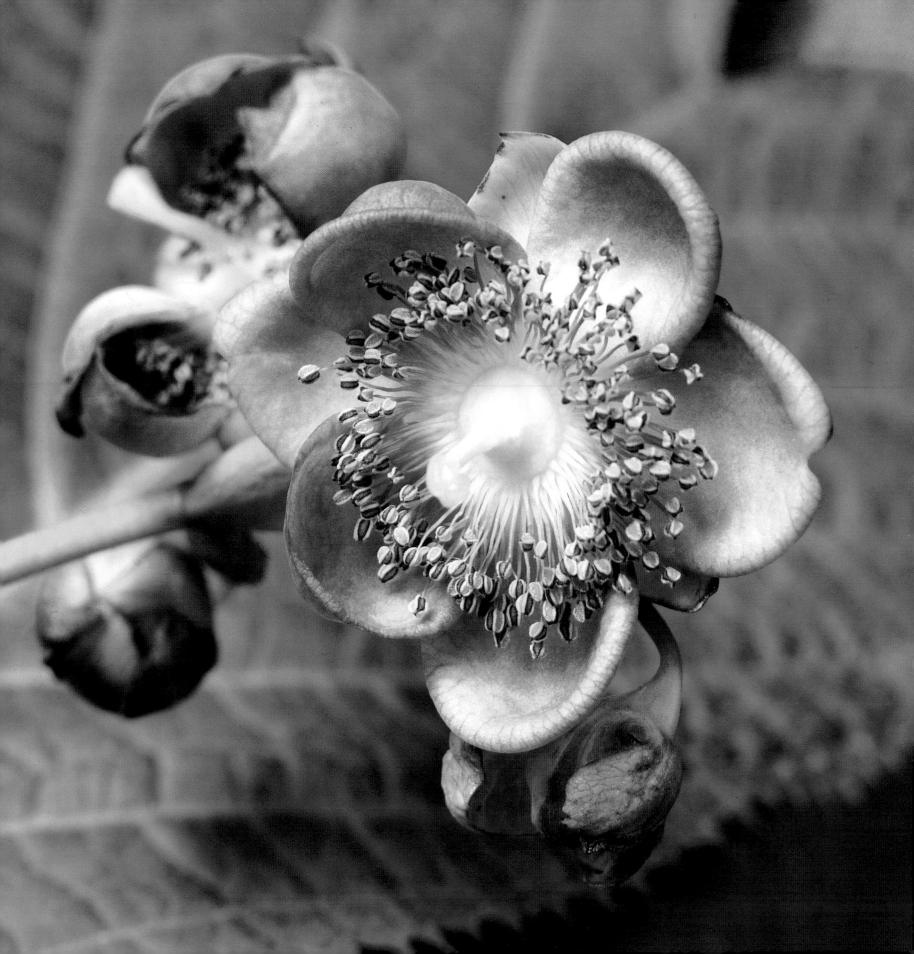

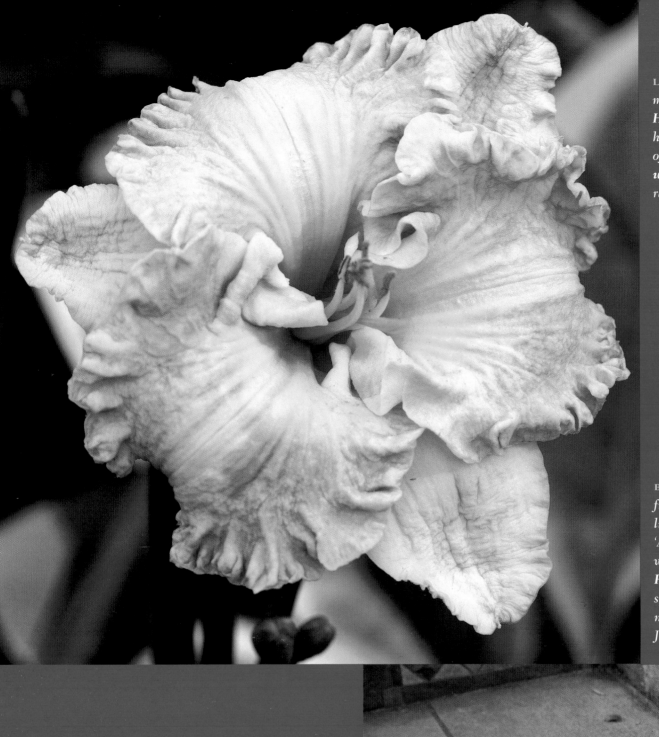

LEFT 'Ed Brown' is one of the most beautiful of all **Hemerocallis**. In my garden, he co-opts the gorgeous foliage of a neighboring **Symphytum uplandicum** 'Variegatum' rather than admit to his own.

BELOW Moist cracks in my front stairs hold treasures. The lilac–blue **Anemone nemerosa** 'Allenii' shares tight quarters with various color forms of **Ranunculus ficaria**. These spring ephemerals ask for nothing, and are dormant by June.

How you compose your plants is the hard part. There are shelves full of books on this subject and this is another one. Combining plants artistically is easier if you know a few basic rules regarding harmony, proportion and contrast. Combining these with good "plant requirement" (basic care) knowledge results in interesting and healthy planting.

Whether in containers or the open garden, plants always group best in triangular blocks. The eye can only drink in so much at a time, so it is best to have a "leader" — a high shape the eye is drawn to — supported by lower, blobbier underplantings on either side or in front. I compose most pots by planting a taller plant at the back first, then working forward, building a slope effect toward the front.

In a mixed planting, never put the tallest plant in the center of the pot. Doing that immediately gives one away as artless. If a pot is to be seen from all sides, plant three tall things in the middle instead of one. They don't all have to be the same, either. Try combining a young New Zealand flax (a **Phormium** cultivar of your choice), a bronze **Carex flagellifera** and a dark-leaved dahlia such as 'Bednall Beauty' or 'Ellen Houston'. This is much more visually interesting than a green dracaena 'spike' (**Cordyline australis**), the last refuge of the truly desperate.

THE SHAPE OF THE ACTUAL CONTAINER SHOULD DICTATE THE end result. Low, wide pots are the most attractive, offering more "tabletop" space to plant in. Pots that are wider than they are tall look more anchored and group themselves more easily. There is nothing wrong with the typical, cone-shaped flowerpot, but why be typical? Limit yourself to one taller pot per grouping, flanked by a cluster of two or more non-identical, lower pots. This is the way to create "eye candy."

When grouping plant containers, don't mix too many textures or materials in close proximity. Stick to one overall theme per cluster: either plain terra cotta, glazed, metallic or wood. Plastic is not an option. Seriously! The plants themselves should overpower every container visually — if they don't, you'd better start over. I remember feeling sorry for the cherub-bedecked, bronze urns at Versailles. Each contained one scraggly pelargonium, dying of an inferiority complex and pleading, "Please take me" to every tourist.

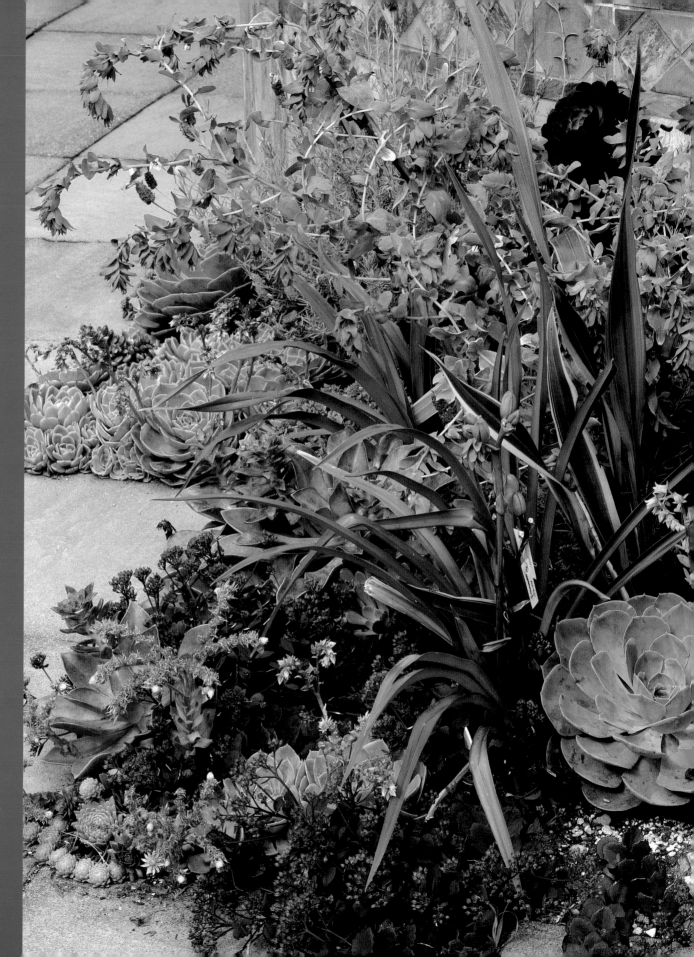

*Cerinthe **major** 'Purpurescens', succulent **Echeverias**, dark purple **Sedum x** 'Bertrum Anderson' and **Phormium** 'Sundowner' on my patio garden. Notice the white tags on my daylily? I am hybridizing them now, instead of orchids!*

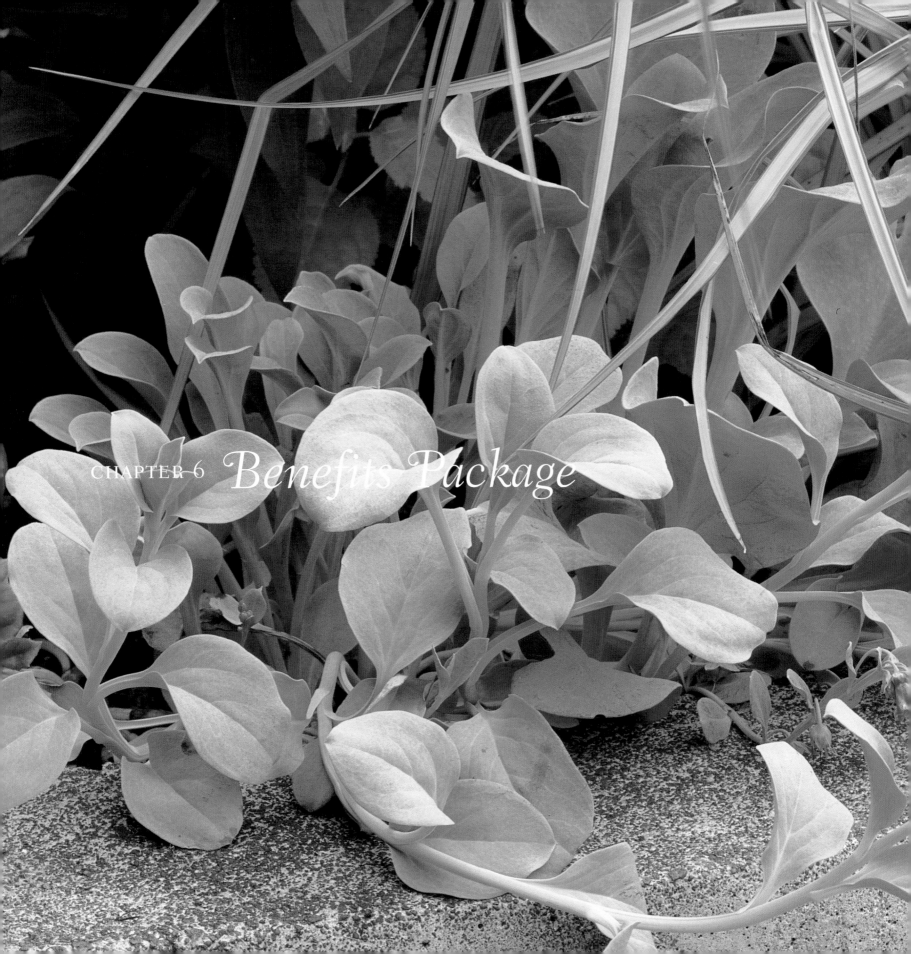

CHAPTER 6 *Benefits Package*

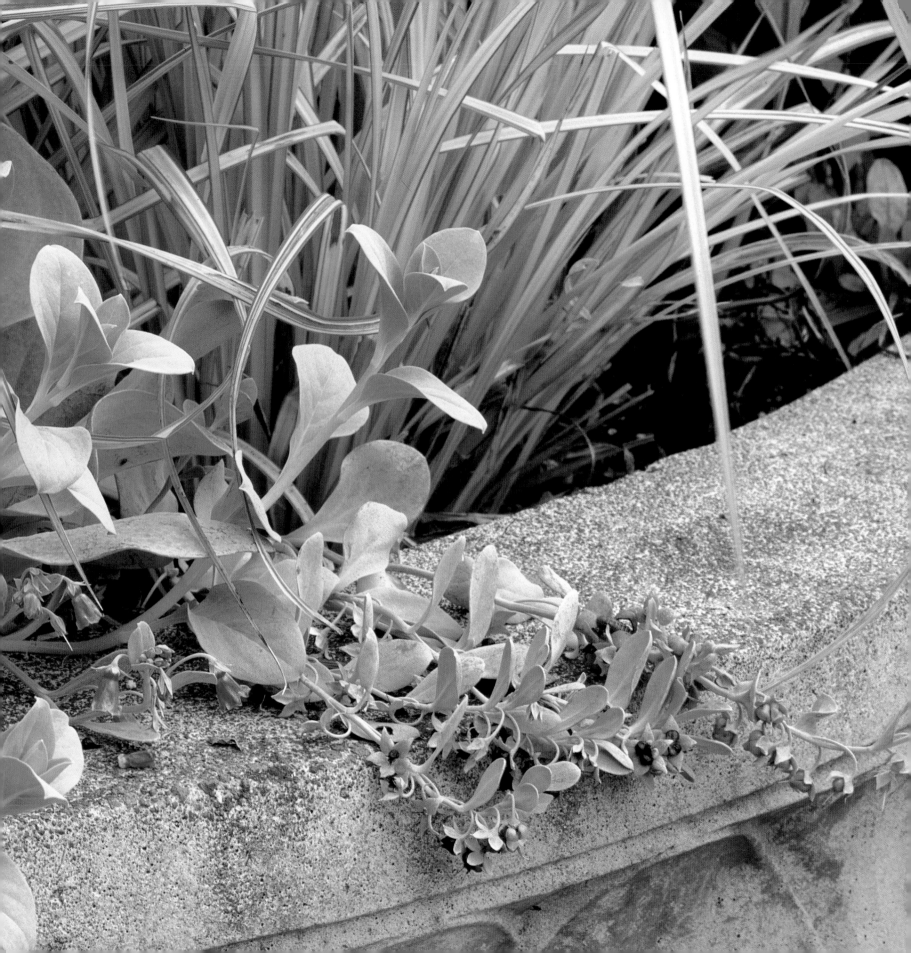

I LIKE TO ASK A PLANT, "WHAT HAVE YOU DONE FOR ME LATELY?" Color, scent and even sound should figure in the reply. I am a sucker for color and am ready to hop into bed (the garden bed, these days) with anything silver, celadon green or violet purple. I also require massive doses of rust, apricot and chartreuse. Interestingly, these colors all look good together in virtually any combination. Celadon green and silver are neutral. Purple is a standout, the alpha wolf of the garden. It dominates but allows rusty and apricot shades to play second fiddle.

Review your own color preference and allow a natural order to occur. If you thrive on red and yellow combinations, you are reading the wrong book. Red and orange is exciting, orange and yellow is tolerable but limited, but red and yellow is artless and screams "Gas Station." There are too many other beautiful combinations out there to ever plant red and yellow together. The glaucous-blue, trailing foliage of *Mertensia simplicissima* (absolute slug caviar) with acid-green *Carex elata* 'Bowle's Golden' grass nearby is pure eye candy. I love blue with green, and rely on this combo as an understudy in my own garden. Hosta 'June' is well behaved and provides a hit of blue with green, as does *Nicotiana langsdorfii* with its amazing robin's-egg-blue pollen and apple-green flowers.

PREVIOUS PAGE *It is important to grow **Mertensia simplicissima** out of reach of slugs and snails, which will quickly destroy its beautiful blue foliage. I was surprised to find how happy it is in containers. **Carex elata** 'Bowle's Golden' makes a screamingly good neighbor for just about anything! Using perennials in pots is not illegal, you know.*

FACING PAGE ***Dicentra** 'Snowflakes' is a perfect color match for slate steps in my garden. Its glaucous-blue foliage takes on a natural tan by midsummer and complements my peachy walls. A polite spreader with crisp white flowers in spring, this hardy perennial is faultless.*

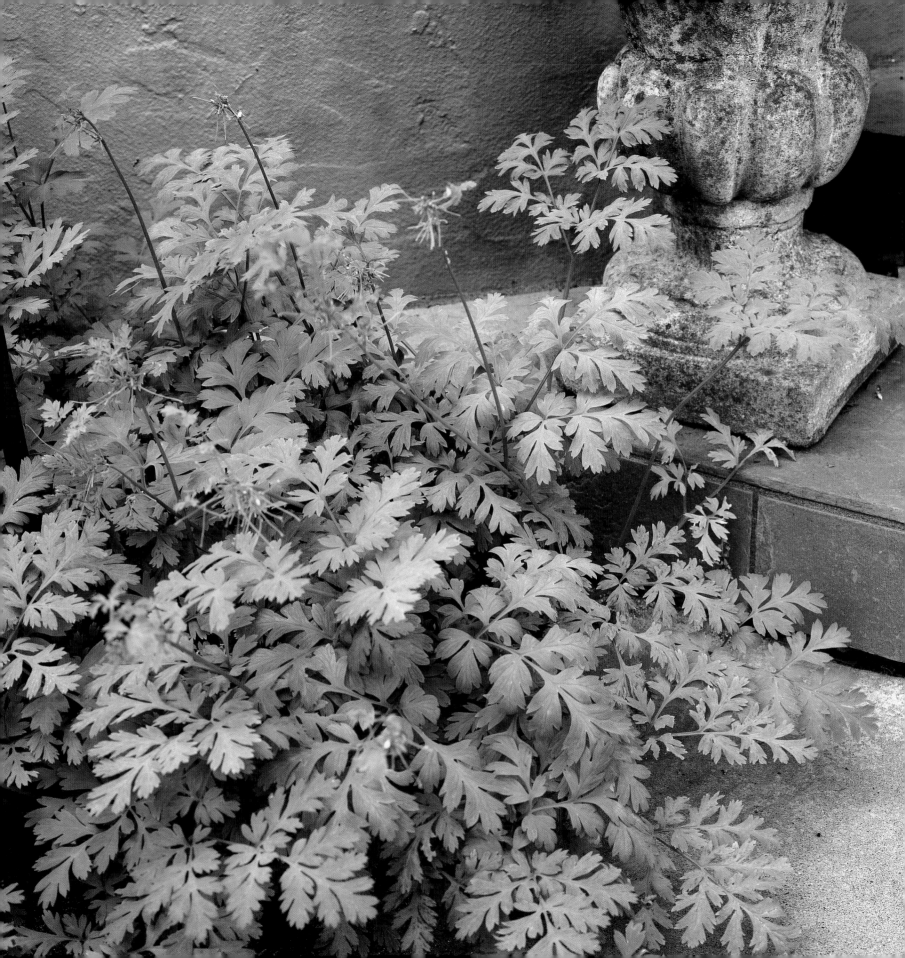

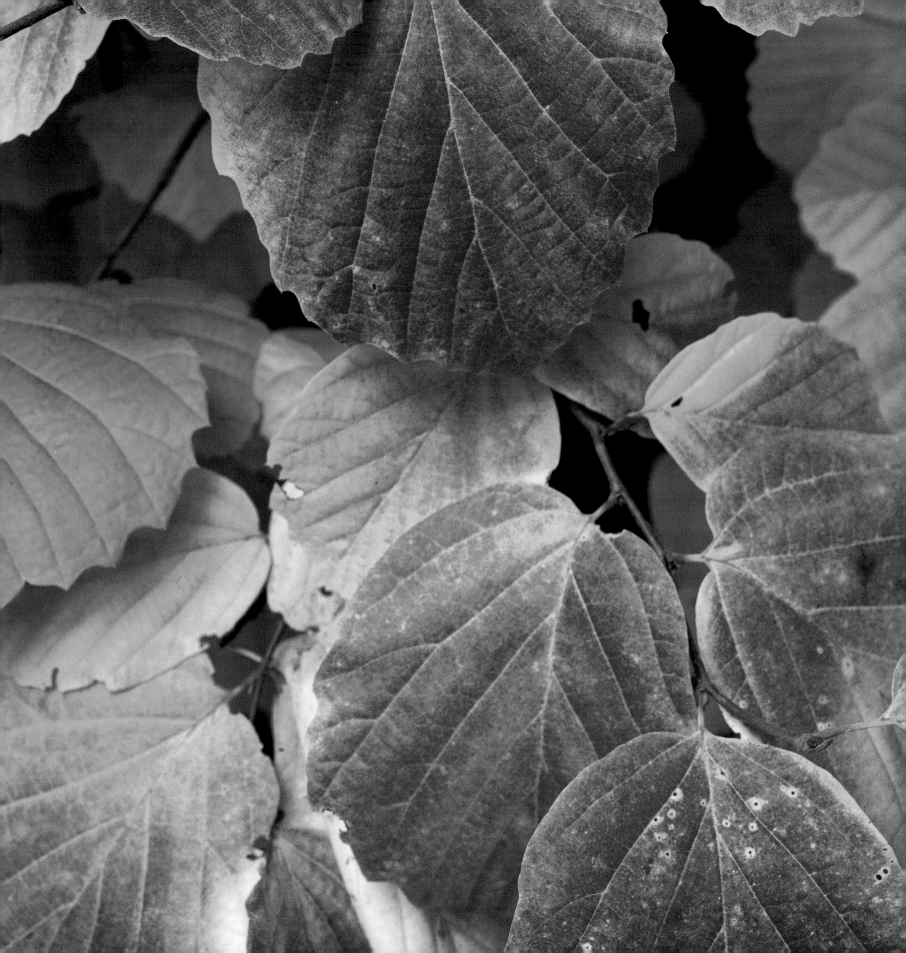

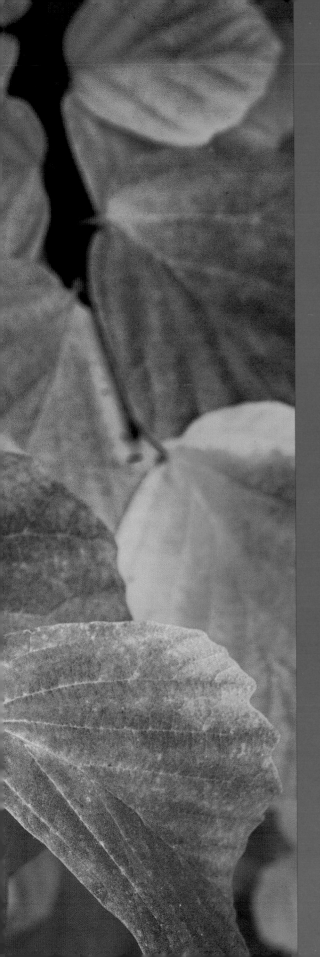

LEFT *Autumn color is a benefit to seek out. The* **Hamamelis** *or witch hazel family includes virtual superstars of autumn glory, such as the coppery-flowered variety 'Jelena', which has superb fall color. Witch hazels become small trees and are perfectly suited for city gardens. Their upright, vase-shaped growth habit allows you to plant woodland treasures underneath.*

BELOW *The pleated leaves of* **Veratrum nigrum** *are beautiful works of nature's art. Reminiscent of origami, they are really designed to funnel and shed rainwater.*

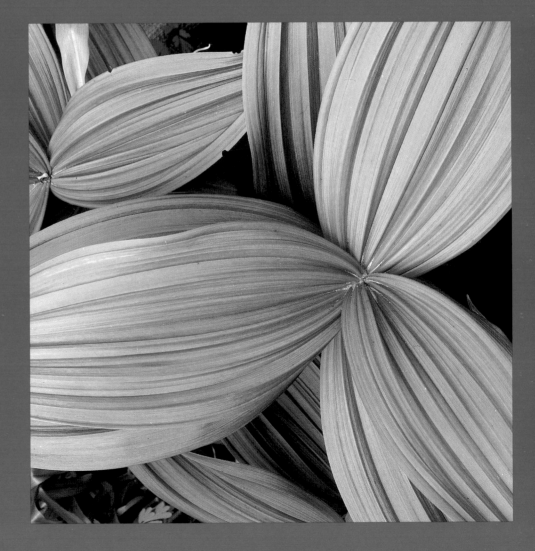

79

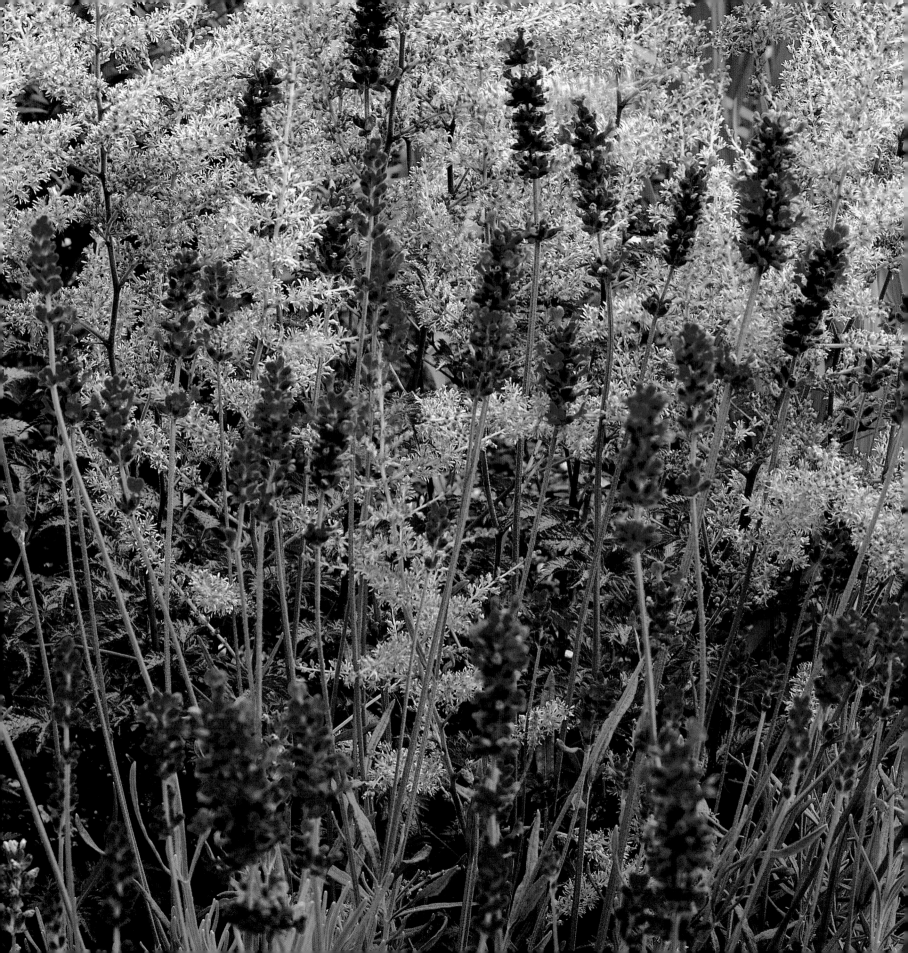

YOU WON'T ACHIEVE THAT "MAGAZINE LOOK" IN YOUR GARDEN until you get the color combinations right. "I'm ready for my close-up" should always be kept in mind when placing a new plant. I assemble plant montages quite slowly. I may find the perfect plant partners two or three years apart. Shifting and regrouping is what gardening becomes; the endless pursuit of perfection. It is hardly drudgery! Playing with plants is safest in spring or fall, but container-grown perennials and shrubs are often irresistible in summer. They don't really feel the move if watered and cared for.

Gardening with limited space should force a high content of "double-duty" plants. Fragrance becomes more important at close range and can instantly alter your mood. Try, if at all possible, to grow a daphne. Daphnes range in hardiness, and almost all are divinely scented. I am particularly fond of **Daphne odora**, whose early spring fragrance carries spicy notes of clove and carnation unusual distances. This broadleaf, evergreen shrub forms a wide, low mound and is happiest when *not* in a pot.

Everyone should grow heliotropes. This favorite of the Victorian era possesses a particularly mood-altering fragrance that immediately cheers people up. It is foolproof as a summer annual and comes in shades of white, mauve or dark purple. I time-travel back to my childhood barbershop every time I smell heliotrope, because the barber used to dust my neck with talcum powder when he was done. Fragrance and memory seem to share shelf space in the brain. Several times I have felt the need to ask total strangers, "What *is* that perfume you're wearing?" Every time it has turned out to be Shalimar by Guerlain. I wish I could grow something even remotely as incredible; the scent immobilizes me.

FACING PAGE *We are all slaves to fragrance, and there is a scent for everyone. Thankfully, lavender has lost its "granny" stigma and is now welcome in even the hippest gardens. Try some in ice cream or crème brûlée!*

THE JEWEL BOX GARDEN

ANOTHER FEATURE TO LOOK OUT FOR IS UNUSUAL LEAF TEXTURE. Not just smooth or fuzzy, but unique qualities like accordion pleating or the way water reacts to the leaf surface. I grow the tropical, palm-like grass *Setaria palmifolia* for its pleated blades, which are very sculptural in themselves. The hardy *Veratrums* also have fabulous folded leaves that clasp the stem; they bring the fashions of Japanese designer Issey Miyake to mind.

I am still amazed when watching water droplets bead up and bounce off the leaves of the elephant's ear plant (*Colocasia*). The black-leaved form, *Colocasia esculenta* 'Black Magic', is especially worth owning. By some kind of evolutionary magic, water becomes mercury-like and rolls off these plants, leaving absolutely no trace of wetness. It's a botanical parlor trick and nature's own Scotchgard!

Sometimes it is necessary to bruise or crush a plant to (hopefully) enjoy its added dimension. The various types of lavender (*Lavendula* species) have never been as popular as they are today. Only a few years ago they were regarded as "granny plants," but no more. Inhaling fresh or dried lavender is immediately beneficial and affects everyone. It also makes fantastic flavoring in plain ice cream! Many people like the peanut-butter scent of bruised *Melianthus major* foliage. I can't stand this scent, but love the saw-toothed, nearly blue foliage of this tender South African native. Another plant I grow but avoid bruising is the bulbous *Nectaroscordum siculum*. This *Allium* relative gets to stay in my garden because of the rigid stems of sophisticated, molasses-striped, beige bells it produces in springtime. If I accidentally break or bruise a bud or leaf when digging nearby, I soon regret it as the gassy odor makes me gag.

FACING PAGE *Watch as leaves change color. This show is free and is often taken for granted. Plants cope with sun just as people do, by adjusting their skin. This aloe is putting on a fine show in midsummer. During periods of less sun, its leaves turn significantly greener.*

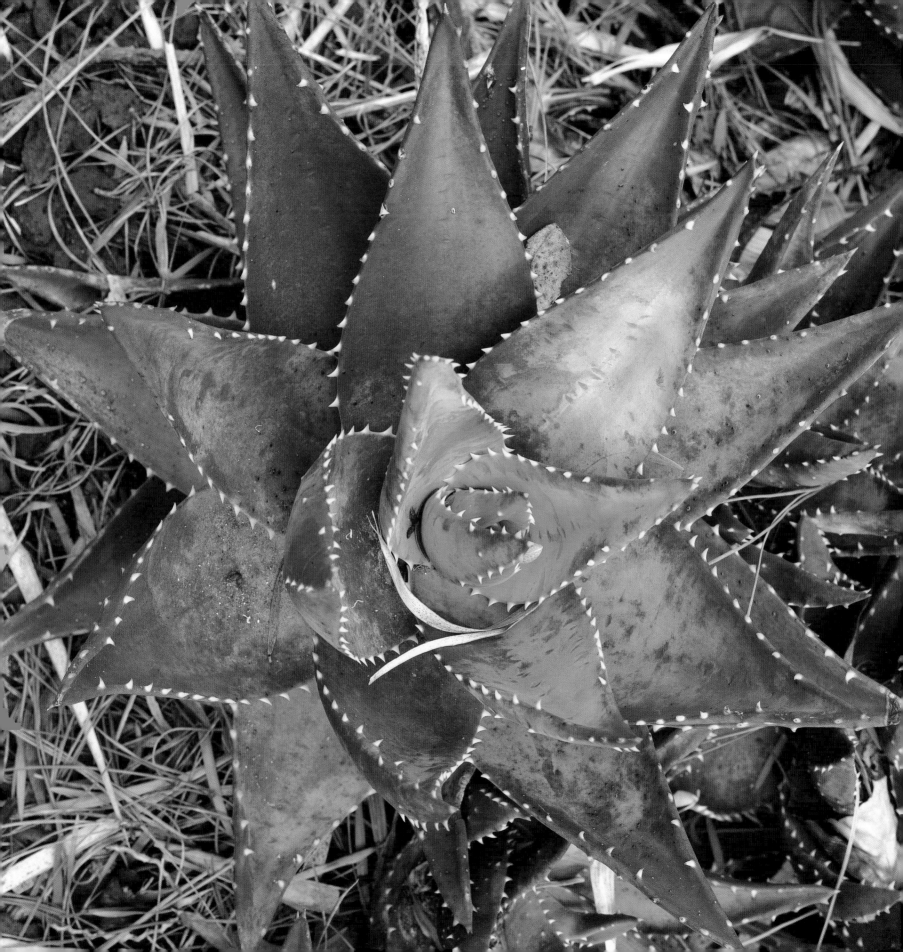

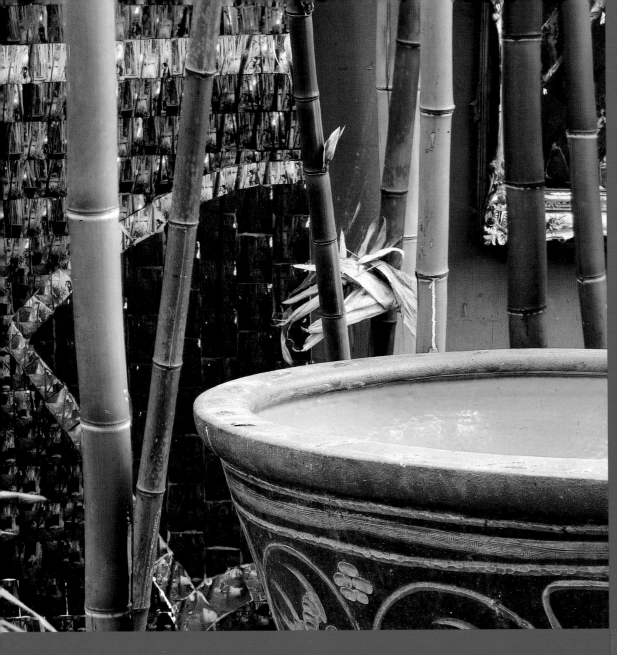

RIGHT *In the* TORONTO *garden of* NANCY AND TOM LAURIE, *a spectacular series of jets forms a stunning backdrop to a formal urn focal point. Such "water tricks" were popular centuries ago in aristocratic European gardens and were often turned on just as guests passed by. I would love to operate one of these by remote control, especially if it shot sideways!*

BELOW *Beautifully tiled in slate mosaic, a small wall niche water feature by my front door holds a few glass fishing floats. Serving no purpose other than visual delight, they move about in an imaginary game of snooker.* **Fuchsia magellanica** *'Molinae' dangles above.*

ABOVE *Unnaturally exciting color is created by kooky background screens in this magic moment by California's* CEVAN FORRISTT. *The brilliant green bamboo stalks are matched in clarity of color by the interior glaze of an intentionally empty Asian pottery bowl. The three elements contribute equally in a perfectly edited vision.*

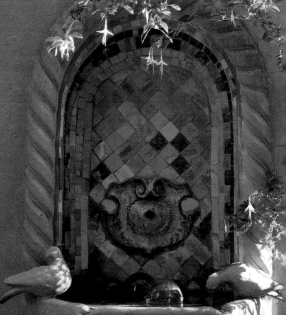

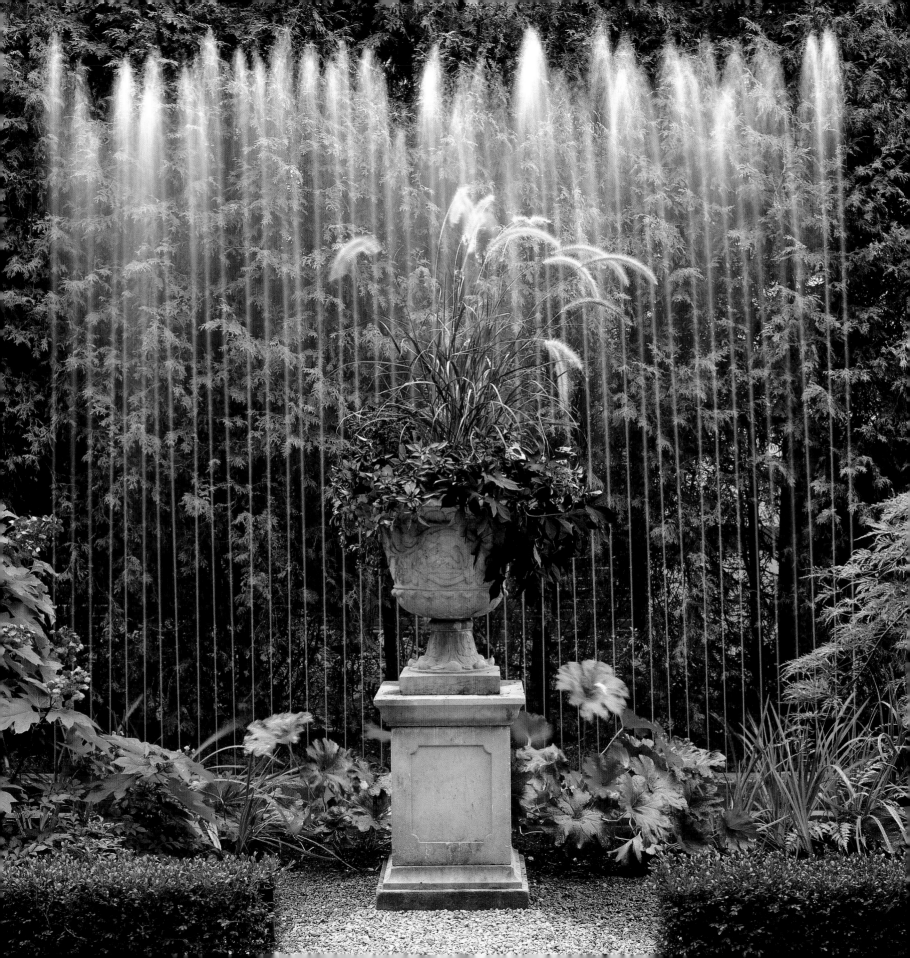

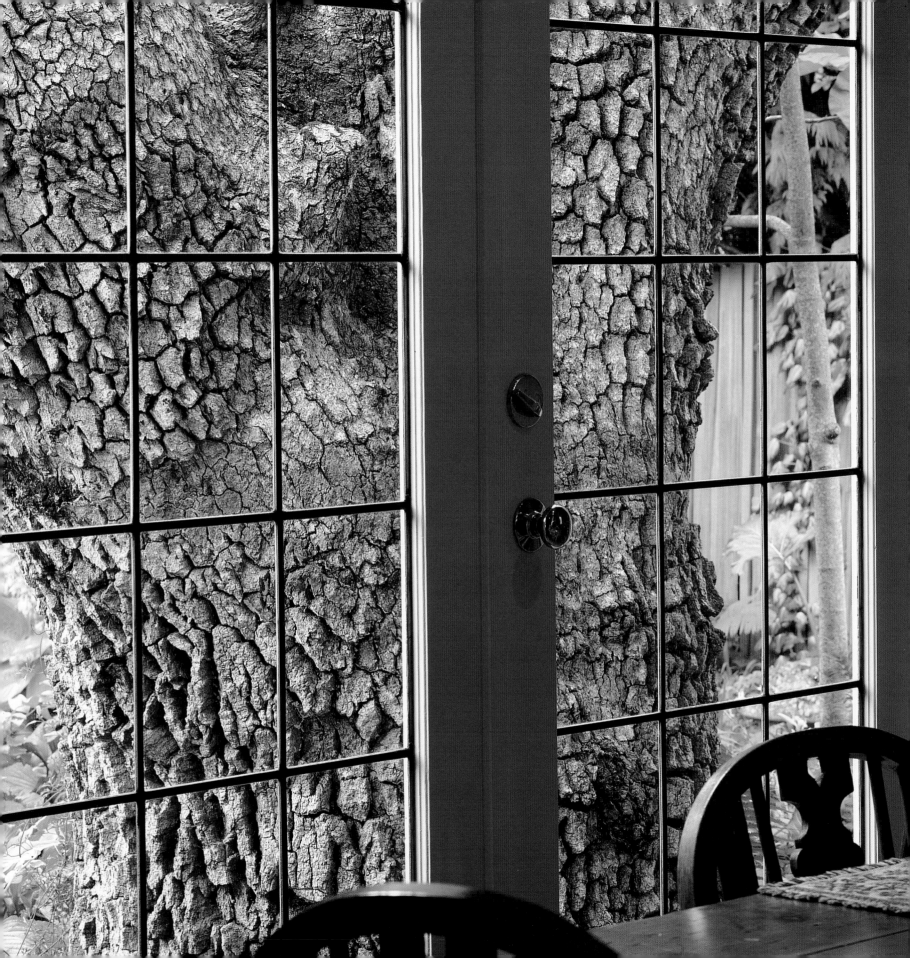

Y OU MAY FIND CERTAIN PLANTS ATTRACT WELCOME VISITORS. Hummingbirds are attracted to tubular-shaped flowers, especially reddish ones. They love **Phygelius**, the Cape fuchsia, and will visit nectar-rich **Cannas**. Many people try to attract butterflies by planting a "butterfly garden," which sounds delightful. In reality, these seeds-in-a-can mixtures result in a weed patch of dull "wildflowers" that only lasts one season. I think butterflies hate people and are better left on their own.

Sound, on a small scale, is very personal. Most plants remain silent their entire lives, though large trees get to rustle in the wind, especially in autumn. We can add limited amounts of sound to our gardens, but it's risky. Wind chimes are dreadful intrusions into neighborhoods: just because you like them doesn't mean the people next door do. I think they are as bannable as leaf blowers.

Water features can bring a pleasantness to a garden, providing a variety of benefits. Large jets cool the air, mask street noise and are always attractive. The simpler, the better. A plain, skyward jet of water should emerge from the simplest possible basin. Homeowners can scale down to suit their space. Even a balcony can feature a small fountain of some type. Pleasant sounds help us escape and *make* us relax, no stereo required. Realizing that creating an outdoor space involves more than just plants is what brings it all together. Don't just fill your needs, include your *desires*.

"My master is the tree outside my window"

ANTONIO GAUDÍ

FACING PAGE *A massive Garry oak,* **Quercus garryana,** *waits outside* TERRY LE BLANC'S VICTORIA, B.C., *kitchen doors. The beauty of its bark and sheer presence is humbling. Our obsession with foliage and flowers seems so shallow when you see a magnificent plant like this.*

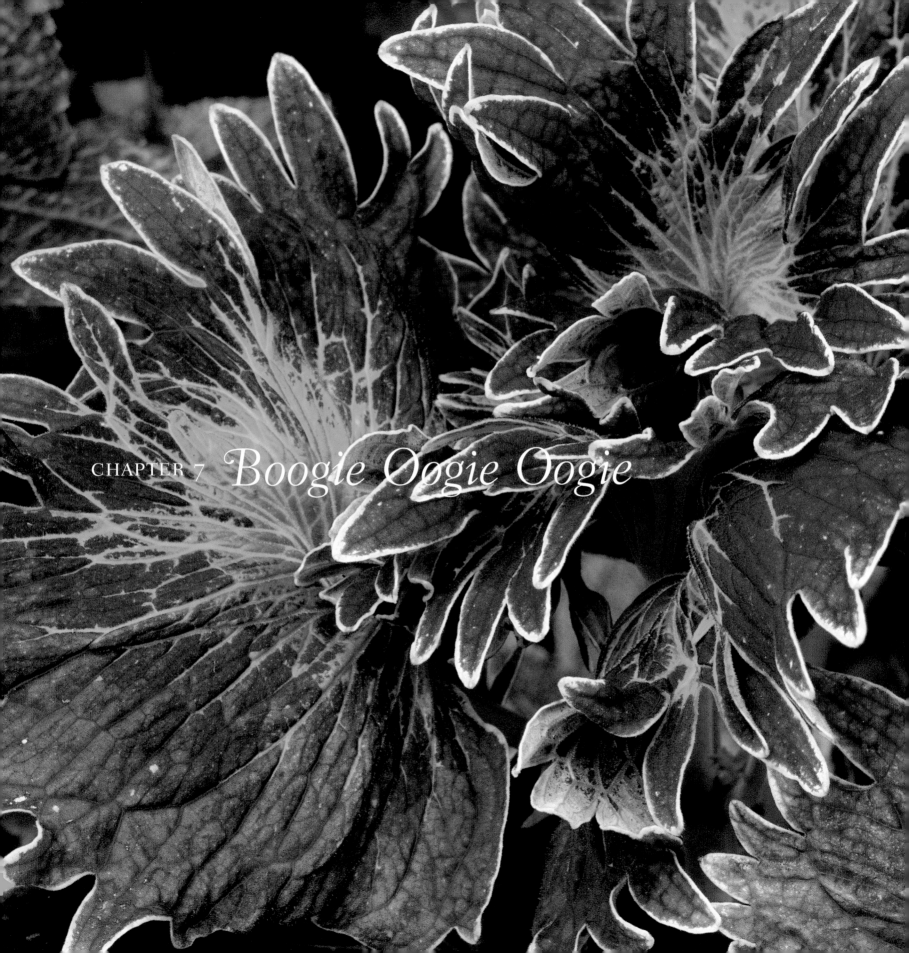

CHAPTER 7　*Boogie Oogie Oogie*

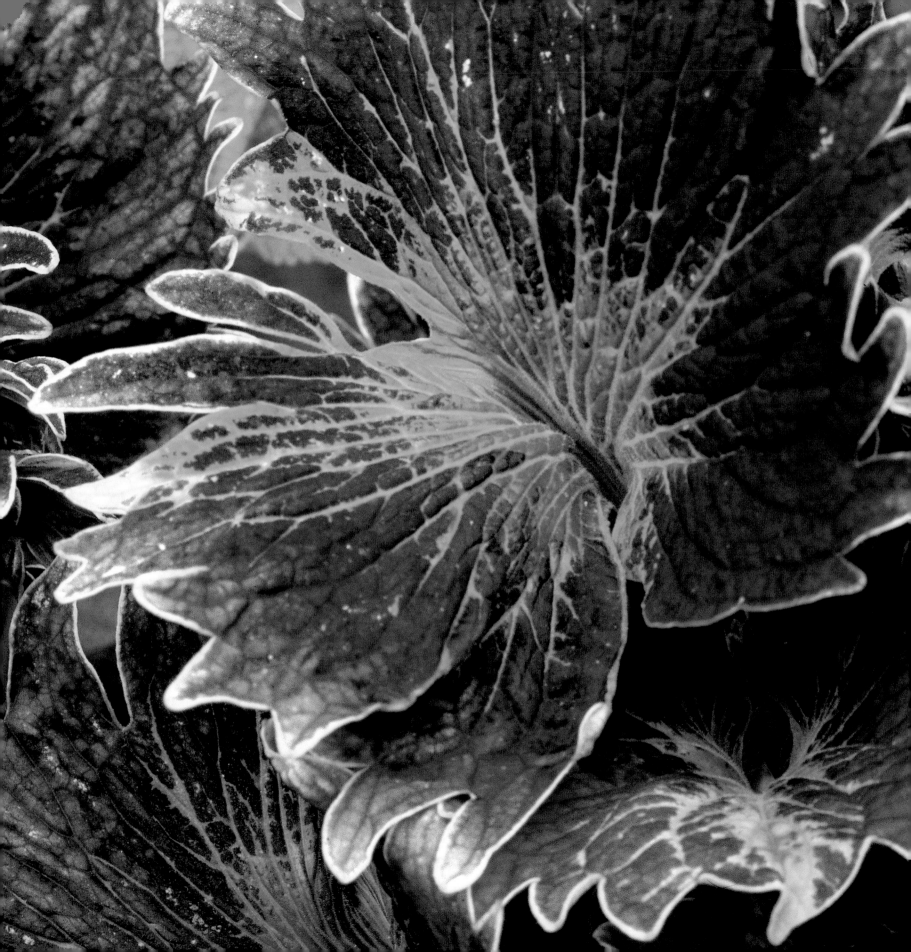

CERTAIN COMBINATIONS ARE HARD TO FORGET. I AM STILL reeling from seeing Kristy McNichol and former TV talk show host Mike Douglas singing "Get Down, Boogie Oogie Oogie" together. They were wearing matching red overalls and descending a blinking, backlit Plexiglas staircase. Twenty-five years later, the damage is still unhealed in my brain. Gardeners have to be careful, too. What was once considered trendy and bold might actually be really ugly.

I feel partially responsible for the recent "zonal denial" craze. Many gardeners found a new kind of liberation by planting just about anything, anywhere. The results were rarely good. Mixing "exotics" with each other is fairly safe, but adding a random bit of "tropicalissimo" into average planting only looks like botanical vandalism. Foliar graffiti.

Creating a *cohesive* plant picture should be your goal. Imagine you are casting a play and each plant is a possible cast member. Will everyone get along? You will need to eliminate plant personality clashes. Dry-growing plants do fine together. Shade lovers unite, and sun-worshippers are happy en masse. Then, looking deeper into each group, you can start to really fine-tune the picture. Noticing foliage's own merit has to come first; flowers, if any, are a bonus. Being able to combine foliage is what earns you respect from other gardeners. This is gardening's highest level of achievement.

PREVIOUS PAGE *Coleus 'Tilt a Whirl' reignited my love affair with this genus of plant playthings. Its exciting leaf shape suggests movement as well as exhibiting gorgeous colors. Multihued leaves offer greater possibilities for playing around when choosing what to plant next to what.*

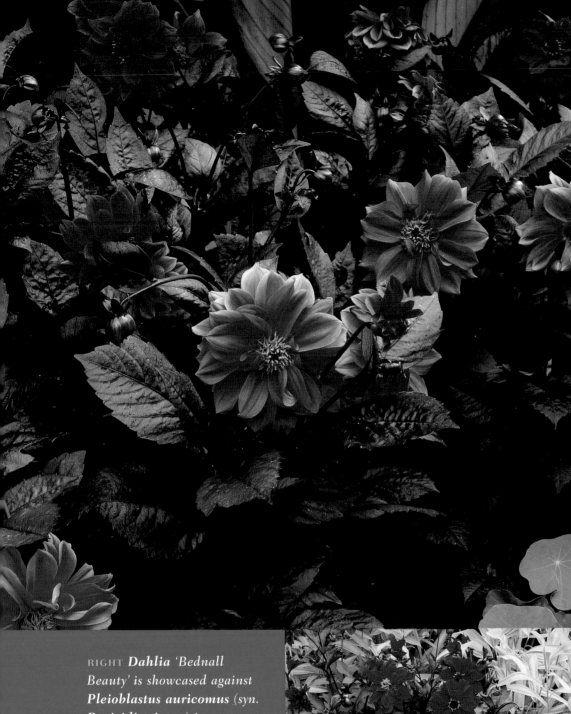

LEFT ***Dahlia*** *'Ellen Houston' is a Canadian-bred variety beloved worldwide. Coppery-black foliage is the perfect foil to its burnt-orange flowers. Limited-space gardeners need to make use of "double value" plants like this one whenever possible: great foliage and great flowers are not common.*

BELOW *Instead of a clash,* STEVE ANTONOW *has achieved a symphony effect with the same* **Pleioblastus auricomus** *bamboo. The acid-green color is amplified by* **Hosta** *'Gold Standard' and a clump of* **Hakonechloa macra** *'Aureola' grass. Even the dreaded, invasive Bishop's Weed (**Aegopodium podagraria** 'Variegatum') looks good, this time!*

RIGHT ***Dahlia*** *'Bednall Beauty' is showcased against* **Pleioblastus auricomus** *(syn.* **P. viridistriatus***) in* STEVE ANTONOW'S SEATTLE *garden. His expert contrast of two very striking foliages allows for better appreciation of each. A touch of silvery* **Plectranthus argentatus** *in the foreground acts as a neutralizer in this pleasant clash.*

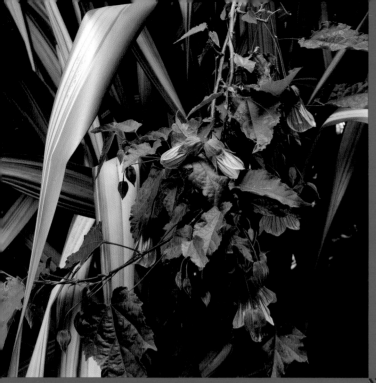

A complete contrast in every respect, the dazzle of **Gingko biloba**'s *autumn farewell is sliced by blades of dark canna foliage in* NANCY HECKLER's *garden near* SEATTLE. *It is an amazing but fleeting lesson in color combination from Mother Nature herself.*

ABOVE *The shuttlecock-like flowers of an* **Abutilon** *pick out the squash-yellow shades in an otherwise peachy* **Phormium** *in* MARCIA DONAHUE's *garden in* BERKELEY, CALIFORNIA.

RIGHT *I like to use coleus to reinforce more subtle neighbors in my own plantings. The peachy stripes of* **Phormium** *'Sundowner' absorb some red from* **Coleus** *'Coral Glo' and look even better.*

92

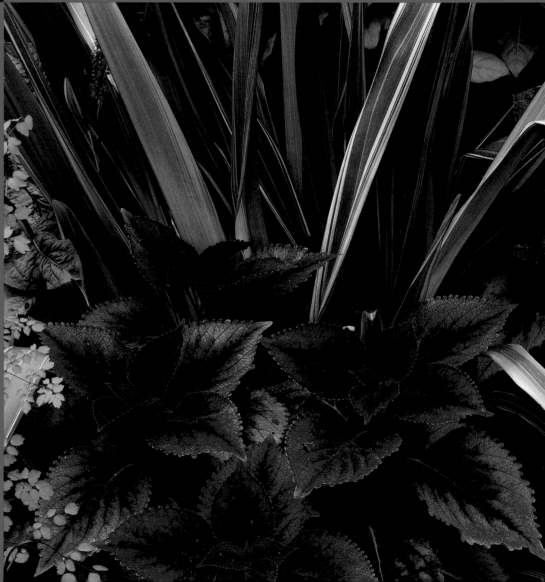

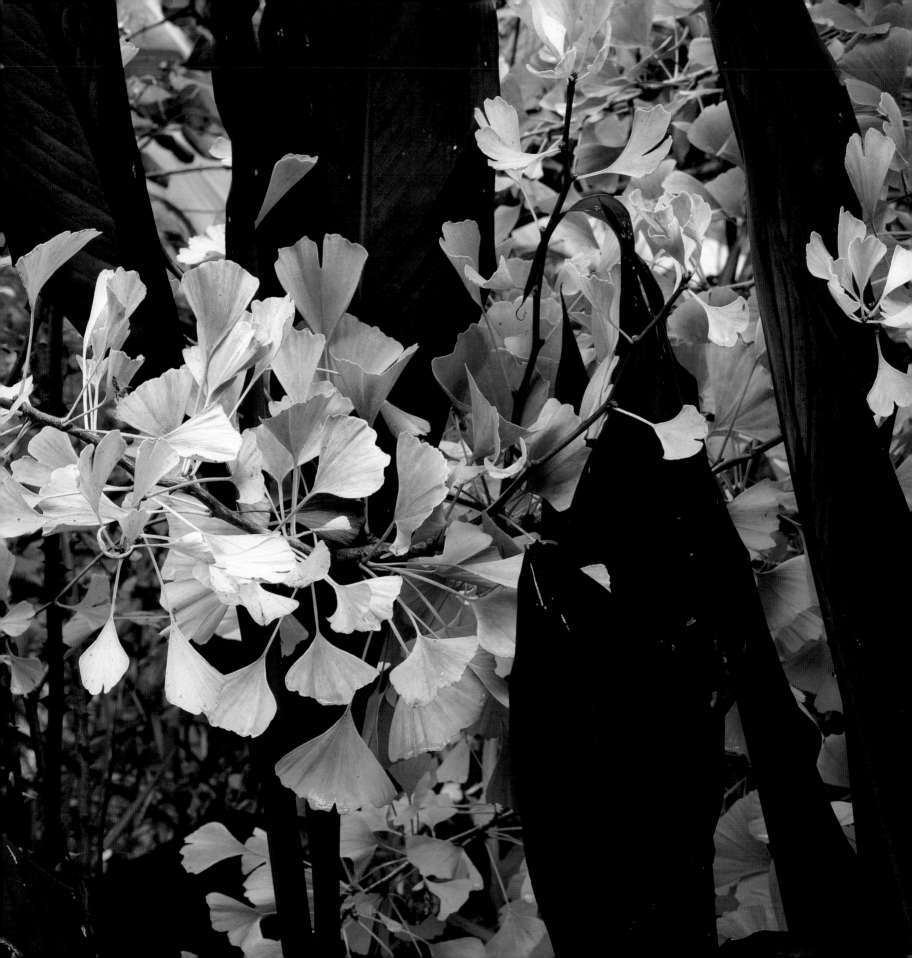

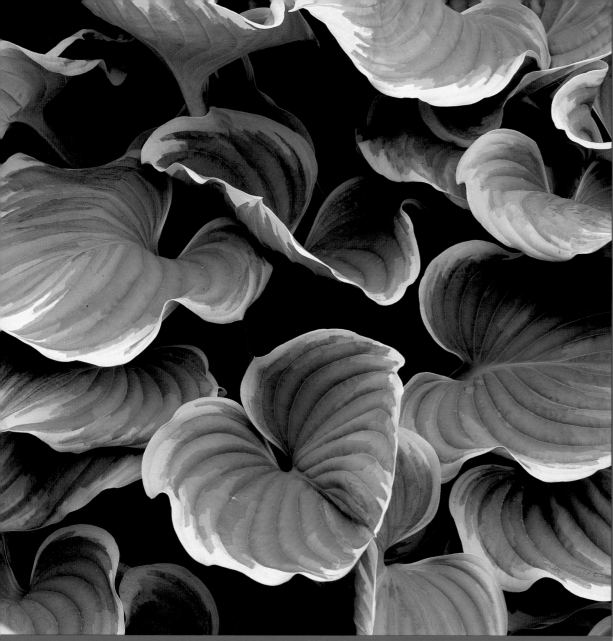

RIGHT **Corydalis flexuosa** 'Purple Leaf' brings a unique hue of flower and foliage to shady garden areas. I like it the best of all the **Corydalis**, as it is vigorous but not invasive. Smoky purple is a color seldom found in flowers. Just a bit mysterious, it combines beautifully with the acid-green creeping foliage of **Lysimachia nummularia** 'Aurea' and the green-flowered primrose 'Francisca' in my own garden.

BELOW 'Bright Lights' is a seed strain of Swiss chard that makes an unforgettable winter ornamental in the Pacific Northwest. Its neon leafstalks thrive in and illuminate the weeks of drizzly rain. Gardeners elsewhere should grow it as a tropical imposter until really hot weather makes it go to seed.

ABOVE **Hosta** 'Sagae' is a big beauty. In moist soil and light shade it forms an imposing and almost slug-proof clump worth every inch of the space it needs! I remove its occasional flower stalks as they only detract from the vision of perfect foliage.

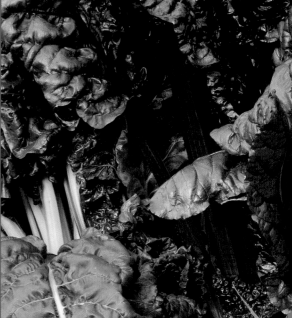

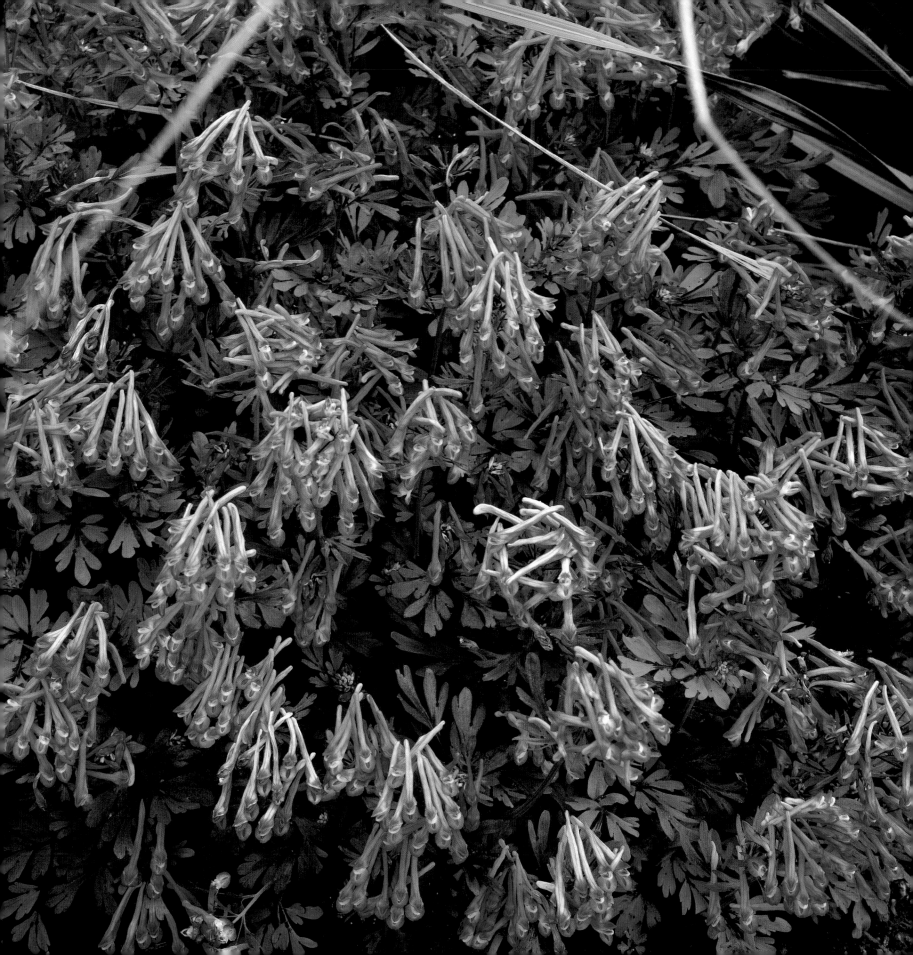

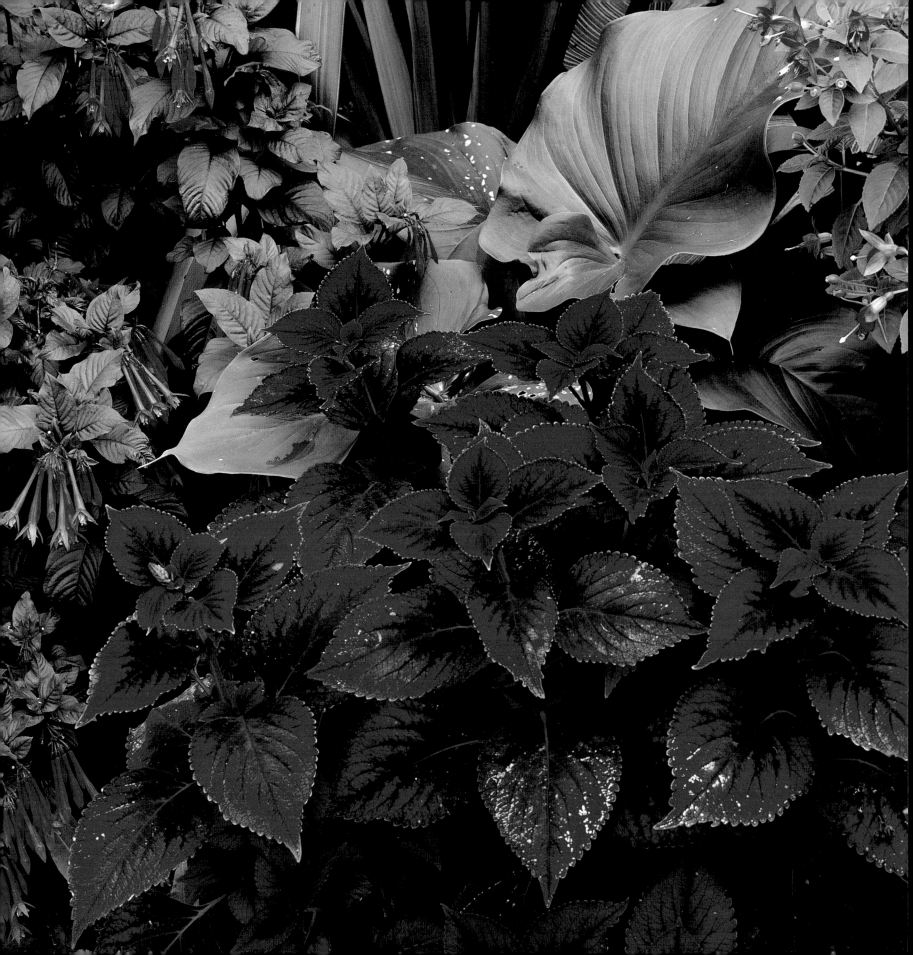

RELYING ON FOLIAGE WOULD BE NO FUN IF ALL WE HAD TO WORK with was the color green. I would only last twenty seconds. We can literally thank God for the multitude of silvers, golds, biscuit browns, purples, reds, celadon greens and mesmerizing variegations he gave us to play with.

Foliage effects last much longer than flowers and are always more subtle. Leaves emerge one shade, expand to another and finally die, often in a spectacular farewell. Often (as with hostas), any blossoms are detrimental. Exceptions are deliberately placed beauties (such as lilies) that appear, do their thing, then go away.

Successful plant pictures will either happen instantly or take *way too long*. Sometimes the "missing link" shows up months later and what was okay becomes *exceptional*. This happens to me every year! Either I can't find a certain shade of **Diascia** or someone has introduced an amazing new **Coleus.** I will attack and redo at any time if something more exciting catches my eye. The missing link!

FACING PAGE *What a difference a plant makes!* **Coleus** *'Coral Glo' steals the scene every time.* **Fuchsia** *'Gartenmeister Bohnstedt' and* **F.** *'Baby Chang' are deliberate color choice "echoes" in my shady border. Keeping the soil very moist produces lush growth.*

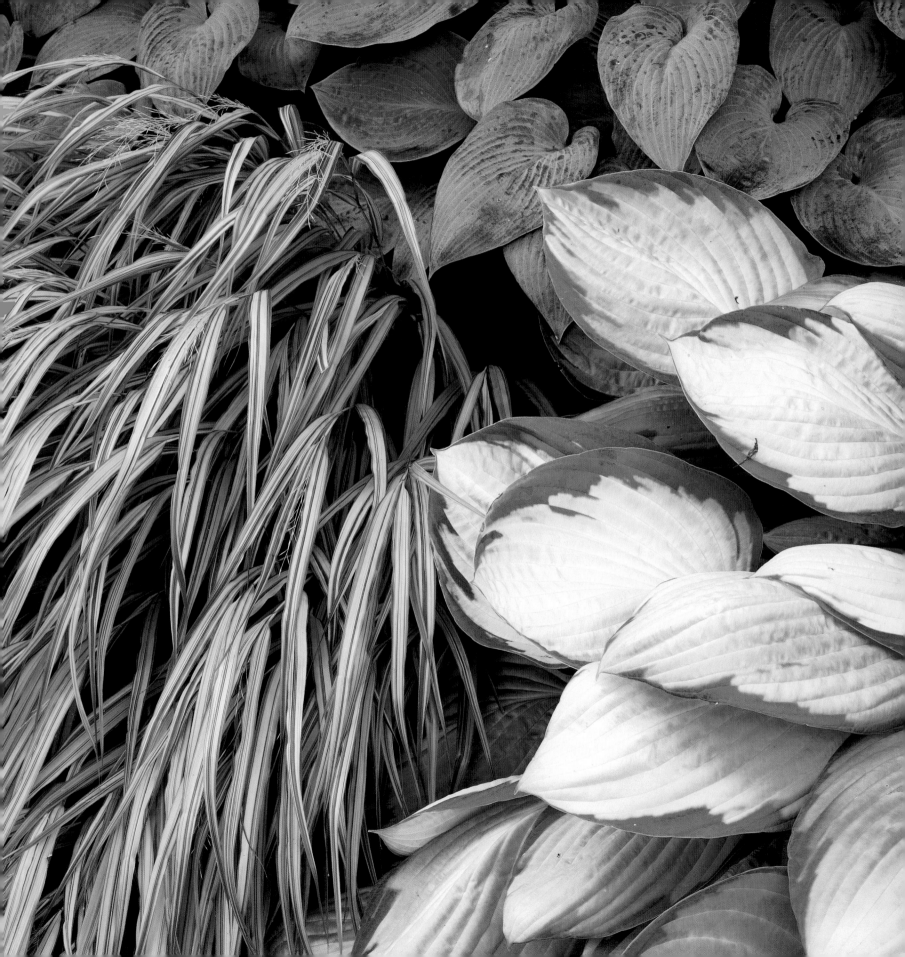

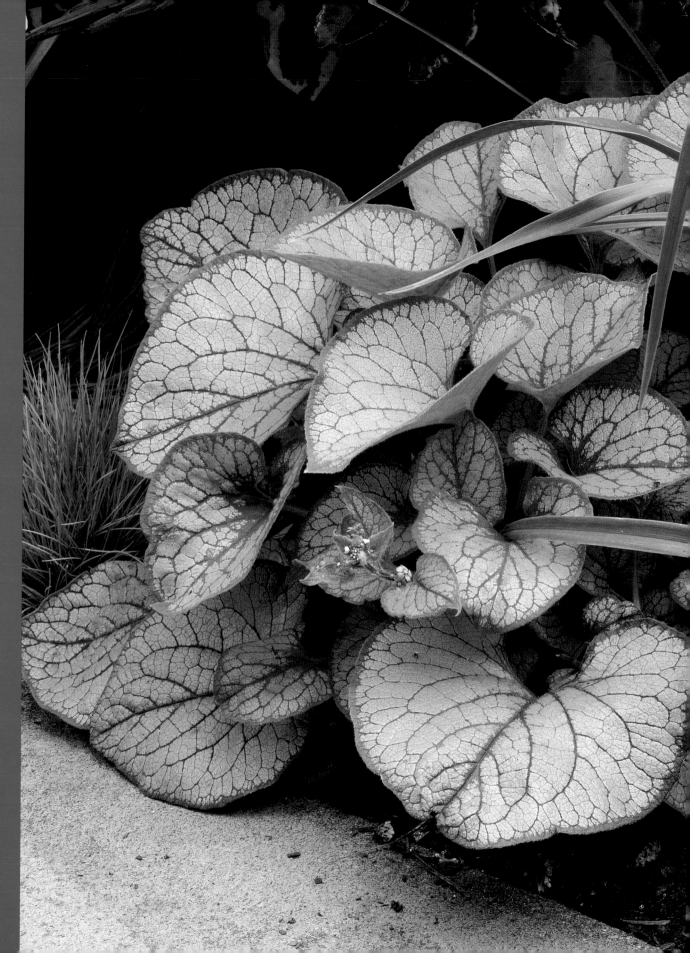

LEFT *A lesson in foliage shapes and color combination in* STEVE ANTONOW's *garden. Golden fingers of* **Hakonechloa macra** *'Aureola' match* **Hosta** *'Gold Standard' in color but not in shape, texture or habit. The neutral blue foliage of* **Hosta** *'Halcyon' helps tone down the wattage.*

RIGHT **Brunnera** *'Jack Frost' is one of the best hardy new perennials. Its silvery foliage looks tropical, but isn't. Summertime sprays of no-big-deal blue flowers are best removed, to maintain a bold effect. Play up the silvery blue by choosing plants such as* **Festuca** *'Golden Toupee' for neighbors.*

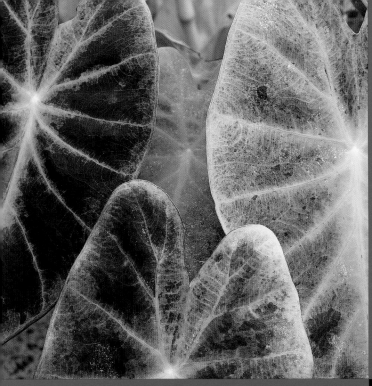

Kalanchoe thyrsiflora
is a scene-stealer. Its cartoon-
like paddles redden in the sun
and are somehow amusing.
Deliberately underplanted
with less interesting **Sedum**
and **Echeveria**, it is displayed
to maximum advantage in a
shallow clay pot.

ABOVE **Colocasia antiquorum**
'Illustris' is an exotic but easy-
to-grow taro with black-suffused
leaves. It loves summer heat
and shallow water. Grow it in
a shiny, glazed black container
to amplify its unique feature.

RIGHT **Pelargoniums** (sold,
incorrectly, as geraniums) can
have incredible foliage. Complex
ring patterns can be cleverly
"separated" using matching but
solid-colored neighboring plants.

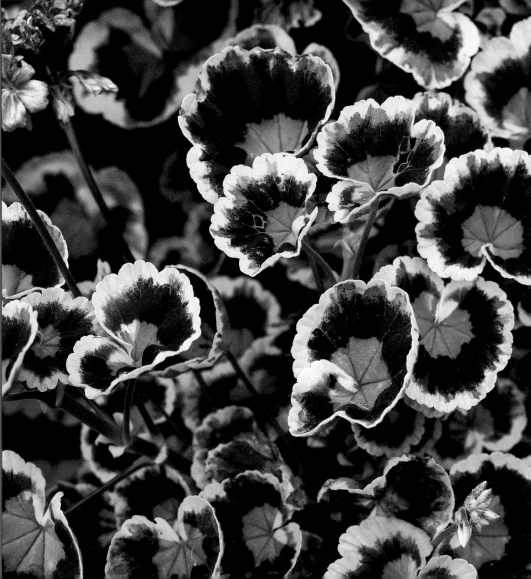

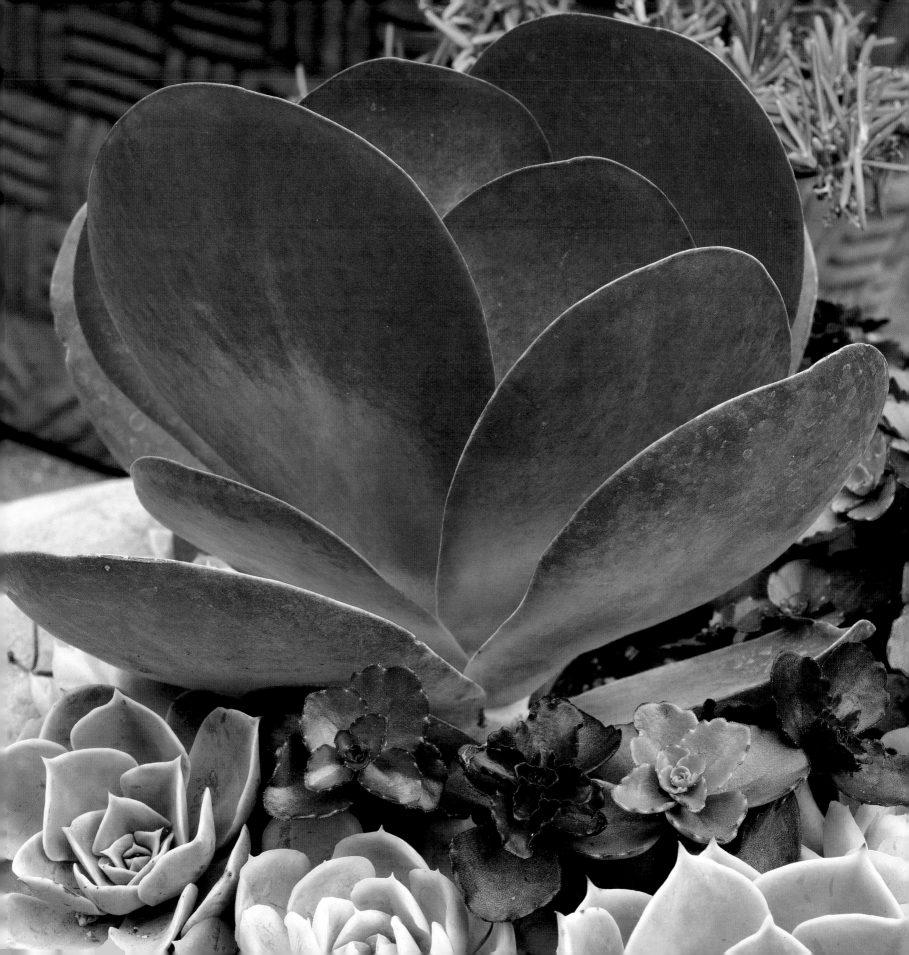

Train yourself to look closely, and notice that all foliage contains patterns. Many are spectacular, so you have to watch what you mix together. Just like getting dressed, there are rules even I don't break. Don't mix checks and spots. Variegation is best in smallish doses. There is a big difference between burberry and the Bay City Rollers!

Spectacular, eye-popping color can really only "pop" if you allow it to. Determine which plant is destined to be "Number One" and build your hit parade around it. Variegated plants hate playing second fiddle. Only a characteristic such as near-black foliage has more power than they do.

Some gardeners will never learn the art of plant assemblage. Try how they might, they are oblivious to what is missing. Things appear healthy and happy, *but dull*. These are the people who keep nurseries in business, their trunks filled with impulse purchases and flats of annuals. As I drive by their predictable efforts, I often wonder, "Is life easier?"

FACING PAGE *Subtlety has its place. Irish moss (**Sagina sublata** 'Aurea') forms an undulating ground cover, but dislikes foot traffic. Not a true moss, it is reminiscent of woodland glades and perfect for a Zen moment in the Jewel Box Garden.*

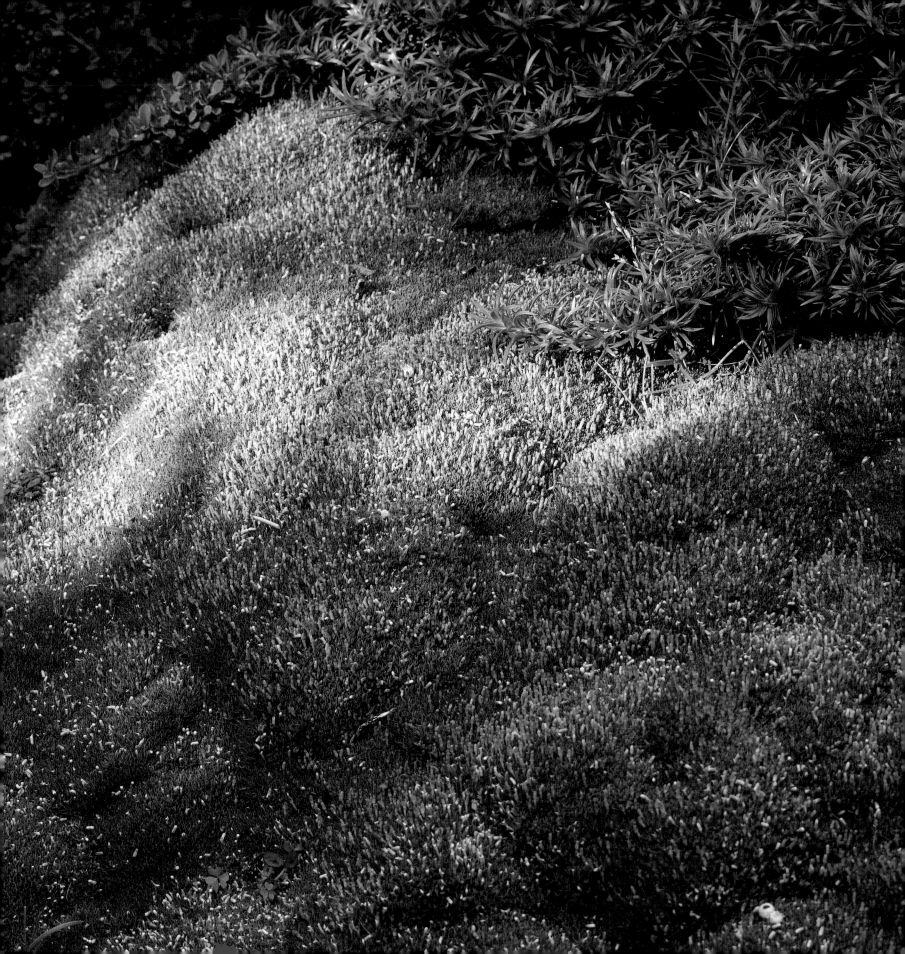

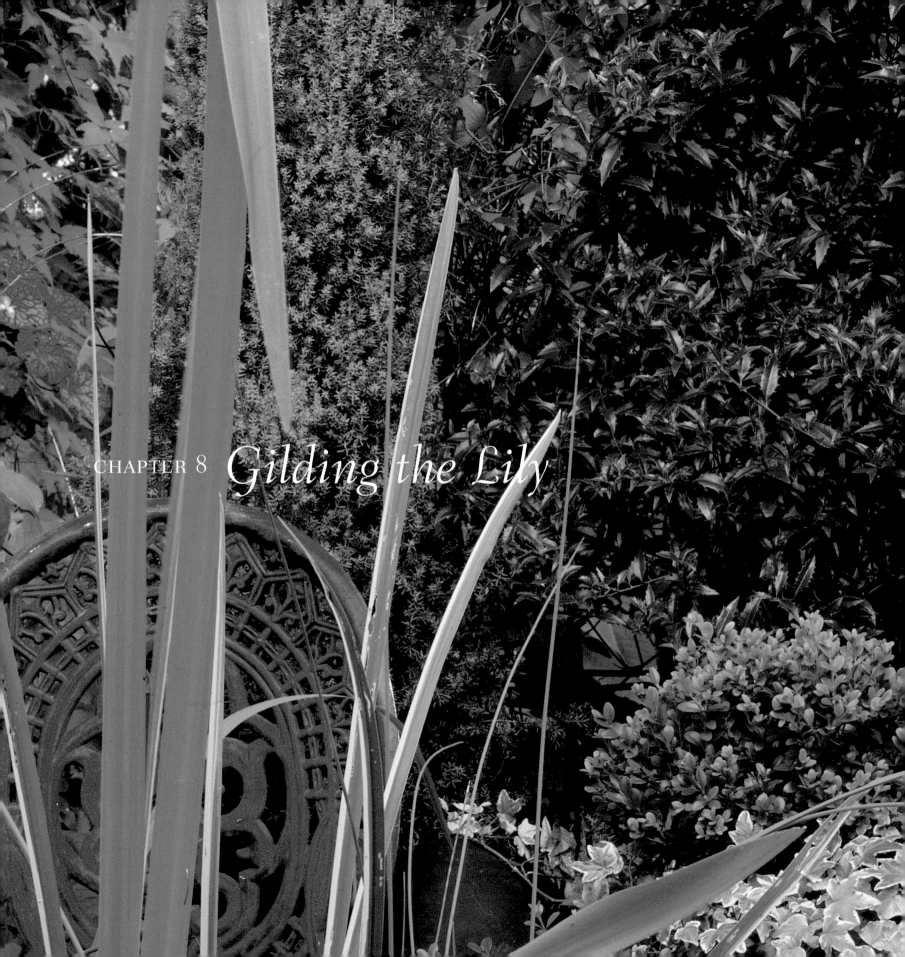

CHAPTER 8 *Gilding the Lily*

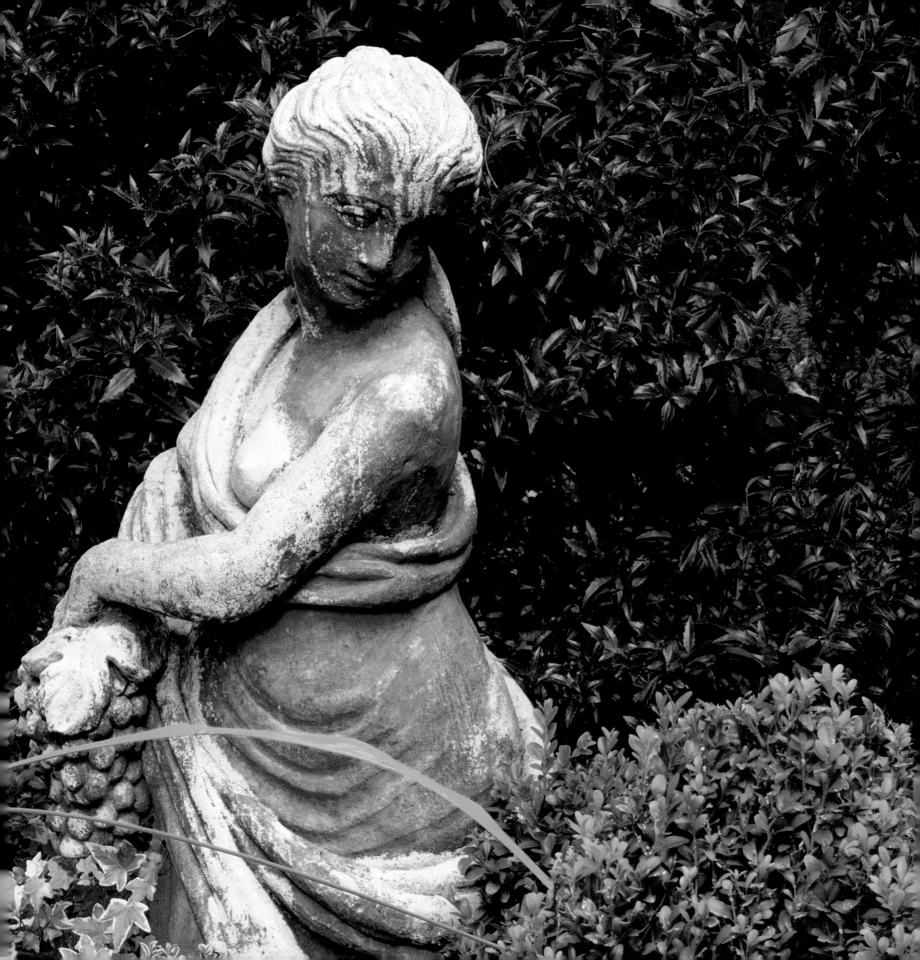

INTRODUCING NONLIVING ELEMENTS INTO YOUR OUTDOOR SPACE is what makes it memorable. Sometimes they can also make it laughable, so you have to be careful. There is an entire industry devoted to tomorrow's landfill: garden décor.

Although I enjoy placing beautiful objects in strategic spots in my garden, I have never deliberately gone out and bought anything to fill that role. It just seems to happen. Adding nonliving elements to the garden is the icing on the cake: it should be done last. Wait until plants have grown in and let them suggest where you have a void. This way, you avoid the "garden makeover" look, where everything is instant and phony looking. Your involvement with any item of garden decoration has to be personal.

I am reluctant to use the phrase "focal point," as it has lost its meaning. Too many homeowners have gone out shopping for one. How about a wishing well or a concrete seal pup with a ball on its nose? Who wants only one?

Any time your eye stops and focuses, you've got a *focus point*, like it or not. It might be a dead rat, or a mildewed rosebush could be stealing the scene in its own hateful way. What is lacking in many otherwise successful planted areas is what I refer to as an "item." This is all-encompassing and neutral enough to mean almost anything except a plant. An "item" is something covetous and slightly valuable. It is code. It means something good.

PREVIOUS PAGE *The refined quietness of green-on-green creates an appropriate setting for a classical statue in* MARK HENRY's *garden. The sculptural shapes of nearby plants are kept simple, to keep our attention focused on the statue.*

MARK HENRY's *dreams of Venice, Italy, flutter in his* SNOHOMISH, WASHINGTON, *garden. Well-tended clusters of pots help marry the house to the garden, and colors are expertly extracted from the flag above.*

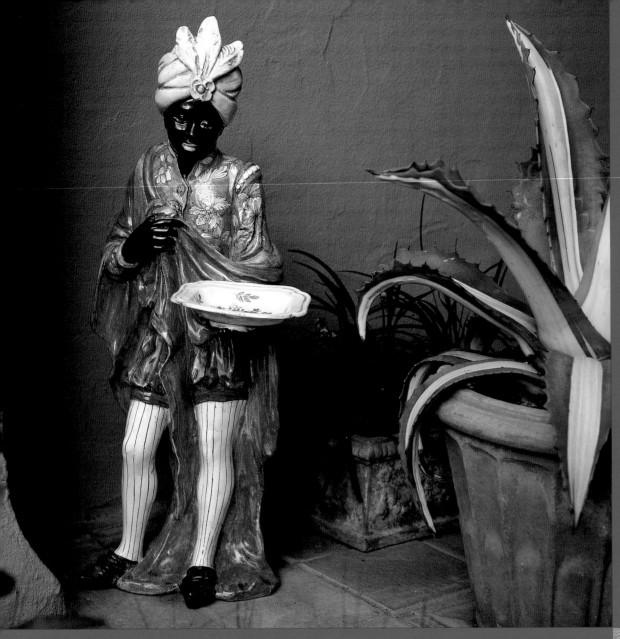

RIGHT A very beautiful Italian terra cotta figure holds a basket of string of pearls (**Senecio rowleyanus**) on her head at SOUTHLANDS NURSERY in VANCOUVER, B.C. Happy in little soil and a perfect match in feeling, this plant is what sold the statue.

BELOW This lead mask from England looks down and over my hot tub, as a reminder not to stay in too long!

ABOVE A glazed figure of a blackamoor from Florence, Italy, waits by my front door. **Agave americana** 'Mediopicta' is beautiful enough to compete, but just barely. Both come inside for the winter.

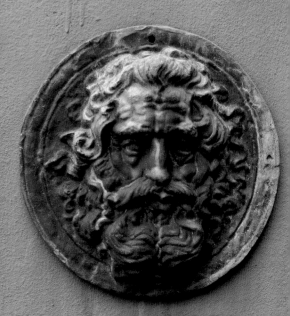

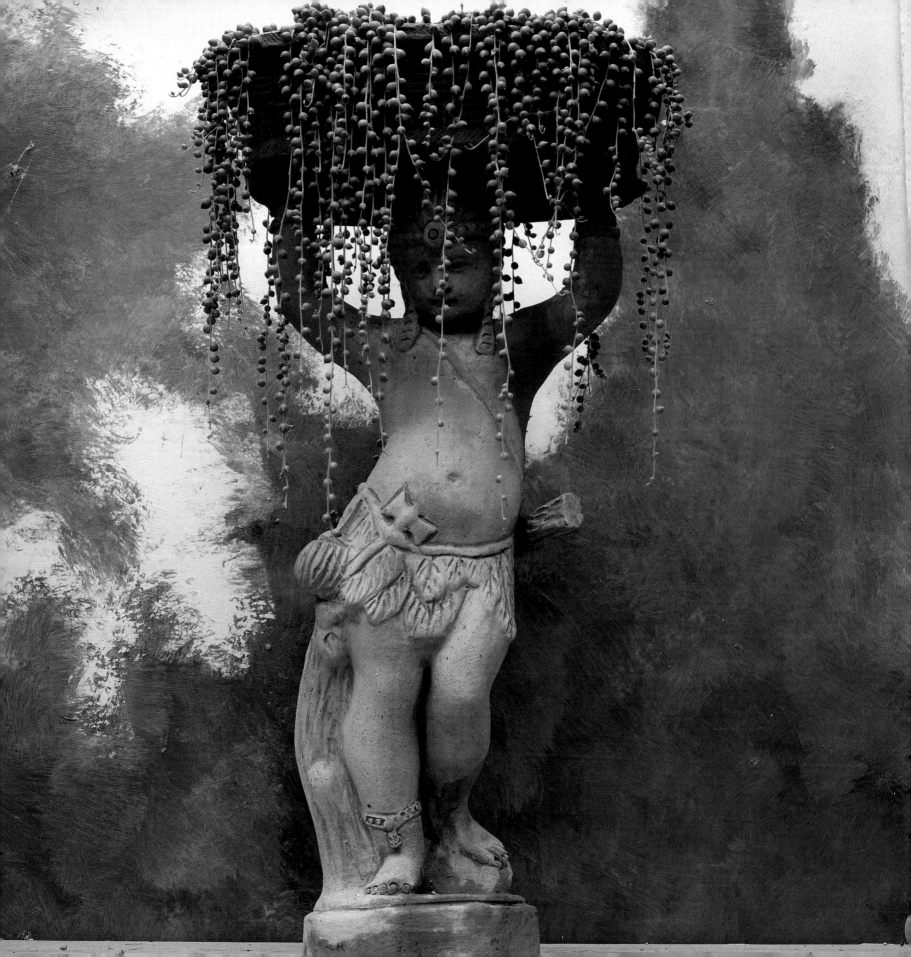

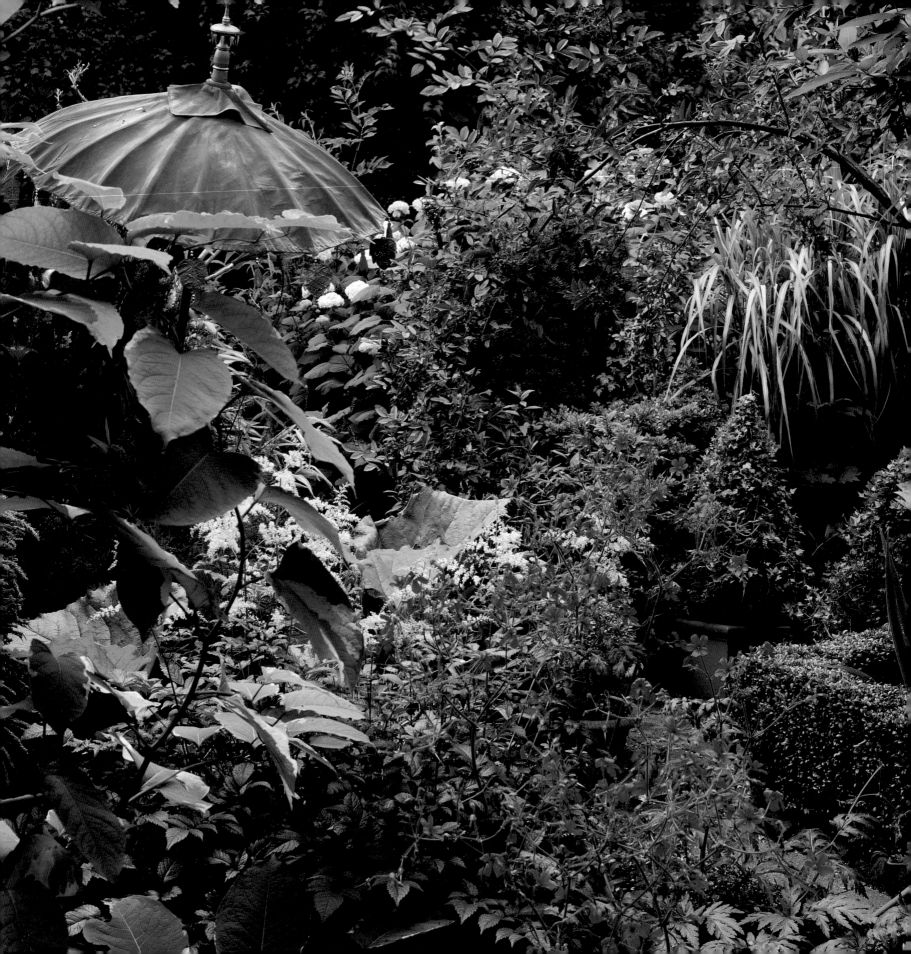

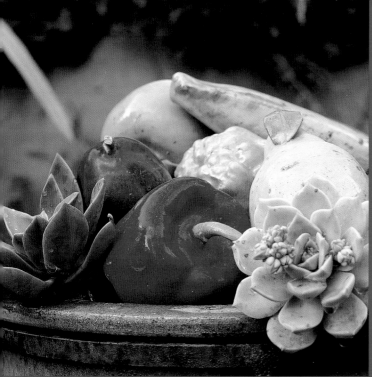

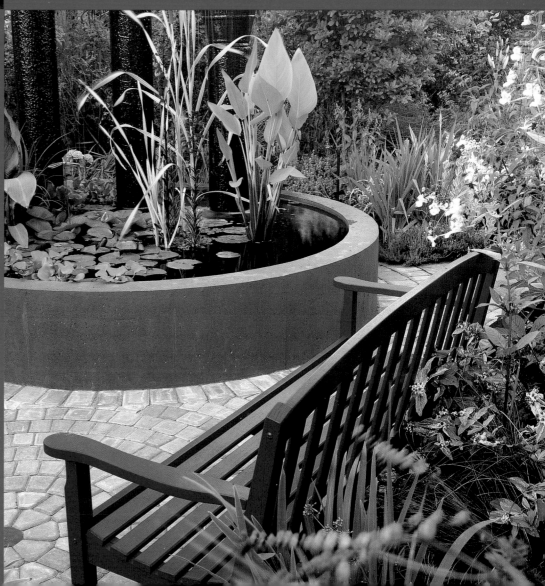

BELOW *Purple paint power!* DANIEL SPARLER *and* JEFF SCHOUTEN'S *use of bold color goes beyond plants in their* SEATTLE, WASHINGTON *garden. Massive doses of in-your-face paint turn what was already eye candy into mind candy!*

ABOVE *A bowl of ceramic fruit in the* RAICHE/McCRORY GARDEN *is made even more interesting by tucking in a few undemanding* **Echeveria**. *What is real and what is not is a mind game that should exclude anything plastic.*

LEFT *A bright purple umbrella from Bali zaps up the scene in another part of* MARK HENRY'S *garden. The magenta blossoms of* **Geranium maderense** *and the gunmetal mauve foliage of* **Rosa glauca** *both seem to draw bonus color from this perky prop.*

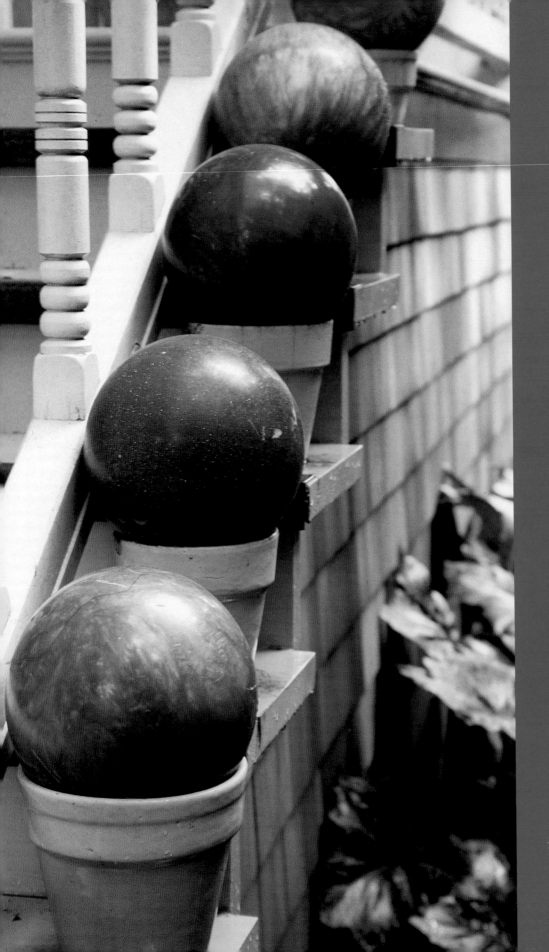

LEFT *Potted bowling balls are hard to kill.* MARCIA DONAHUE *welcomes visitors to her* BERKELEY, CALIFORNIA, *home with a row she grew from seed.*

BELOW **Sempervivums** *surround weird little Tiki gods in* BOB CLARK *and* RAOUL ZUMBA'S GARDEN. *A sense of humour makes visiting a garden much more fun.*

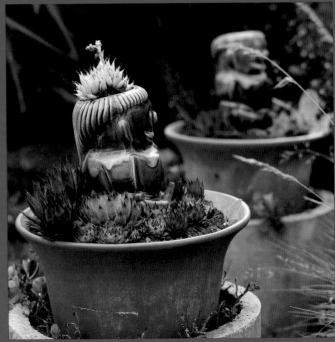

TARTING UP THE GARDEN WITH TOO MANY YUM-YUMS IS A PITFALL not just reserved for the rich. Although I have winced at more plastic in gardens than anything else, bronze has recently become mentally toxic to me. How can I delete visions of cast-bronze children chasing a frog, or Grandma welded to a park bench?

Mass-produced items also lack appeal. Concrete *anything,* unless dripping with plants, is too ordinary. There is something less desirable about products when you know a factory is shipping them everywhere. It keeps them out of my garden: I would rather buy something out of town and have it shipped home, to remind me of my holiday. Garden ornaments, "items," have to be, in some way, works of art. They don't have to be museum quality, but they have to involve emotional *thought*. It should be *you* floating glass fishing floats in a pool of water, deliberately staging something beautiful. Make your own birdbath instead of buying one.

Placing your treasures should be a gut reaction. Obvious homes for "items" are on walls, steps and nestled amongst plants. My rule is that I should only be able to see one non-plant treasure per glance. Keep things apart, so you will appreciate their beauty and the contribution they make to your personal oasis. The less space you have, the more you have to really treasure your garden accessories. Only use the meaningful.

We all admire antique garden statuary in European gardens. It is *appropriate to time and place*. Remember that, and apply it to your own space. Bowling balls are appropriate in Marcia Donahue's garden/gallery in Berkeley, California, because *she did it first*. It's a wacky place, and if your garden isn't, no bowling balls for you!

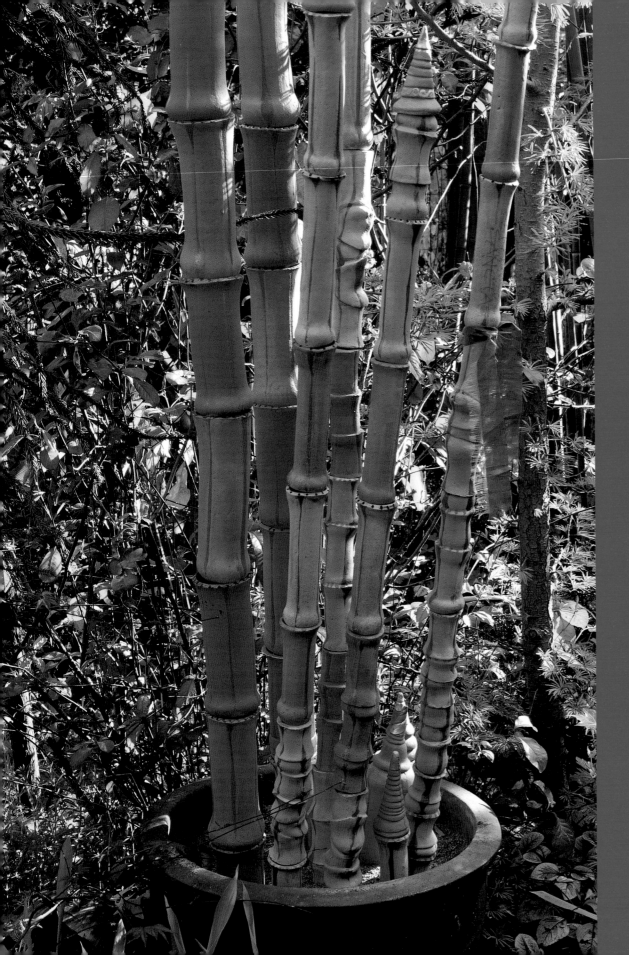

LEFT *Although there are many beautiful bamboos in nature, none are quite as colorful as Marcia's own ceramic creations. This potted fantasy is too good to be true; part plant, part sculpture and no care required.*

RIGHT *I realized my home's blank stucco walls were potential canvases, waiting for dabs of ornament. This cast stone cherub keeps aging and improving in appearance. My very own Portrait of Dorian Gray?*

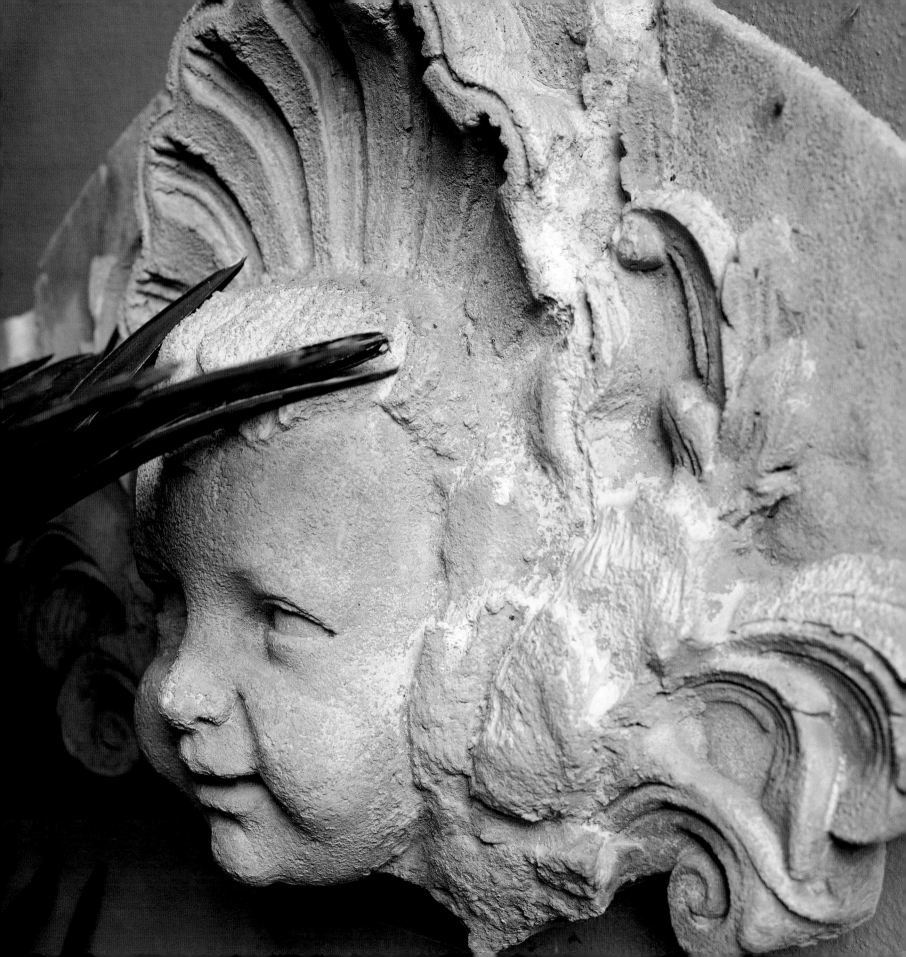

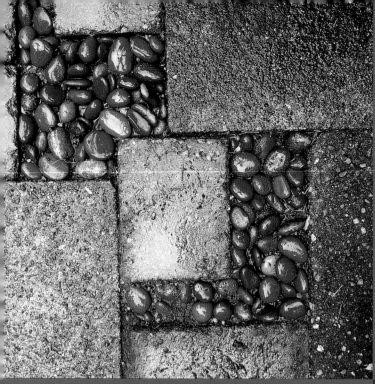

RIGHT *A "mulch" of rocks is so much more interesting than bark chips would have been in* NANCY *and* TOM LAURIE'S TORONTO *garden. The smooth trunk of a dwarf Japanese maple (**Acer palmatum** cultivar) benefits visually by association.*

ABOVE *Remember, surfaces are often underfoot, but not invisible. In* JOHN RAMSAY'S VANCOUVER, B.C., *townhouse garden, designer John Minty created a patterned surface. Dark, smooth pebbles fill deliberate voids in a recycled concrete-paver terrace.*

RIGHT *Granite cobblestones in* NANCY KENNEDY'S TORONTO *garden set a formal rhythm in motion. Clipped balls of ever-green **Euonymus** and collars of English ivy create a sophisticated sculpture court.*

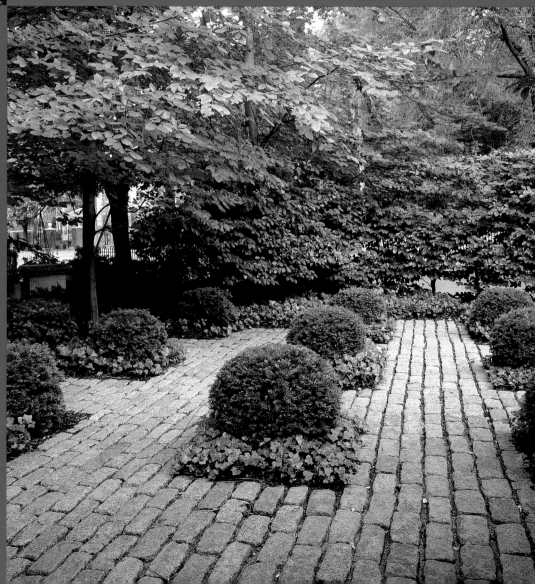

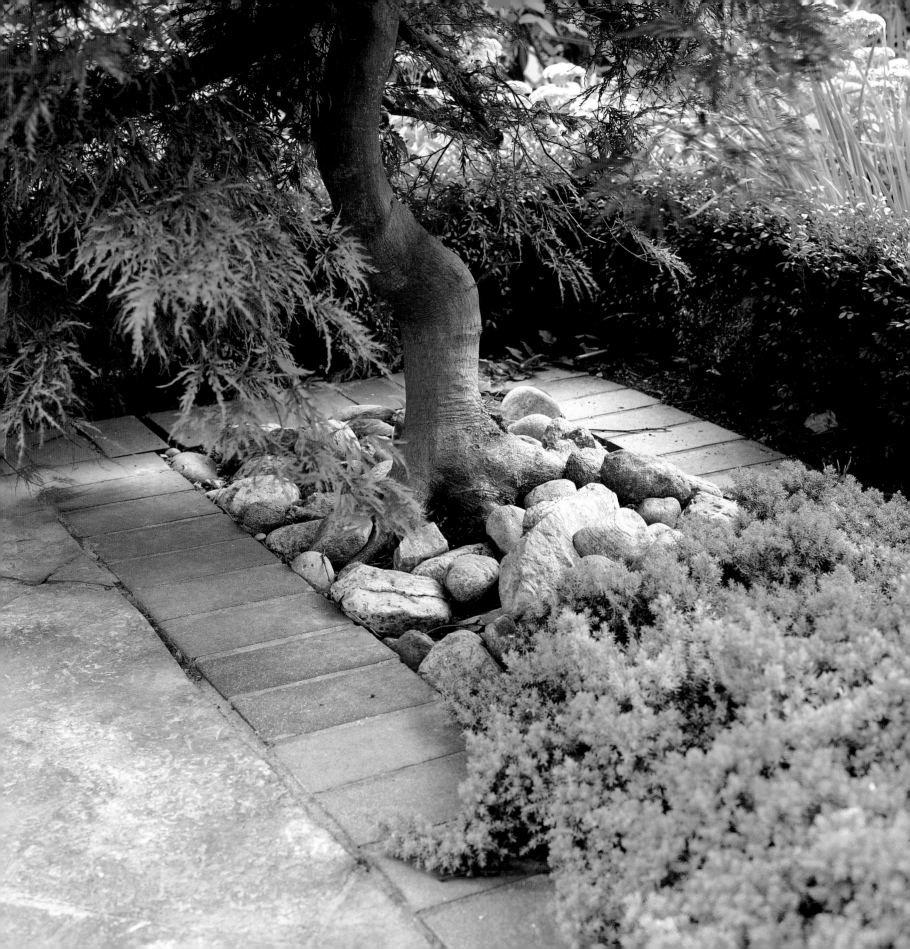

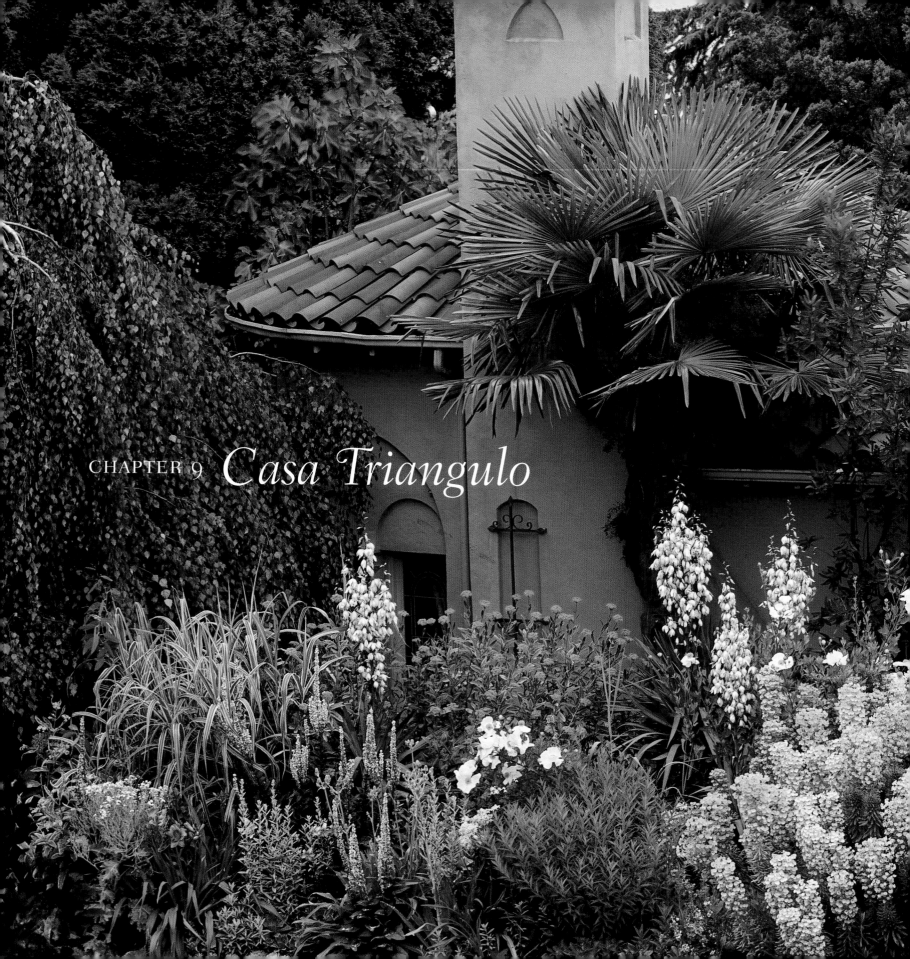

CHAPTER 9 *Casa Triangulo*

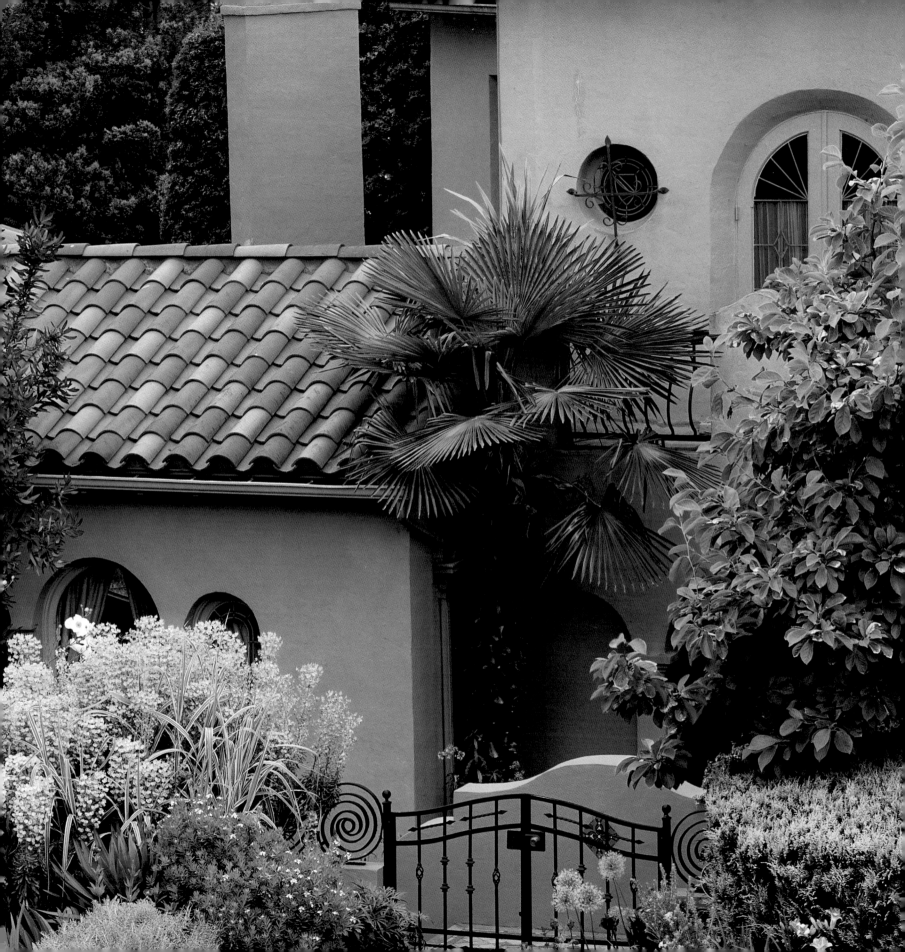

NESTLED ON A STEEP HILL HIGH ABOVE A BEACH KNOWN AS Spanish Banks sits one of Vancouver's best examples of an architectural style known as Mission Revival. Built in 1933, the house was the home of Dr. Joseph Kania, who was also its architect. He moved to British Columbia from Los Angeles during the Depression, when the only job he could find was "up here" at a securities firm. He decided to recreate an L.A. dream home in Vancouver.

I first saw "Kania Castle," as it was known in the neighborhood, in 1975. A friend drove me by in his sports car, knowing I would be enchanted by its faded Hollywood awnings and intricate tile roof. I was more than enchanted: I nearly got whiplash. The house was surrounded by huge trees, many of which had been "topped" to improve neighbors' views. The street was still unpaved at that time and hard to find, and the house looked almost abandoned. Strings of old Christmas lights were falling off the eaves and a stuffed pheasant stared out of the living room window. On the cliff side, concrete stairs with rickety wooden handrails rose through blackberries. I returned occasionally to sneak around. There were three underground garages! I imagined Norma Desmond's car was still in one of them; "Max" was probably watching me from the living room.

PREVIOUS AND FACING PAGE *Giant **Chamaecyparis lawsoniana** trees dwarf my house in Vancouver, B.C. Many similar ones are dying of a deadly phytopthera organism in the groundwater. I hope my steep hillside's excellent drainage saves them. **Trachycarpus fortunei** palms, **Euphorbia characias** 'Wulfenii' and the white spikes of **Yucca recurvifolia** enhance the Spanish architecture. **Magnolia** 'Forrest's Pink' appears as a green blob, but in spring is a complete knockout with its bubble-gum-pink blizzard of 10-inch blossoms.*

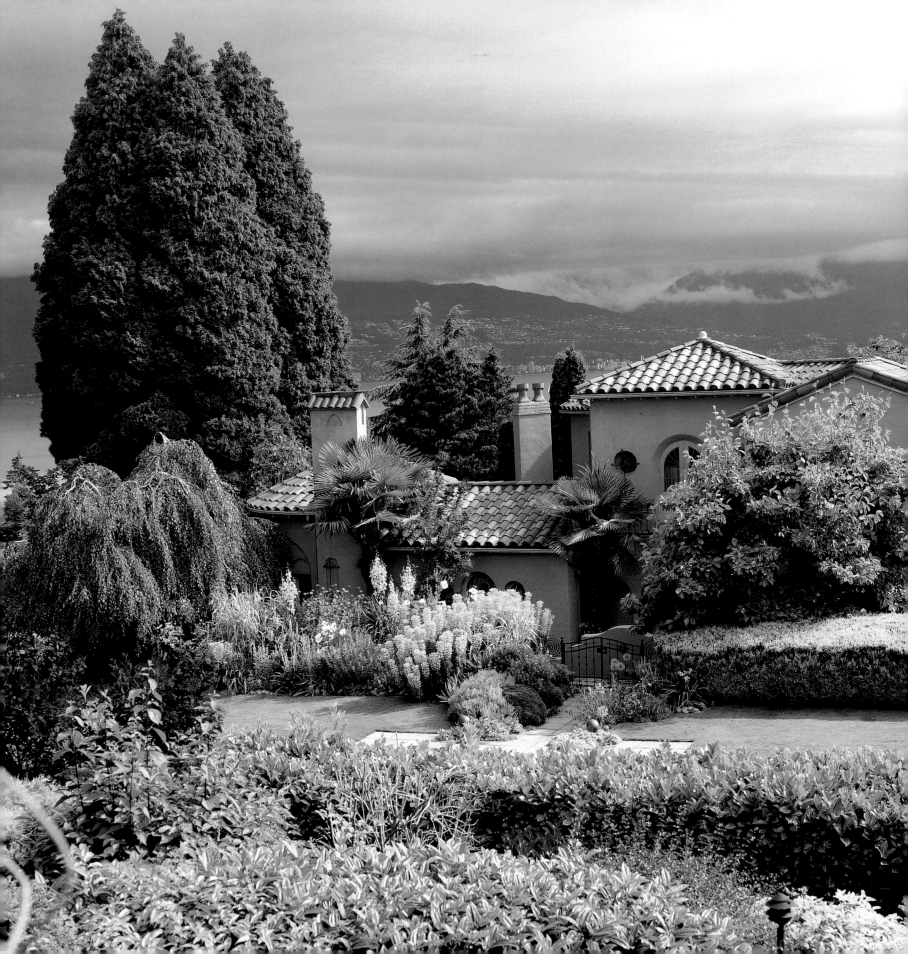

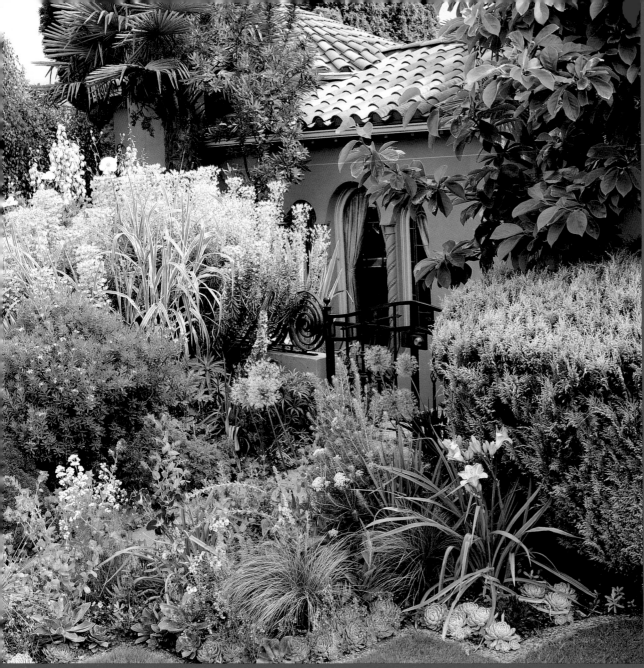

LEFT *My front walkway is planted with muddy colors and includes favorite daylilies. The gold-edged purple 'Scott Fox' and peachy 'Pizza Crust' bloom with bronze **Carex flagellifera** and bluish **Echeverias**.*

BELOW *Along my front walk, the dried orb of **Allium schubertii** appears to have landed from another galaxy. The self-sown purple bells of **Cerinthe major** 'Purpurascens' are always welcome, but dry up by late July. **Hemerocallis** 'Scott Fox' and an unusual white-flowered **Calceolaria alba** from Chile welcome me home.*

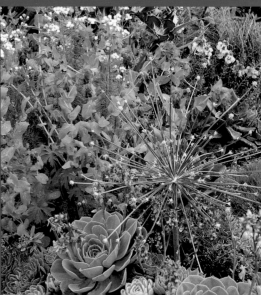

122

I BECAME OBSESSED WITH THE HOUSE AND BEGAN STALKING IT. I was terrified someone would buy it and tear it down. It had spectacular views of downtown, the mountains and the harbor. I returned many times to make sure it was still there. The pheasant in the window never moved. I could tell "old" people lived there. *Nothing* ever changed.

By this time my young flower shop was getting on its feet. I had no money, but every top real estate agent was using me to send flowers to their best clients. I gave one of them the address and asked her to find out what she could about the house. She did, and I felt hopeless. It was way out of my wildest dreams dollar-wise. I kept the piece of paper anyway. I remember staring at it, thinking how odd it would be to garden on a triangular lot, living in a triangular house ...

Several snoopy visits later I decided to write a letter to the house. It was 1977, and I was 23 years old. I said I was in love with the house and hoped, one day, to be able to afford it. I also said that I was worried that someone else might tear it down. I would never do that. I would restore it and protect it.

Ten years later my florist shop phone rang. A little old man introduced himself as Joe Kania, and asked me point blank if I still wanted to buy his house. I said, "the *Spanish* one?"

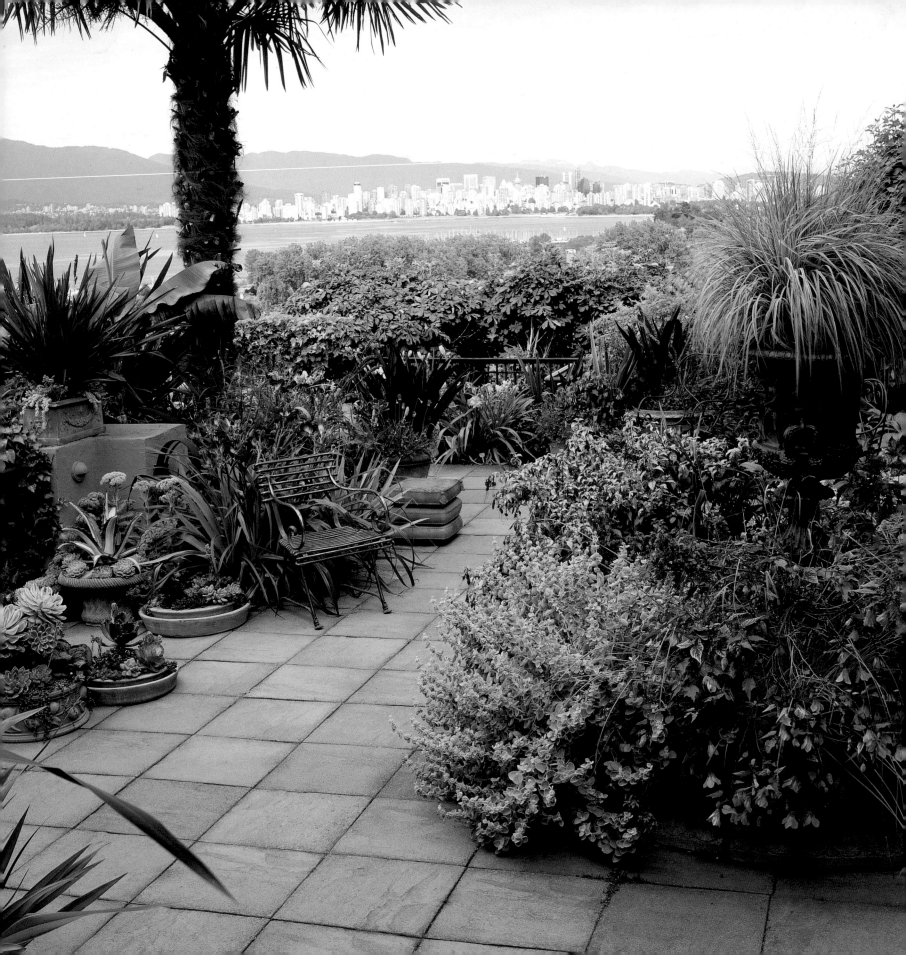

LEFT *We built this sweeping terrace to maximize our views of downtown Vancouver. A planting pocket holds an ever-taller **Trachycarpus fortunei** palm. Uplit at night, it is easy to imagine oneself on the Riviera. I soon stopped wrapping my palms for the winter as they have proven to be totally hardy. Gold-leaved **Fuchsia** 'Genii', **Ballotta pseudodictamnus** and **Abutilon** 'Melon Delight' spill out of a raised, circular planter. **Molina caerulea** 'Variegata' fills an antique iron urn and adds another vertical element.*

RIGHT *Comfortable patio furniture is a must. Low planters of **Echeveria** and a big pot of the dark-leaved **Cimicifuga simplex** 'Hillside Black Beauty' are all there is room for on a small raised patio.*

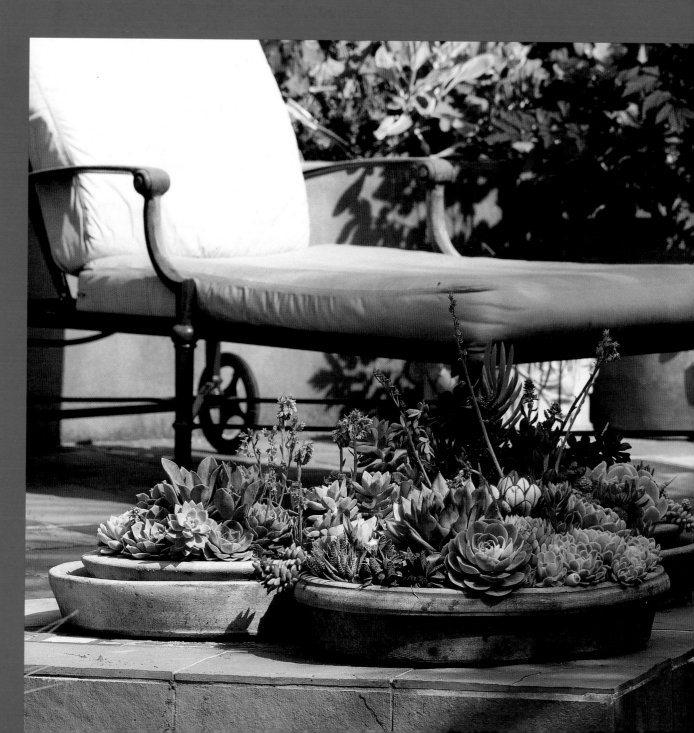

IN THE TEN YEAR INTERVAL BETWEEN WRITING THE LETTER AND receiving that phone call, there had been no contact between us. I didn't even know his name. I had met my partner Brent, and we had a tiny but perfect little seven-hundred-square-foot shingle cottage in one of the city's less glamorous areas. The exodus from Hong Kong was hitting Vancouver hard. Countless older homes and many mansions were razed to make way for "International Style" monster homes. I knew what I had to do.

Dr. Kania said to come over right away. I asked if I could bring my "brother" — I didn't want to blow this opportunity to see inside the house! I will never forget ringing the doorbell, expecting "Max," or at least Harvey Korman dressed as "Max," to open the door. Instead, a very short Alfred Hitchcock type greeted us, with a badly-wigged woman peering over his shoulder. The first thing he said to me was, "I've spent ten years checking you out. You are the only person I will sell my house to."

To make a long story short, he was serious. He considered me an "artist" and he believed his house, his pride and joy, would be in safe hands. He was almost ninety, and the time to pass it on had come. Luckily, I had a great bank manager! I drove him past the house and he said "Don't worry." Brent and I managed to finally sell our tiny cottage, skip several steps and move into a house ten times bigger. The past fifteen years have been spent working on the house and the garden, trying to put beauty everywhere.

FACING PAGE *Abutilon* '*Huntington Pink*' *and* **Hedera helix** '*Goldheart*' *follow the curves of a garden wall.* **Stipa arundinacea** *froths about, while succulents in a shallow moss-and-chicken-wire nest adorn the top of the wall. A peel-and-stick waterproof membrane went down first, with everything else resting on top.*

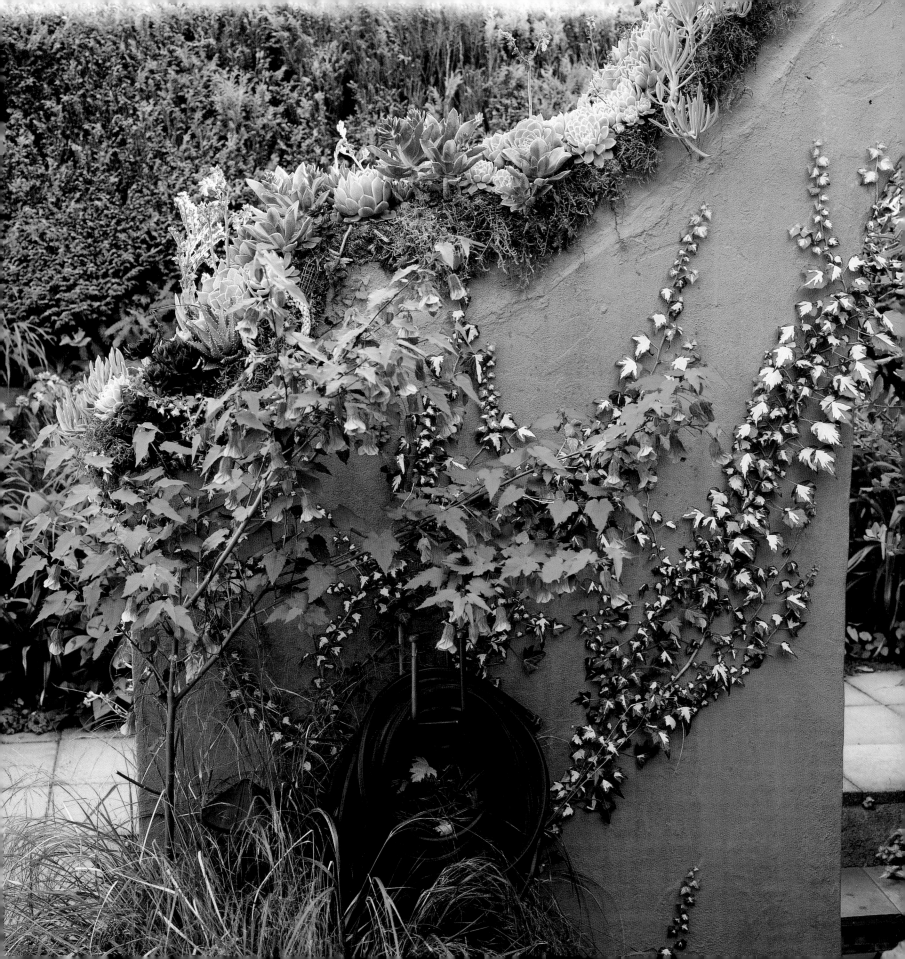

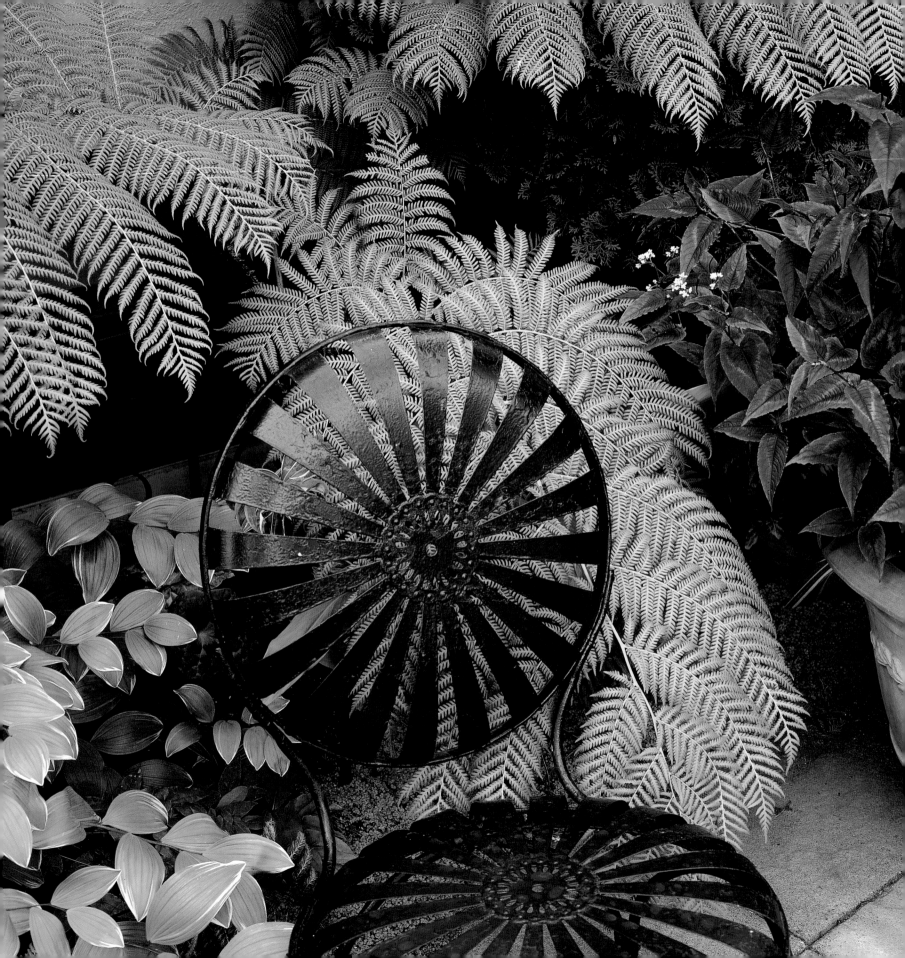

M Y STYLE OF GARDENING OWES A LOT TO THIS HOUSE. THE whole look of the place became much more dramatic when we painted it a rich salmon. I tried thirteen colors, and remember a neighbour saying "You're not *really* painting it that color, are you?" After being white for nearly sixty years, it was a dramatic change. Now everyone loves it. It has mellowed, and I like the mottled effect of algae, sun and shadows on its rich surfaces. Plants pop out against my peachy walls.

The garden is actually very small. It encircles the house, and a path of cast-concrete pavers that look like mellow Yorkstone allows you to see it all without much effort. Beds are accessible from this path, and pots decorate the odd set of steps and two sunny terraces. I splurged on a very large hot tub/plunge pool, but it too is beautiful.

Dealing with such a major plant addiction has made me ruthless in tearing things out. There is actually very little still here of what Dr. Kania planted. Two groups of enormous *Chamaecyparis x lawsoniana* date back to when the house was built; they are now at least seventy feet tall, and break the wind from the bay below. My already warm garden is a microclimate because of them. I also kept a huge fig tree, *Ficus carica*, that produces delicious figs every August. A weeping birch, *Betula pendula* 'Youngii', got to stay only because it creates privacy.

I view the rest of the garden as a big plaything. Like a child, I wander outside with no mission on my mind, then suddenly and randomly find something to do. Something to play with. I rearrange pots, cut back *Eryngiums* and *Verbascums*, or dig out a peony that doesn't bloom. I garden.

FACING PAGE *I expected it to succumb to our regular but light frosts, but an Australian tree fern, **Alsophila australis**, has survived year round in a sheltered corner. An antique garden chair competes for pattern against its magnificent fronds.*

CREATING A "MEDITERRANEAN STYLE" GARDEN TO GO WITH MY house's architecture hasn't stopped me from indulging in woodland plants. I love them, too. I unknowingly created a shady walk between my house and the neighbors. Here I grow many jewels that would look inappropriate out front in my "burglarproof" border of yuccas and other spiky plants. I am trying to collect as many forms of hart's tongue fern, **Phyllitus scolopendrium**, as possible. This evergreen has undivided leaves (fronds) that come in a number of forms. My favorite is totally ruffled, like a tacky tuxedo shirt. I adore these ferns so much, I had a sofa upholstered in botanically accurate fern fabric! No one can sit on it.

I use my garden as a laboratory, to see what new trends I can come up with for my nursery. Daylilies, succulents and ways to integrate them artistically seem to be where I am now. Such odd bed-fellows make it quite a challenge. And *that* is exactly what I need.

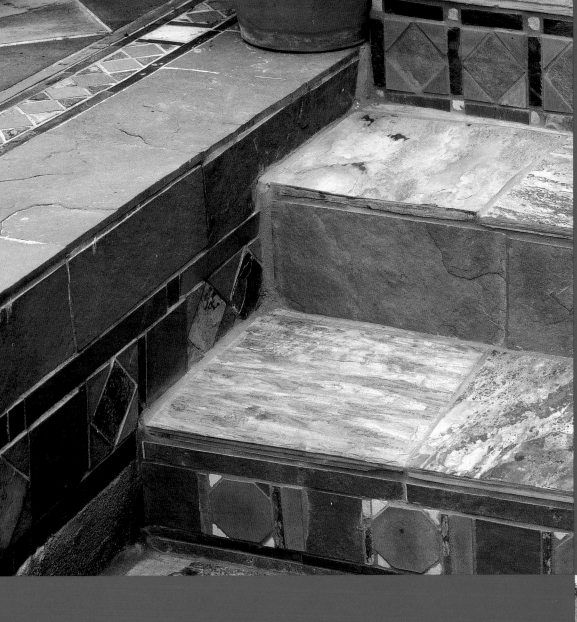

*When I come home I often say,
"I'd like to see the wizard,
please." My partner Brent is
the wizard of many things, one
of which is cutting up tile and
pieces of slate. Our garden
benefits immensely from his
decorative treatment of all
hard surfaces.*

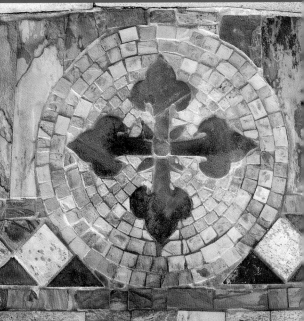

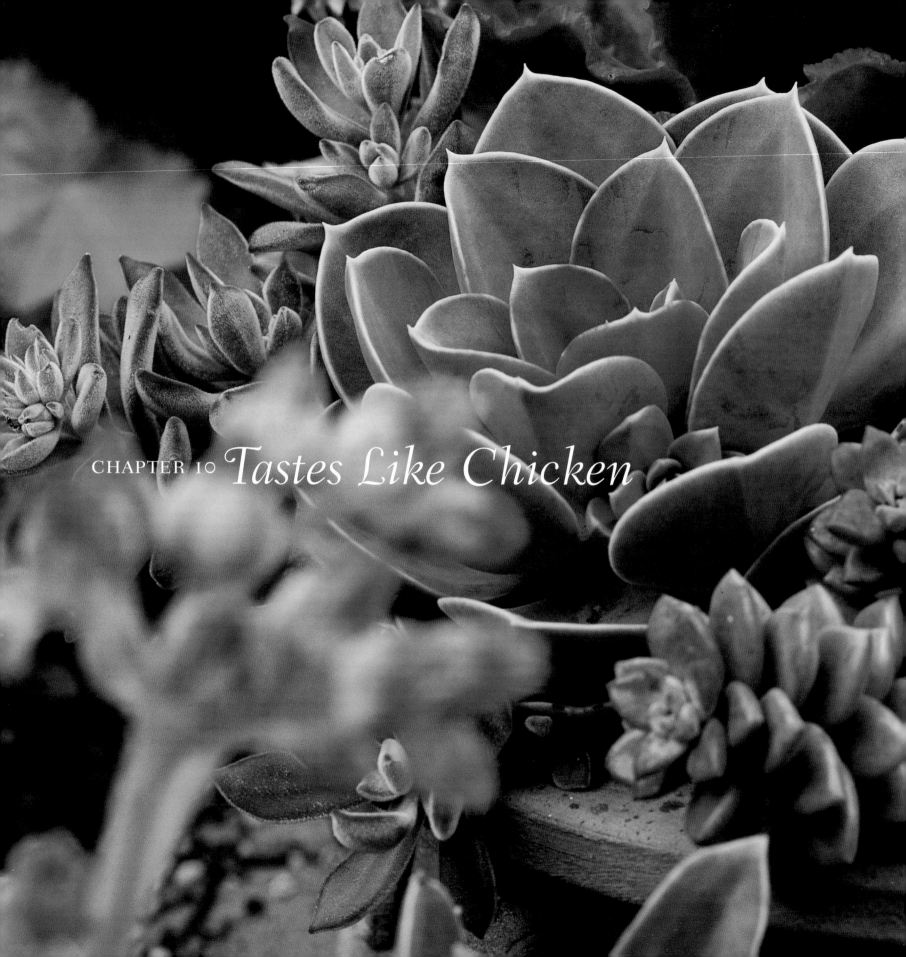

CHAPTER 10 *Tastes Like Chicken*

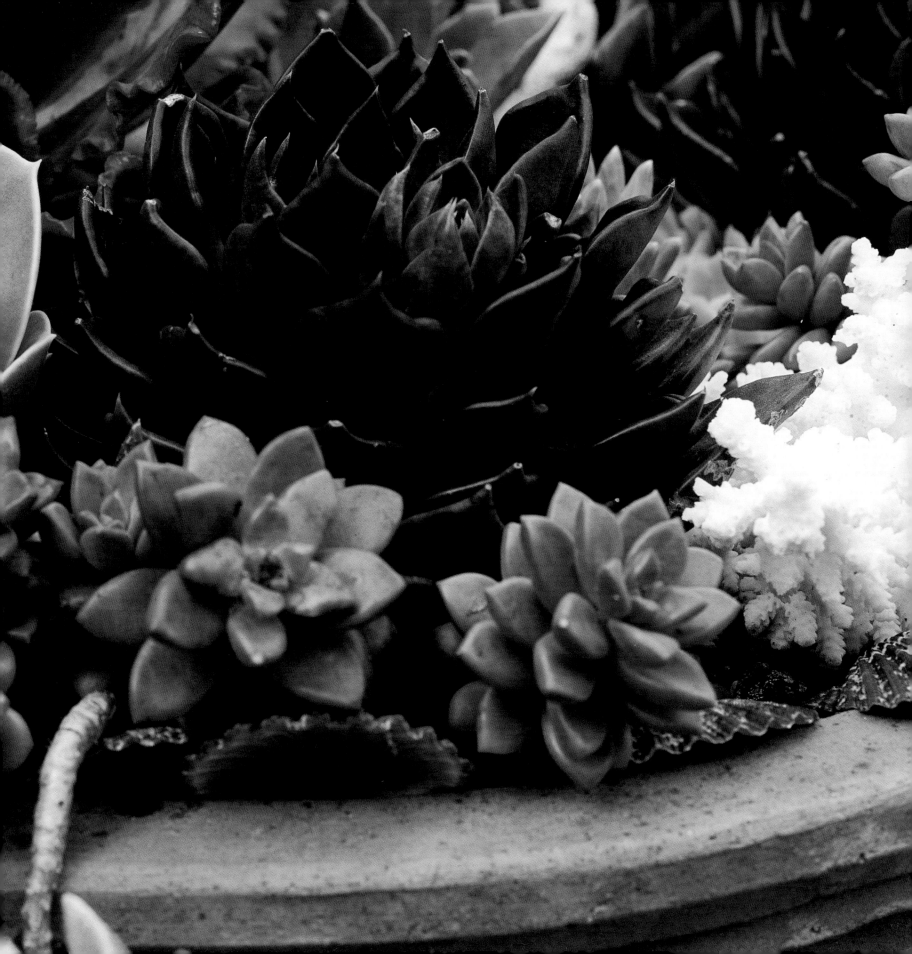

IF THE WORDS "TENDER" AND "SUCCULENT" IMMEDIATELY MAKE you think of chicken, this chapter should change your life. Tender succulents are to today's hippest gardeners what *Canna* and *Colocasia* were five years ago. They are the epicenter of a new botanical quake of creativity. Their ease of culture and fabulous variety of form allow *anyone* to create something fairly amazing their very first try.

My adventures with tender succulents began in the late 1980s, when my partner Brent bought a few flats of surplus *Echeverias* at our local botanical garden's plant sale. They were leftovers from the parks department's elaborate summer bedding schemes, and a real bargain at $5 per *flat!* Since Victorian times, civic crews have used the tight rosettes of *Echeverias* to spell out words and edge formal beds. Although not winter hardy in our mild Pacific Northwest climate, we began using them as garden plants anyway. At first they filled odd empty spaces at the fronts of borders, mixing well with perennial grasses and hot, spiky favorites such as *Eryngium* and *Dierama*. We always made sure to lift them before any real danger of frost, and overwintered them in a heated but cool greenhouse.

PREVIOUS PAGE *Potted succulents really are the treasure trove. Here, bits of coral add stark contrast in an arrangement by my partner, Brent Beattie.*

FACING PAGE *The handmade terra cotta pots from Impruneta, Italy, are perfect for holding a collection of* **Echeverias**. *The very dark* **Echeveria** *'Black Prince' contrasts well with a chunk of coral and creates an undersea vision.*

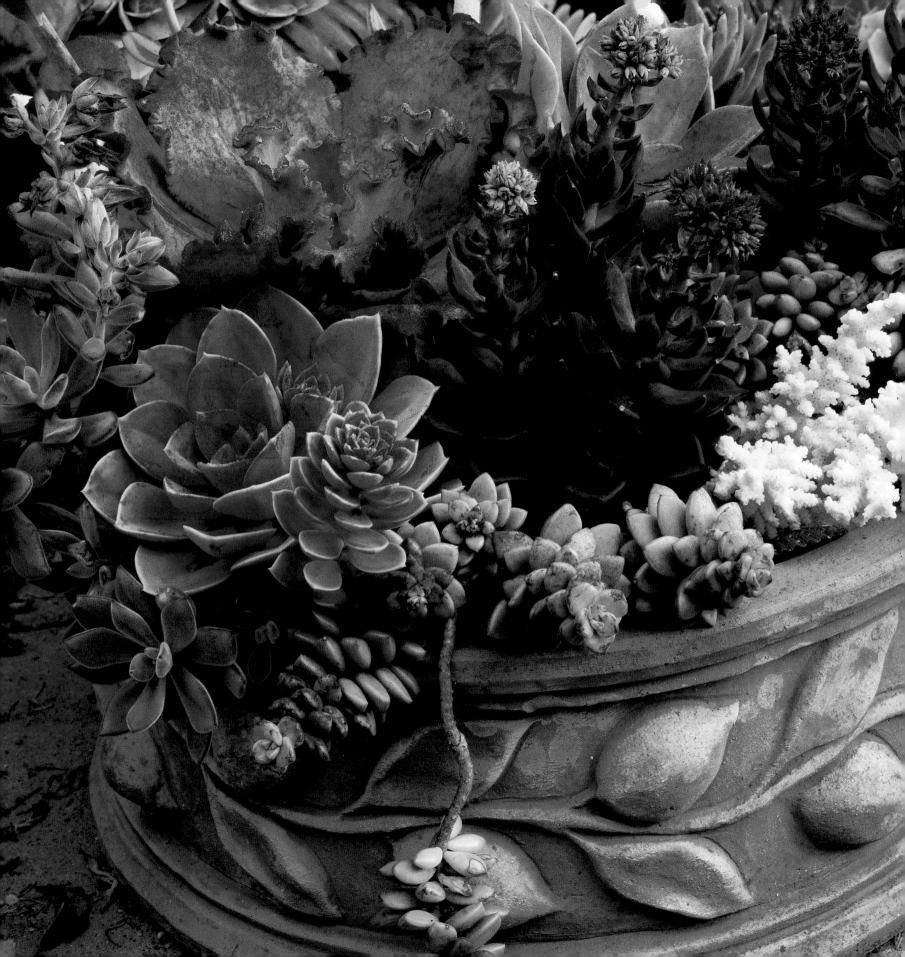

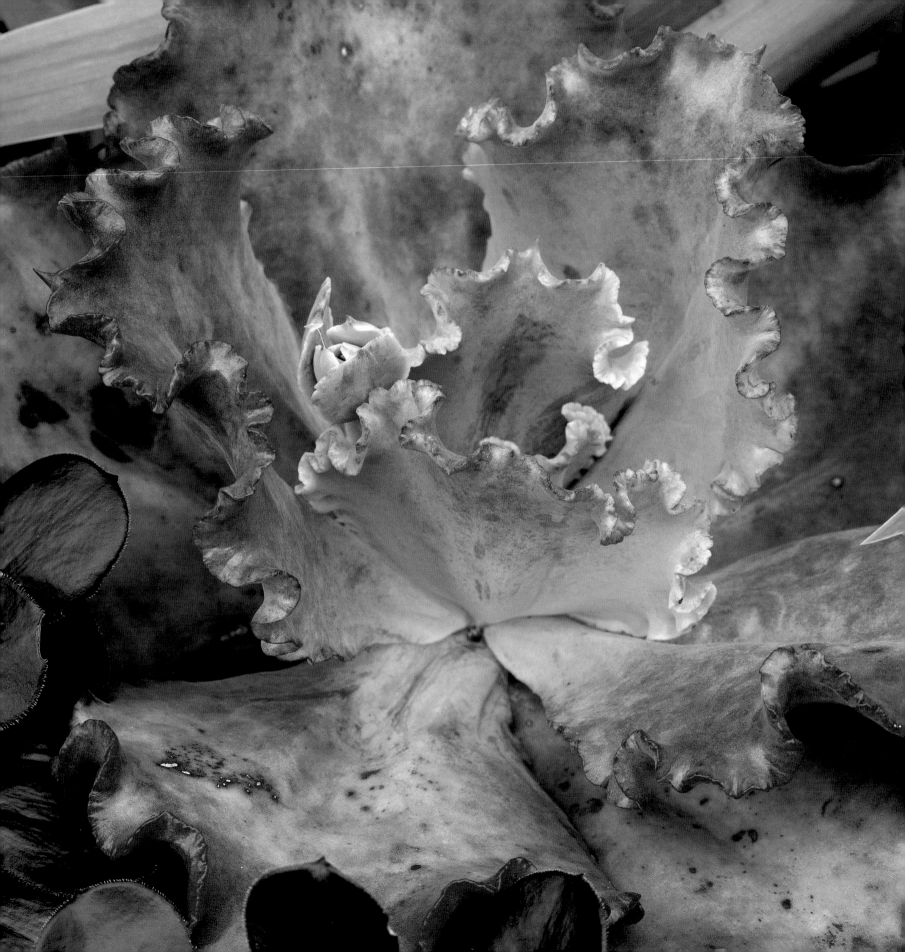

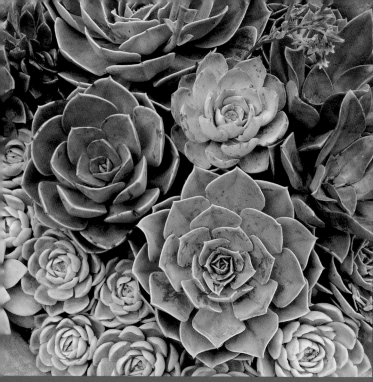

BELOW *A mixed pizza of blooming, completely hardy* **Sempervivum**, *the fabulous-but-tender* **Kalanchoe thyrsiflora** *and a few* **Echeverias**. *The* **Kalanchoe** *takes on a vibrant foliage "tan" the more sun it gets, then completely loses it in the greenhouse each winter. The container is an unusual double-rimmed "ant saucer" from Italy.*

ABOVE *A completed "Echeveria Pizza" in a low clay saucer. Be sure to jam-pack it or it won't look right.*

LEFT *The frilly* **Echeverias** *are mostly unnamed hybrids. They are also the hardest to find outside of California. But isn't that what overhead bins are for on domestic flights?*

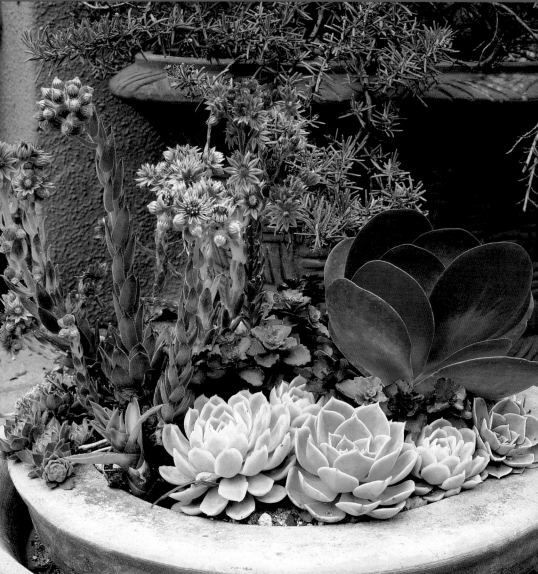

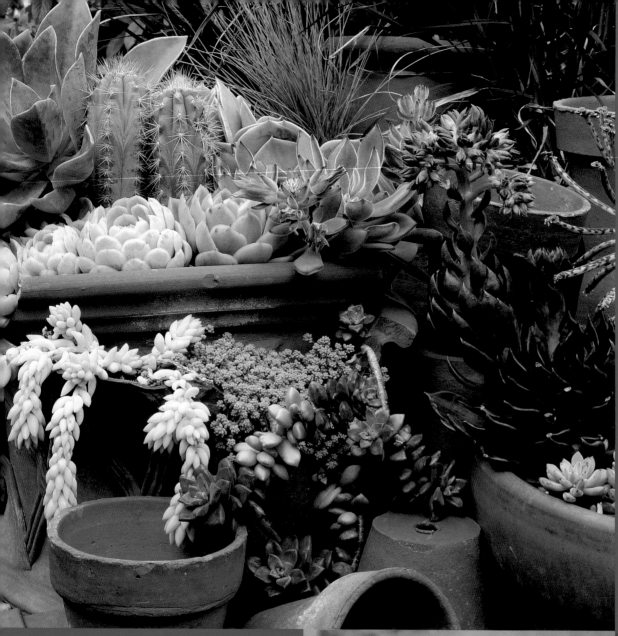

LEFT *In this display at Southlands Nursery,* TYLER MERKEL *uses a broken, but still beautiful terra cotta pot by Whichford Pottery. The popular houseplant burro's tail (**Sedum morganianum**) cascades from a created crevice of broken clay.*

BELOW *Tiny terra cotta pots hold tiny **Sempervivums** on my patio. Although they look Italian, these cute "knock-off" pots are made in China.*

RIGHT *If you can't find enough **Echeverias**, use **Sempervivums**, which are widely available and come in many rich colors. They are also very tolerant of extreme winter cold, and thrive in baking summer heat!*

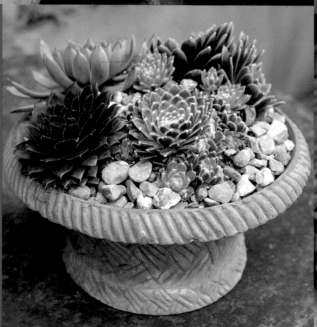

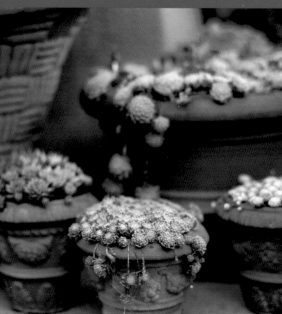

138

I SOON BEGAN NOTICING MORE UNUSUAL FORMS AND COLORS OF these charming little cuties in the cactus selections at our "big box" stores. Every so often I would rescue an exceptionally blue or mauve *Echeveria* from the dreary tables and add it to our selection. Then I found black ones, wavy ones and one with blistery warts ('Paul Bunyon'). These were too special to place in the open garden and needed to be featured in shallow pots. The "Echeveria Pizza" was born!

Knowing that these Mexican natives like full sun and excellent drainage, we began potting them in shallow containers. Clay saucers are perfect for this, but first need to be drilled to create drain holes. Terra cotta has an appropriate texture for housing succulents, as its natural roughness contrasts well with their crisp smoothness. It is better to plant your pizza tightly right from the start; I butt each root ball up against its neighbor's root ball for a full look. Usually one or two plants are a little bigger or more special than the others: these will be the focal point of the arrangement, and you have to place them as such. Don't place them in the center — that is too obvious and unartistic — but off to one side, for a less "man-made" look. Group supporting plants around and fill any crevices with potting medium.

SUCCULENTS ARE NOT FUSSY ABOUT SOIL. AS LONG AS EXCESS water drains out and the sun shines, they are happy. I like to top dress succulent creations with a small pea gravel. If you look hard enough you will find lovely biscuit-brown gravels for sale; they certainly look better than grey crushed rock. You may want to add non-living accents such as bits of coral or seashells to create an underwater illusion. The resemblance to sea creatures is striking and a bit of a mindbender when well done.

Succulents used as summer ornamentals should be fertilized occasionally. They respond gratefully by plumping up and getting much larger than expected! I water them every few days in hot weather, and once a month I treat them to a liquid feed of 20-20-20 fertilizer at a higher than recommended dose. I put about two heaping tablespoons of this powdered fertilizer in my one-gallon watering can and deliberately sprinkle the entire rosette of leaves and the soil, to feed both foliage and roots. I know that their succulent leaves allow them to survive droughts in the wild, but I have seen them shrivel and lose the will to live when treated like cacti. They *love* moisture as long as it comes — and *goes*.

FACING PAGE *Seashells deliberately pick up the burgundy tones of this* **Sempervivum***. Notice that the gravel mulch is a pleasant biscuit brown, not grey or, worst of all, white!*

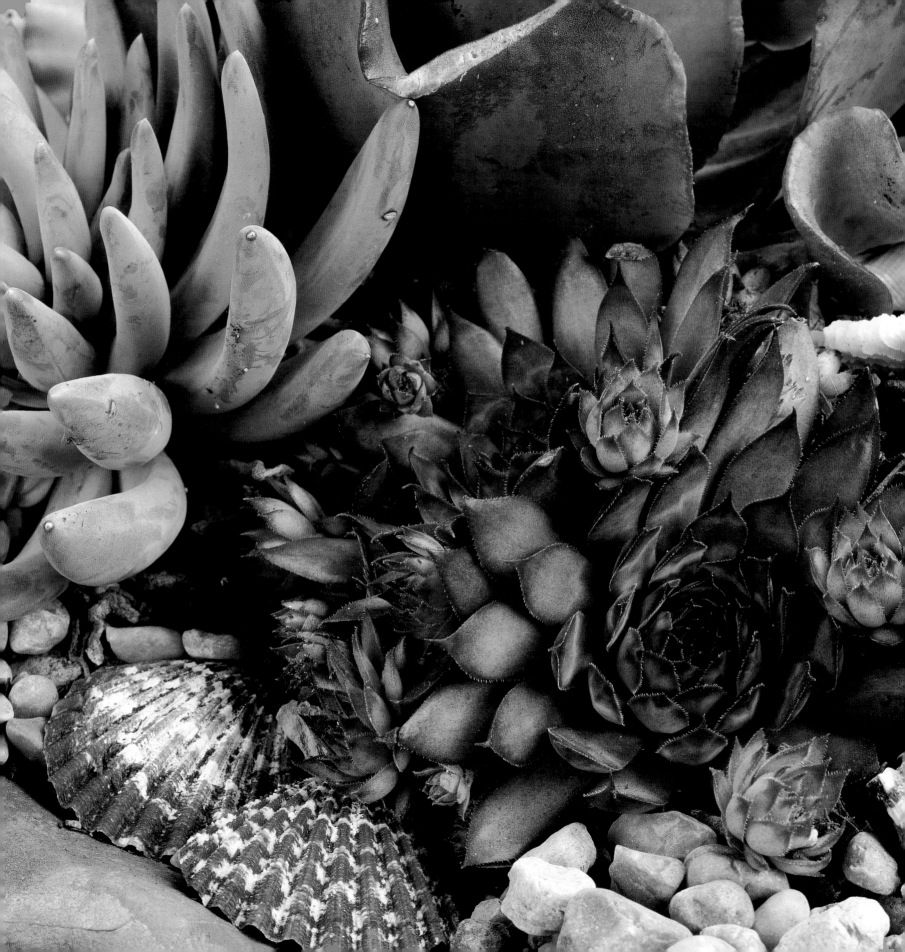

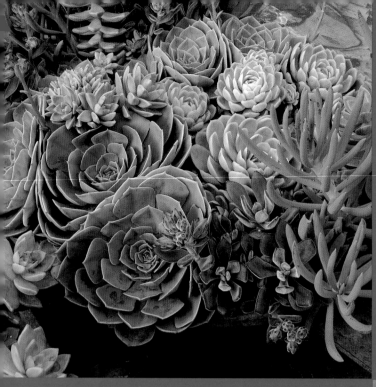

LEFT *By late summer, my planters are bursting but happy. The icy "blue chalk sticks,"* **Senecio mandraliscae**, *adds textural interest to this otherwise "one topping" pizza. An occasional dousing with 20-20-20 fertilizer in the water creates lush growth.*

BELOW **Aeonium arboretum** *'Schwarzkopf', a frilly* **Echeveria** *hybrid.*

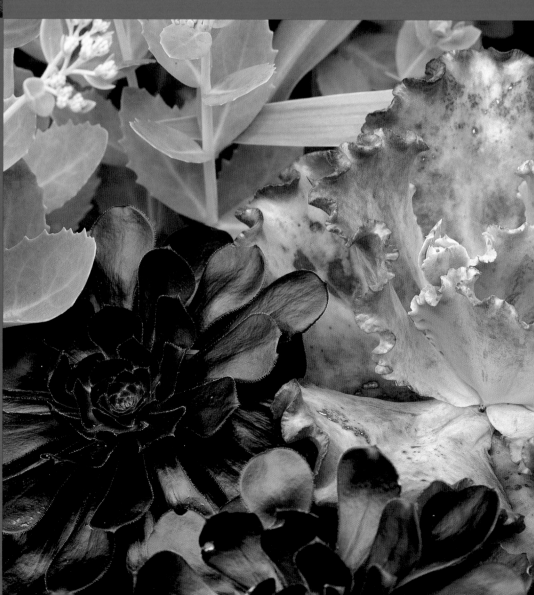

THE TREND OF GARDENING WITH MASSES OF NON-HARDY succulents is limited by the fear of winter. What do you do with them then? They are too beautiful to be considered disposable. All they need is bright light and an above-freezing windowsill to hang in there until spring. Lack of light in winter will result in stretched growth and very unattractive plants. Lower leaves will turn yellow, then papery and need constant removal. If you cannot provide a very bright location for winter storage of your succulents, give them to someone who can, or set up a grow light in the basement or an unused area. Keep the plants very close to the tubes if these are fluorescent, and watch for stretching.

Gardeners with hundreds of *Echeverias* (they multiply like rabbits!) stash them in plastic flats, not pots. At my house, I call this "Operation Echeveria Lift." Around Halloween, helpers from my nursery come with our big truck and we begin scooping them up with our bare hands. We place them tightly beside each other in plastic nursery flats and spend the next month cleaning them up. We check for insect grubs, slugs and rot, then group the plants by variety and place them, root ball and all, in flats. They spend the winter in semi-hibernation in a barely heated but bright greenhouse. They receive much less water (maybe once a week) and are allowed to rest.

Around March 1, I begin fertilizing again. A liquid feed of 20-20-20 at half my usual strength wakes them up. The increased light that spring brings really turns these plants on! Struggling specimens suddenly perk up and look happy. Once all danger of frost has passed, I place the flats of *Echeverias* out in the sun to "harden off" for a month or so. This direct sun brings out the subtle coloring and individuality of each variety. Then it is time to play!

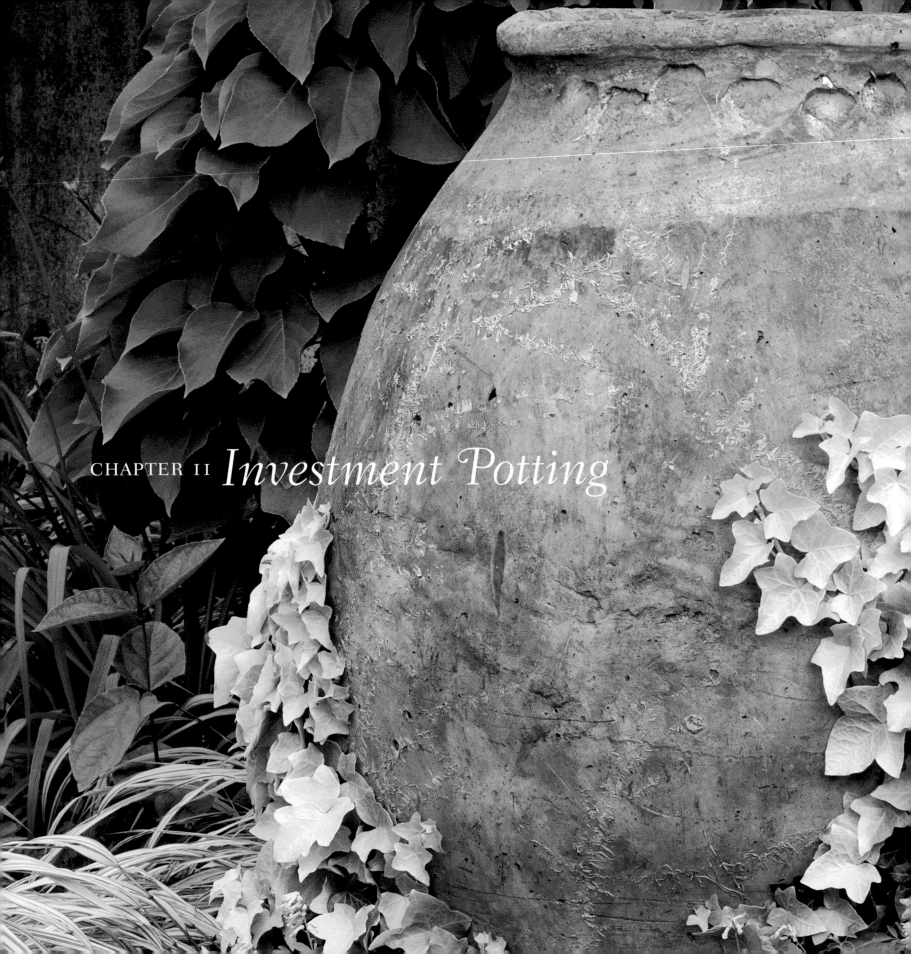

CHAPTER II *Investment Potting*

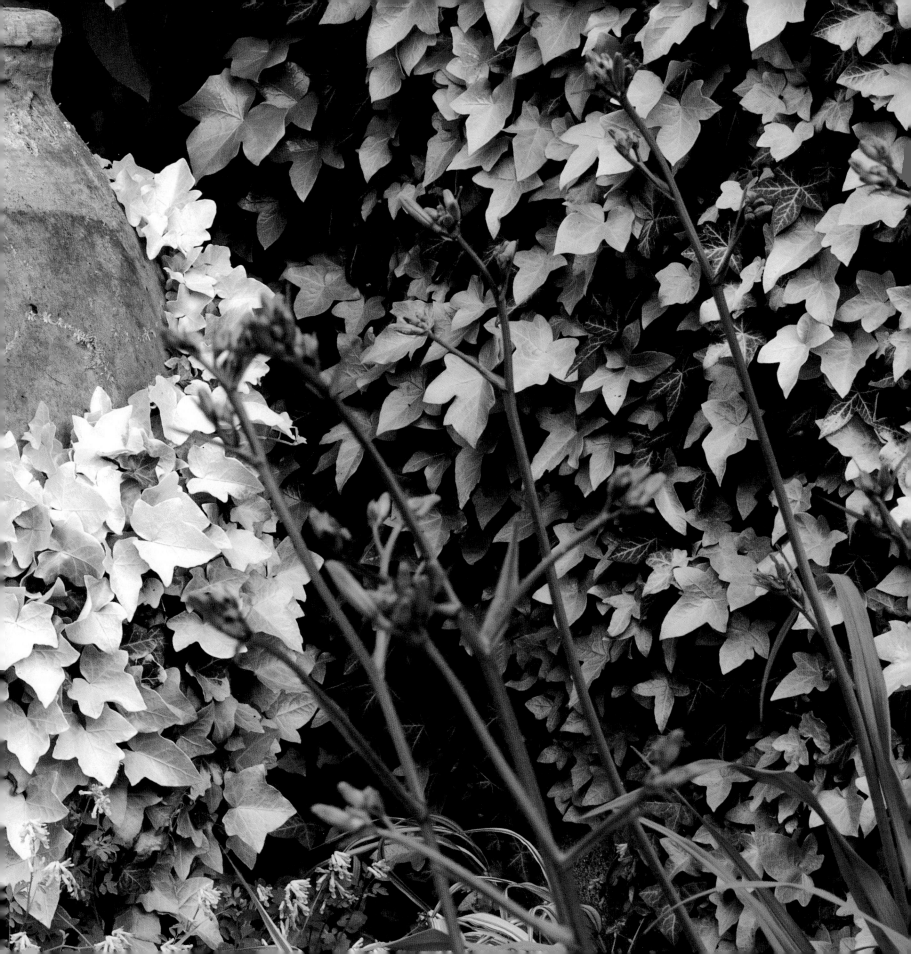

MOST GARDENERS WOULD NEVER PUT THE WORDS "INVESTMENT" and "potting" together. But potting has a lot more in common with banking than you might think. Your pots and containers should pay an *aesthetic dividend,* as well as contain your plants. In other words, buy some good pots!

I find I am inspired by my containers themselves. I once lugged home an antique cast iron *jardinière* from the Paris flea market, and I am not about to fill it with meaningless impatiens; its weathered, metallic patina deserves better. The tiny celadon-green leaves of *Hebe* 'Quicksilver' and a dark apricot *Diascia* 'Coral Belle' made a lovely combination for this pot. Another year I filled it with the coppery foliage of *Haloragis erecta* 'Wellington Bronze'; this easy-from-seed New Zealand weed behaved well for me, though I've heard it is a terrible self-sower elsewhere.

For an increasing number of people, container gardening is their only choice. Housing prices only go up and balconies keep getting smaller. What used to be the size of a bank vault is now more like a safety deposit box. All the more reason to use it wisely. Your choice of containers is an *aesthetic milestone.* Think of it as a major hurdle that will decide whether or not you are even in the race.

PREVIOUS PAGE *Hedera helix* '*Buttercup*' *marries this aged olive jar to its bed of* **Hakonechloa macra** '*Aureola*' *grass at* CHANTICLEER GARDENS *in* WAYNE, PENNSYLVANIA. *By keeping the ivy under control, the beauty of the jar is not lost. It looks like it has always been there.*

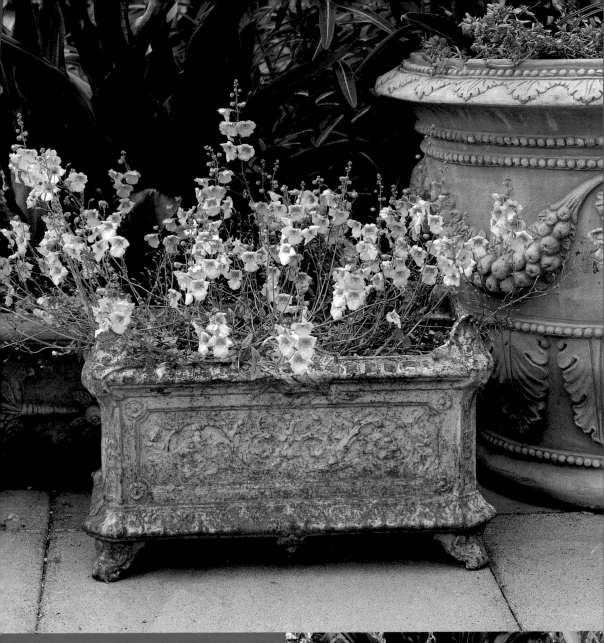

LEFT **Diascia** 'Blackthorn Apricot' fills a French antique iron planter on my patio. Behind it, the dark spears of **Eucomis** 'Sparkling Burgundy' rise. A particularly fine Italian terra cotta pot is deliberately left without trailing plants, as I want to appreciate its decorative detail.

BELOW A handmade terra cotta olive oil jar and column from Impruneta, Italy, serves as sculpture in my own garden. I cut down an evergreen magnolia tree to make room for them, and don't regret the decision. **Hosta** 'Sum and Substance' and **Dienanthe bifida** play back-up roles and allow the jar to star. **Parthenocissus quinquefolia** 'Engelmannii' forms a delicate tracery and adds interest to the background wall.

RIGHT **Fuchsia** 'Autumnale', **Cuphea ignea** and **Setcreasea purpurea** spill and **Eucomis** 'Sparkling Burgundy' rises from a pot on my patio. I like to assemble plants for their foliage value rather than any flowers they may produce.

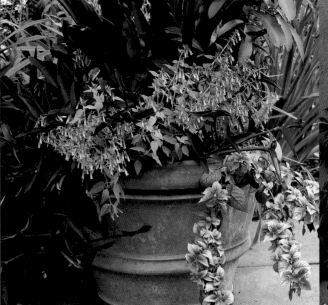

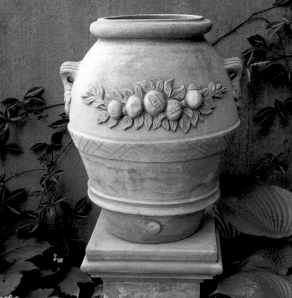

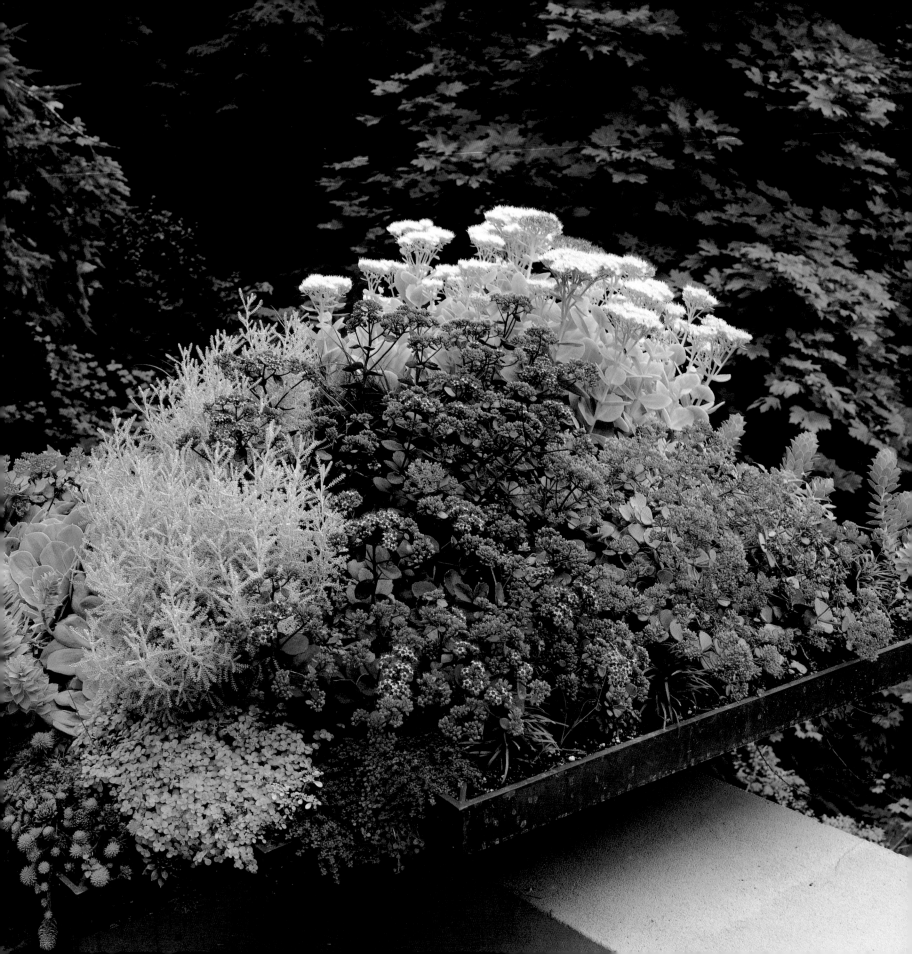

In the VANCOUVER, B.C., *garden of* MAUREEN LUNN, *custom-made bronze planters hold a different and dazzling display each year. Their wide, open shape allows for a mounding of soil and a non-flat final composition of pure artistry. Plenty of succulents mix with a touch of purple from* **Setcreasea purpurea** *and* **Sedum** *'Bertram Anderson'. Silvery* **Santolina chamaecyparissus** *and lime green* **Sedum makinoi** *liven things up in one planter, perched high over a ravine.*

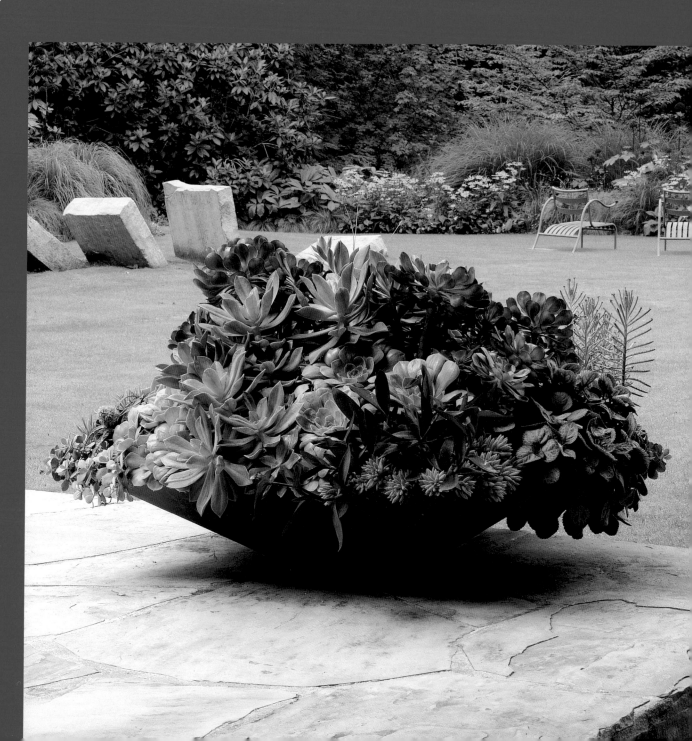

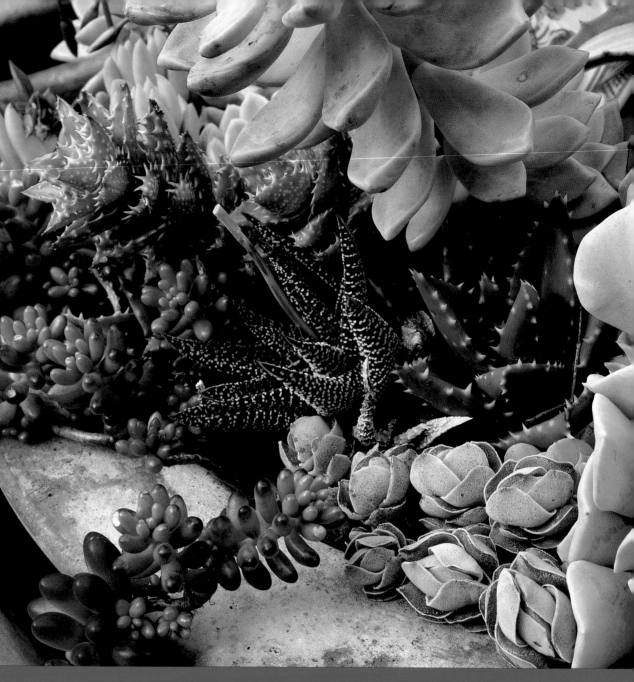

*Echeveria Pizzas — once you make one, it is hard to stop. The very dark **Echeveria** 'Black Prince' combines with a few spiral seashells and a touch of burro's tail (**Sedum morganianum**) in an Italian "ant saucer."*

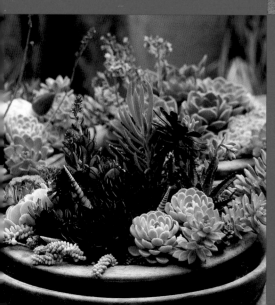

ARDENING IN CONTAINERS IS ANOTHER FORM OF SELF-expression. Like painting or taking a pottery class, you are revealing things about yourself every time you put two plants together. Psychiatrists study people's doodles, so what do your containers say about you? Does a giant concrete boot *and* a plastic swan planter suggest arrested development or cruelty to animals? I have been tempted to knock on strangers' doors and ask them if they even knew they had a hanging basket out front. If so, why is it dead?

The ship has literally come in for small space gardeners. Containers of containers from Vietnam, the Philippines and China are flooding all markets with great-looking, inexpensive glazed pots. Available in many colors, some of the best looking ones are also dirt cheap. I particularly like the tawny brown and mustardy tones. These solid, neutral colors often have a matte or even rough finish that appears almost unglazed. They combine particularly well with simple plantings of grasses: tufts of **Nassella** (formerly **Stipa**) **tenuissima**, sugary brown **Carex flagellifera** and the dried blood-red **Uncinia rubra** are enough on their own. Such simple pots look best in groups of three to five, and one tipped on its side and half-buried looks great!

There is something mesmerizing about blue glazed pots. I think we simply don't get enough blue in our lives. There is a true short-age of blue flowers in the world, so we have to compensate. Cobalt glazed pots deliver a throbbing fix — they make nearby foliage appear more glaucous, and succulents housed in them look icy and cool. When working with strongly colored containers, limit yourself to just one part of the spectrum. Additional pots have to be neutral, terra cotta or something similar. A grouping of containers should look like a gallery exhibit, not a garage sale.

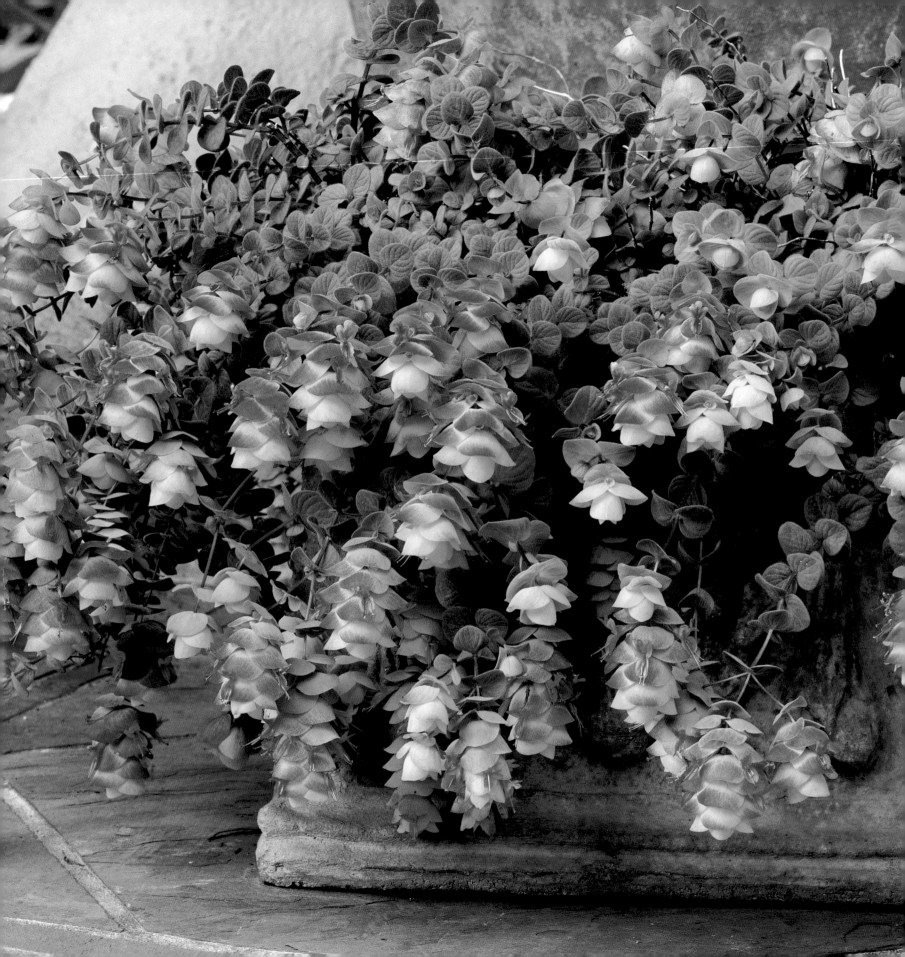

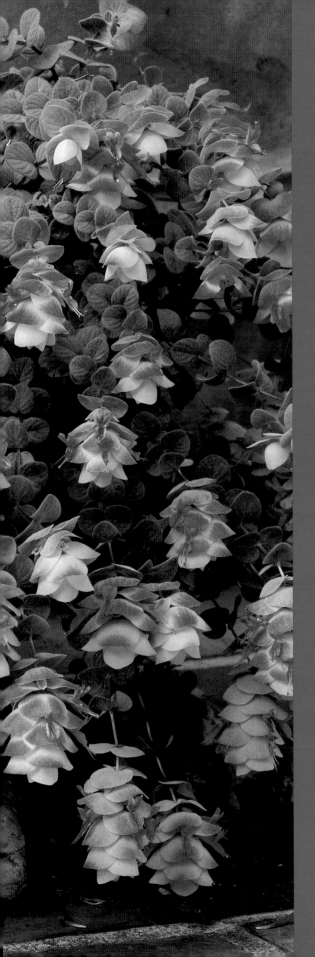

LEFT *Little Miss Muffet? Actually it's a happy pot of* **Origanum** *'Barbara Tingey'. Very special and favorite plants are often shown to best advantage on their own. This sun-lover has proven to be much hardier than I thought, and now spends all year outdoors.*

BELOW *Oxalis spiralis ssp. vulcanicola cascades from a mixed pot in* ROGER RAICHE *and* DAVID M^cCRORY'S *garden. This recent introduction produces coppery-tinged new growth that fades to shades of lime. Notice the rock, which adds greatly to the plant composition.*

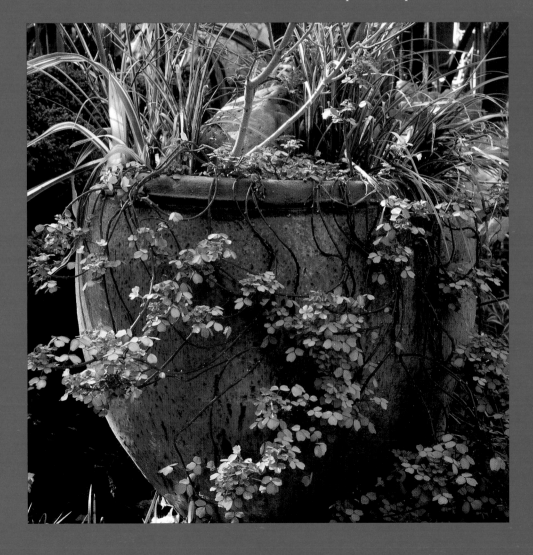

GLAZED POTS ARE RARELY FROSTPROOF AND NEED TO BE OVER-wintered inside. Glazes trap water and will often crack or chip from cold. Cold-climate gardeners should not risk losing containers by leaving them outside all winter, even filled with soil. Gardeners in milder areas can keep on using their pots in winter and usually plant them seasonally. I own several hand-made Italian terra cotta pots from the famous Impruneta potteries. For centuries, this small town near Florence has produced the most beautiful clay pots in the world. Family-owned businesses hand press a particularly iron-rich local clay into molds. After firing, this clay turns a distinctive peachy-rose shade that is instantly recognizable as an "Impruneta pot." Their high iron content and surprisingly heavy weight make these pots more frostproof than other clay pots. And their design and ornamentation are so timeless that any plant benefits aesthetically just by association.

By purchasing a few "investment pots," you automatically raise the bar. What you put in them now matters. They become receptacles for botanical treasure, no longer utilitarian vessels or coffins of misery. Owning a few "important" pots also makes plant shopping more fun. Now you will want to evaluate whether or not a plant is *worthy*. You establish a balance between plant and container, and in doing so create a Jewel Box Garden.

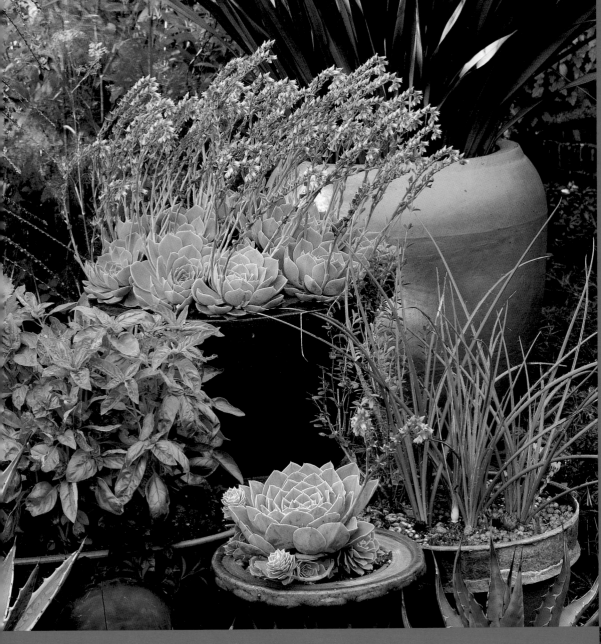

In VICTORIA, B.C., VALERIE
MURRAY *clusters pots of sun-
lovers together. The bronze
blades of New Zealand flax
(**Phormium tenax**
'Atropurpureum') gain some
additional height by being
grown out of the ground. A
plain Asian pot keeps the
focus on the plant material.*

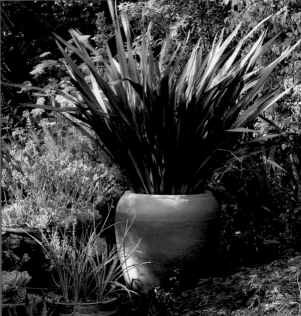

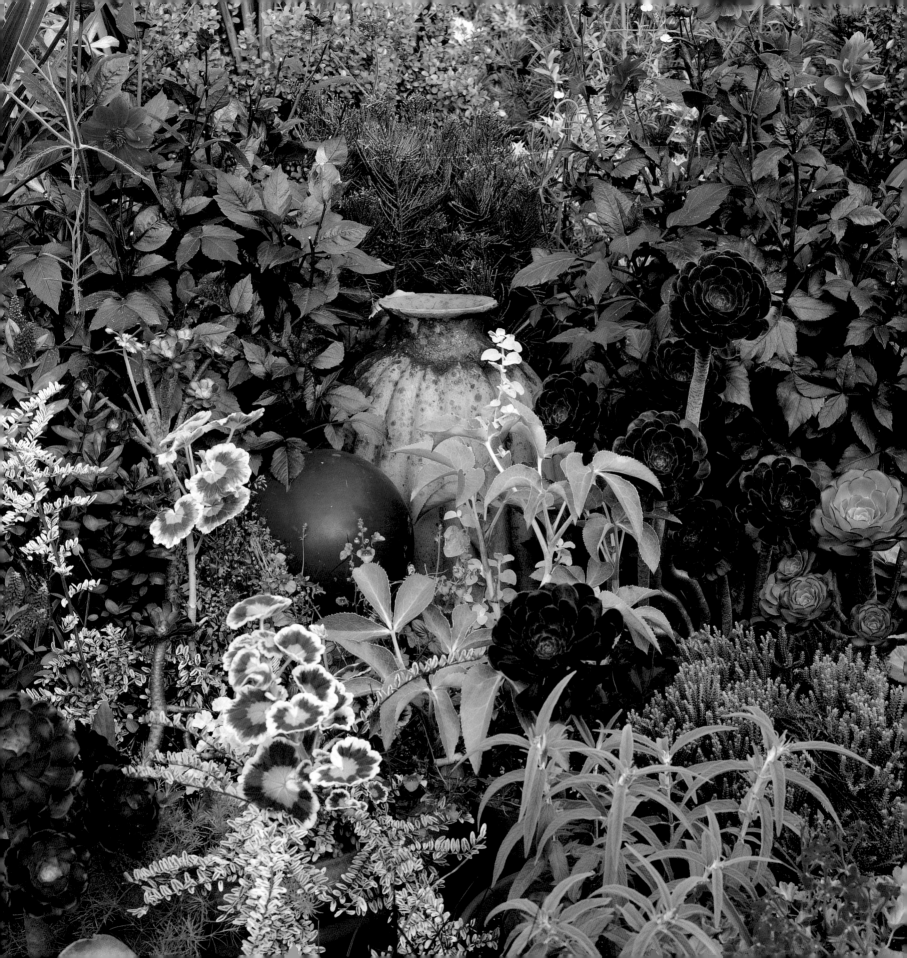

THERE ARE ENDLESS OPTIONS WHEN CHOOSING A CONTAINER theme. But make plastic your last resort: it announces budget constraints loudly. For the same outlay, you can easily find alternatives in wood, clay or metal. Zinc has become popular. Its contemporary, smooth shapes are perfect for holding "modern-looking" foliage plants such as *Elegia capensis, Chondropetalum, Equisetum* and grasses. The almost black rosettes of *Aeonium arboretum* 'Schwarzkopf' always arouse plant lust and do well outside in pots. Don't obsess over "hardy/not hardy" or you won't have any fun and certainly won't be creative. Most of the fun stuff is not hardy except in the mildest areas, so get over it! For decades gardeners have been brainwashed into planting "annuals" as dictated by the dullest nursery conglomerates possible. Luckily, there is a plant resistance movement. Come, join us!

After a while, some plants become special to you. In the world of Jewel Box Gardening, these are your estate jewels. If there was a fire, you would grab them while your CDs and clothing burned. I once carried three *Agave americana* 'Mediopicta' plants across North America in the overhead bins on airplanes. I told fellow passengers they were wedding bouquets, and nobody squashed them! They are the Tiffany of agaves, and I still treasure them. Each leaf has a pure white stripe down its center and the whole plant has a tailored, geometric growth habit. I know not to mix them with "lesser jewels" and allow them to star in their own pots on my terrace.

FACING PAGE *Dark leaves of* **Dahlia** *'Bishop of Llandaff' and* **Aeonium arboreum** *'Schwarzkopf' frame an exciting tableau in* VALERIE MURRAY'S *garden. The duo of a well-placed blue bowling ball and a pottery vase makes a perfect focal point.*

MY GOOD FRIEND HELEN DILLON, A PLANTSWOMAN FROM Dublin, Ireland, refers to her favorite plants as "tots." I suspect they know it: every temperamental treasure thrives for her. Good gardeners establish a rapport with their plants, and container plants need this the most. *They depend on you* — I think this is an unwritten rule of gardening. By isolating a plant from contact with the earth itself, you are taking on the responsibility for its welfare. Container gardening leaves less to chance — you really are in charge.

Much depends on what you use for "soil" in your pots. Most packaged "soil" is largely peat and a horrible fraud. I would never use it as is. Buy some if you must, but amend it liberally with actual organic matter. Composted manures are easily available: I like well-rotted steer manure and aged mushroom manure. I create a more "living soil" for my pots by mixing these at a proportion of about one third each! That means that for every bag of "potting soil," I blend in a similarly sized bag of each of these two manures. I end up with a yummy, friable, water-holding mix that my container plants love. I also find it unnecessary to change container soil. Summer annuals receive monthly applications of 20-20-20 delivered by watering can. This gives them a quick fix that produces lush growth and more bloom.

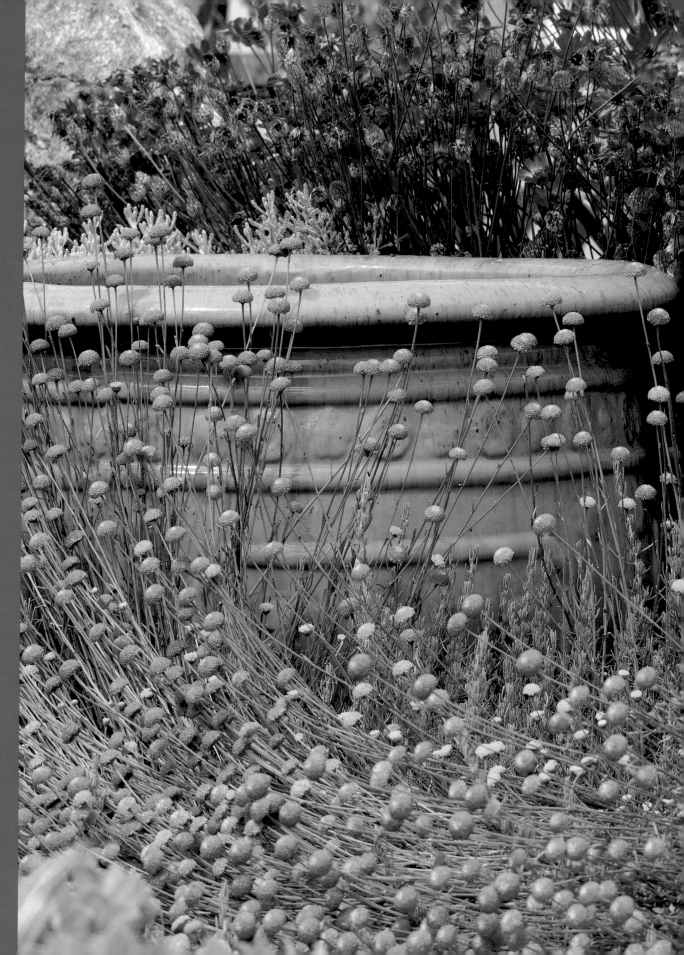

A punch of color in MARNIE
MᶜNEILL'S VICTORIA, B.C., garden
comes not from plants, but from
an empty pot. This unusual
shade of teal blue combines
well with neighboring cupid's
dart (**Catananche caerulea**)
and the straw-yellow buttons of
Santolina chamaecyparissus.

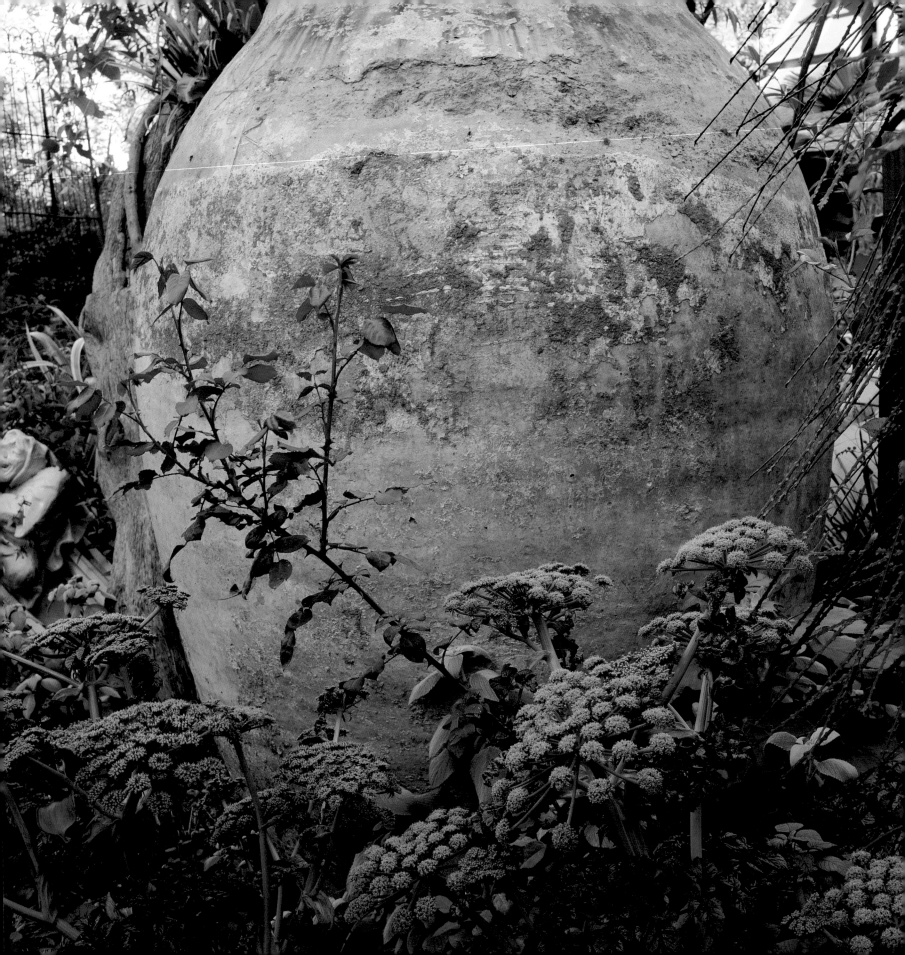

D RAINAGE IS AN IMPORTANT ASPECT OF CONTAINER GARDENING. Plants really can drown, and excess water must escape from all pots except water gardens. If you *must* use saucers, raise your pots up out of them by filling them first with gravel. This not only looks better, but allows air to flow in and out of your soil. Roots needs this. There are exceptions, but most plants do not enjoy sitting in water.

A lot of what you can grow is determined by your light and exposure. Most failures are a result of placing plants in inhospitable or completely foreign new homes. They hate it, and die. Shop according to what you have to offer at home. Is it a baking-hot rooftop or a shady balcony? Do some research and find out where a plant came from. Plants that evolved in South Africa will probably like your blazing deck; Japanese woodland ferns will not. Real gardeners always make the effort to satisfy a plant's genetic programming.

By selecting inspiring containers and trying exciting, off-beat plants, *you have won half the battle*. Throw in the secret ingredient — commitment — or nothing much else is going to happen.

FACING PAGE *The apple-green umbels of* **Angelica pachycarpa** *anchor an enormous jar in* ROGER RAICHE *and* DAVID MᶜCRORY'S *old garden in* BERKELEY. *Why is scale a toy most seem afraid to play with?*

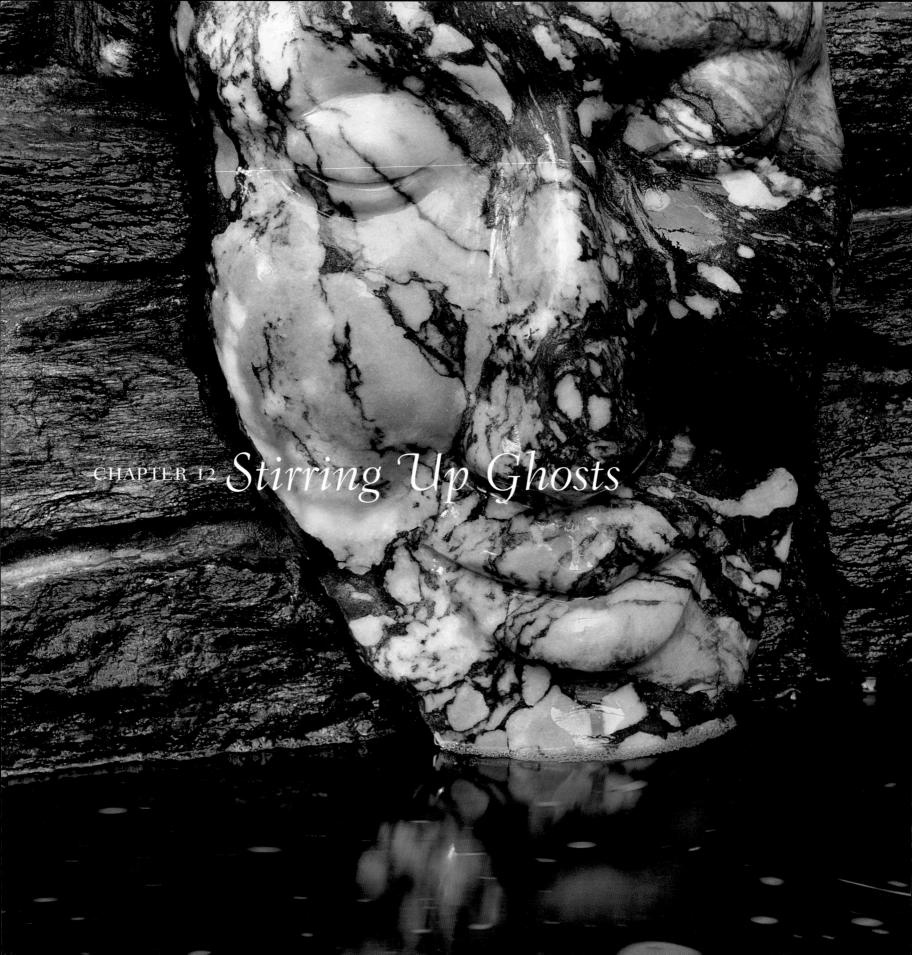

CHAPTER 12 *Stirring Up Ghosts*

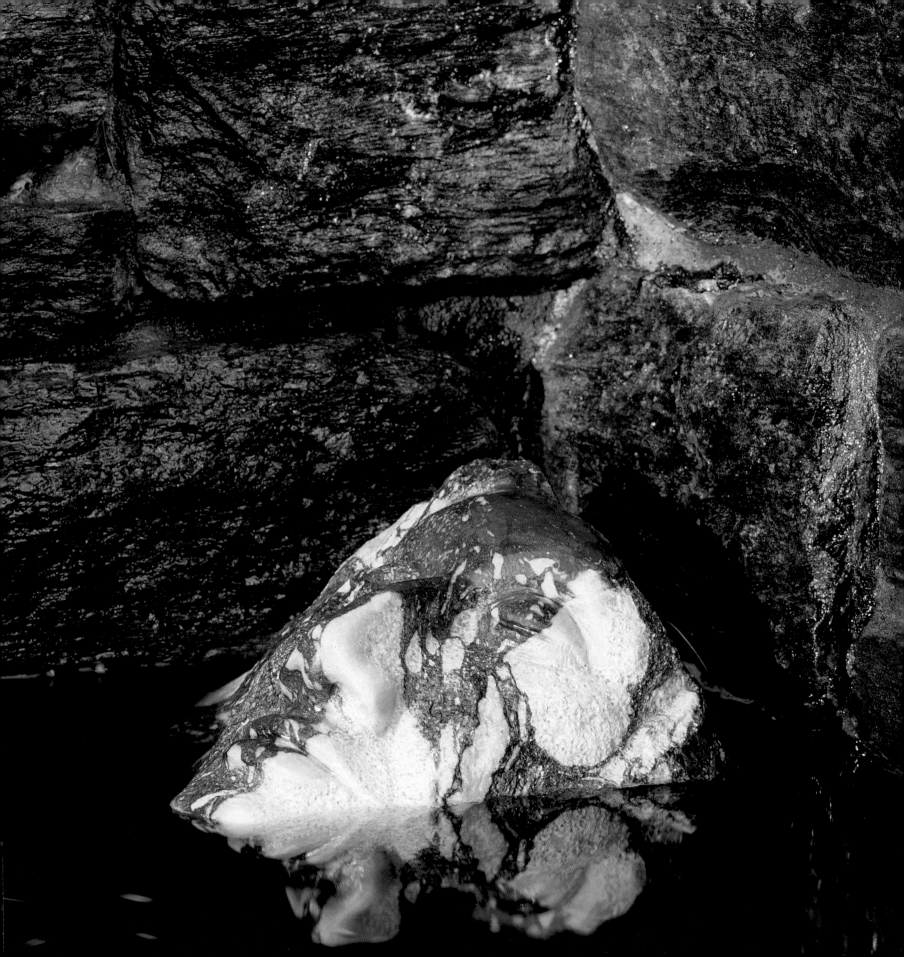

I LIKE THE CONCEPT OF TRYING TO MAKE GARDENING A LITTLE more spiritual. I do my best thinking while weeding, away from life's distractions. I know I am more vulnerable while gardening — my defenses disappear. Therapists now use gardening as medication, whereas we have always administered our own doses.

In this doped-up state of gardening euphoria, it is possible to become very melancholy. This is when we are most creative. Think of all great painters, and what they painted *from*. Creativity comes from adversity, not from art school. Maybe your garden isn't exciting because you haven't suffered. What is interesting about any landscape plan? It is time to look deeper and find the door to your well of creativity. *Access the scary side of your personality.* I like listening to *very* sad songs by Jane Olivor, Helen Schneider or Jackson Browne. I absorb the lyrics, to be rehashed later in my mind as I plant. I feel lucky, and blessed that I have not had to go through most of what they sing about. For me, this audio fertilizer is a form of sensitization. My mind has now tuned in to a higher channel, where like spirits dwell.

The results are certainly better than mindless "landscaping." One only has to drive by any new housing complex or commercial project to see a lack of spiritual connection to plants. Like abandoned puppies, plants are stranded in mass graveyards. For true gardeners, it is our personal bond and actual concern for their welfare that keeps our plants happy, if not healthy.

PREVIOUS PAGE *Kiss the pretty picture? I don't think so. Some life force seems to inhabit the dark waters of an amazing ruin in these unsettling carved marble heads by* BERKELEY, CALIFORNIA, *artist* MARCIA DONAHUE. *A fairly recent addition to Chanticleer Gardens in Wayne, Pennsylvania, this gutsy folly stands alone in public or private horticulture. For now.*

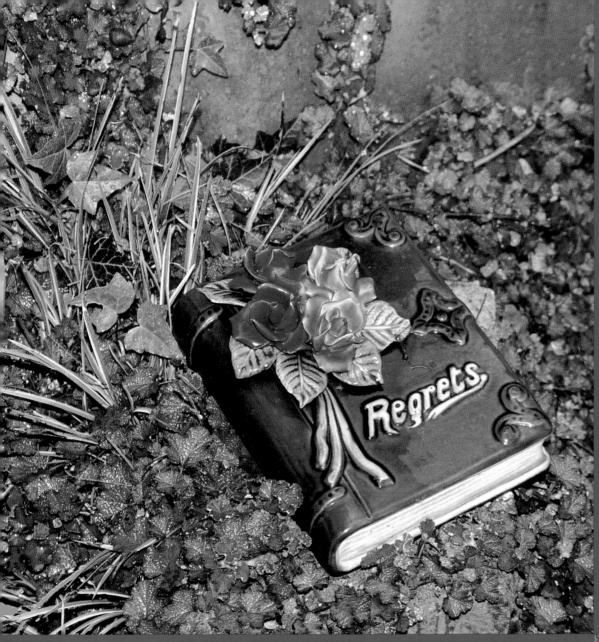

LEFT *Mysteriously placed in* ROGER RAICHE*'s former garden in* BERKELEY, CALIFORNIA, *this ceramic book stopped me in my tracks. That is the sign of good garden ornament.*

BELOW *In her own* CALIFORNIA *garden,* MARCIA DONAHUE*'s carved stone leaves soften the fall of an artistic accident. A sad and broken little man lies at the feet of the sculpture* **Big Beauty***, as art imitates life once again.*

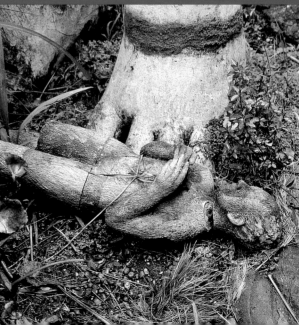

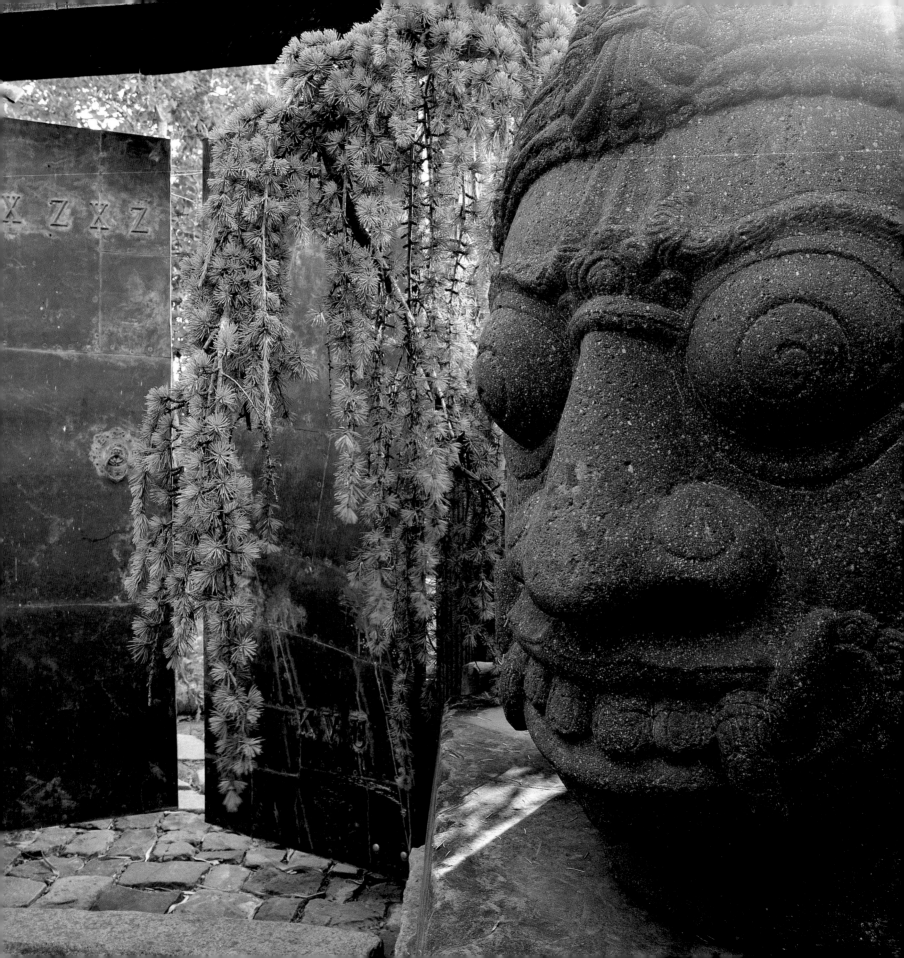

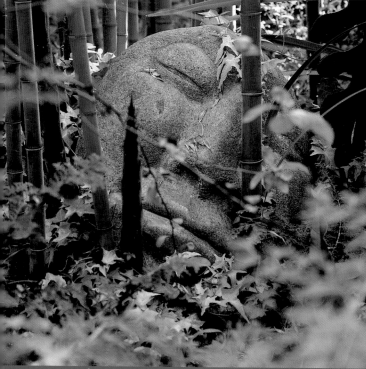

BELOW *The insect-eating pitcher plant,* **Sarracenia rubra**, *waits silently while ceramic slugs frolic around a carved granite skull. It could only happen at Marcia's.*

ABOVE *Protected by her bamboo fortress, sleeping beauty (a non-Disney version) rests in* MARCIA DONAHUE'S *private theme park in* BERKELEY, CALIFORNIA.

LEFT **Cedrus atlantica glauca** *'Pendula' softens copper entry doors in* CEVAN FORRISTT'S SAN JOSE, CALIFORNIA, *garden. Its verdigris needles echo in a cryptic message while an intimidating stone head from Thailand keeps the timid at bay.*

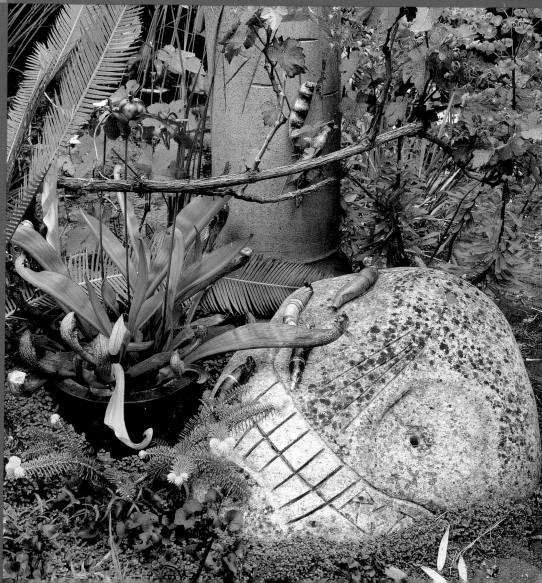

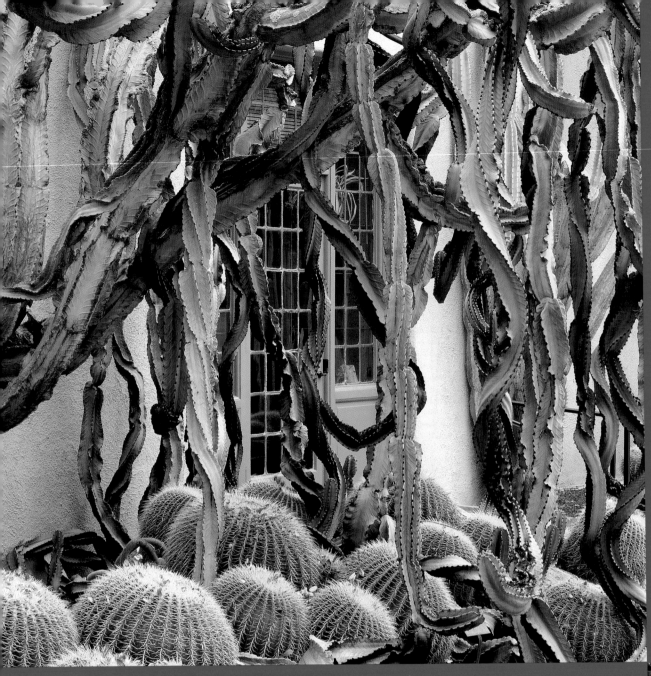

LEFT *At Lotusland,* GANNA WALSKA'S *realized dream in* MONTECITO, CALIFORNIA, ***Euphorbia ingens*** *tries to protect the house from visitors. Forming a terrifying curtain, this plant fills an important role, and I am sure Ms. Walska's spirit directs its every move. Golden barrel cactus* (***Echinocactus grusonii***) *acts as ground cover.*

BELOW ***Echeveria elegans*** *surrounds a mysterious hole in* BOB CLARK'S OAKLAND, CALIFORNIA, *garden. I like to think of this as a portal — is something coming out, or do we go in?*

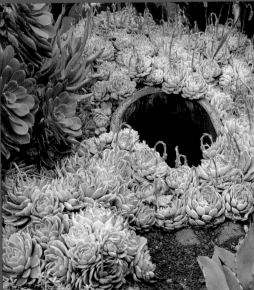

168

W HITE CALLA LILIES (*Zantedeschia aethiopica*) HAVE AN intrinsic sadness to them, and many people avoid them. I think they are the stars of the arum family and at their best close to a water feature. Bearded iris (**Iris germanica** hybrids) come in the most amazing, hypnotic colors. I grow them in odd shades of brown, near-black and rust. They are happy in full sun and seem to like no competition. Keep them unshadowed by neighboring perennials and replant the rhizome tips often. I always place a handful of bone meal under each rhizome when replanting. This group of plants is unfairly snubbed by nearly all gardeners. No other genus contains such magical colors and impossible beauty.

Other "forgotten" groups of plants, botanical ghosts, include dianthus, **Primula auricula**, ranunculus and chrysanthemums. At some point, these and many more families of plants were enormously popular. Entire societies and exhibitions were devoted to them. Centuries before the present age of DVD and video, collectors in England built "Auricula Theatres" onto their homes. Here they would stage their prized collection of primulas. Are we de-evolving?

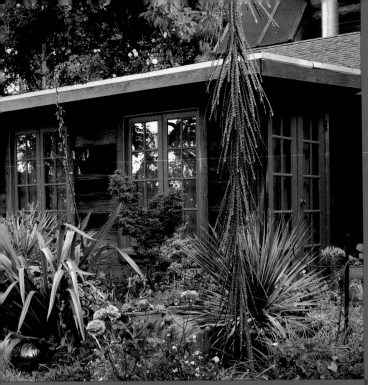

RIGHT *Allium christophii* always dries perfectly in situ. Here it is surrounded by the extra-lovely cut-silver foliage of *Centaurea gymnocarpa* in the late STEVE ANTONOW'S SEATTLE garden.

ABOVE *In* ROGER RAICHE *and* DAVID McRORY'S *former* BERKELEY, CALIFORNIA, *garden, it is the bright blue painted window trim, not the plants, that matches the glazed decorative objects. This bonus color intensifies the scene, which otherwise belongs to a strange New Zealand native,* **Pseudopanax ferox**. *Trying hard to look dead, its jagged juvenile leaves feel like plastic and emerge in a terminal blob of clear goo!*

RIGHT *The deciduous* **Catalpa bignonioides** *'Aurea' forms a living sculpture in* LINDA COCHRAN'S *garden near* SEATTLE. *Notice the way a hint of color on the pottery vessel ties it to the color-washed concrete wall.*

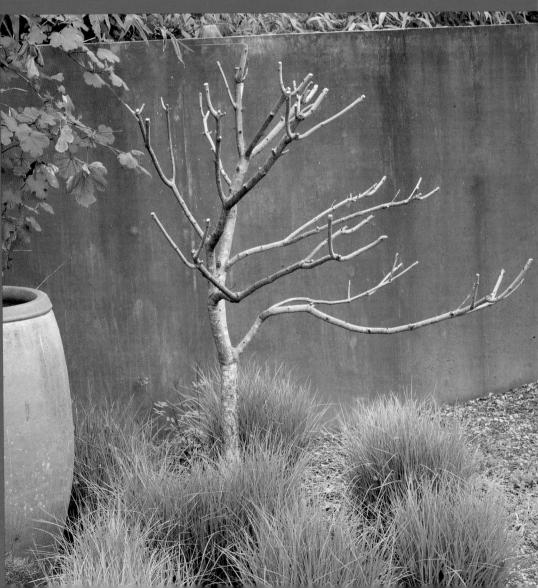

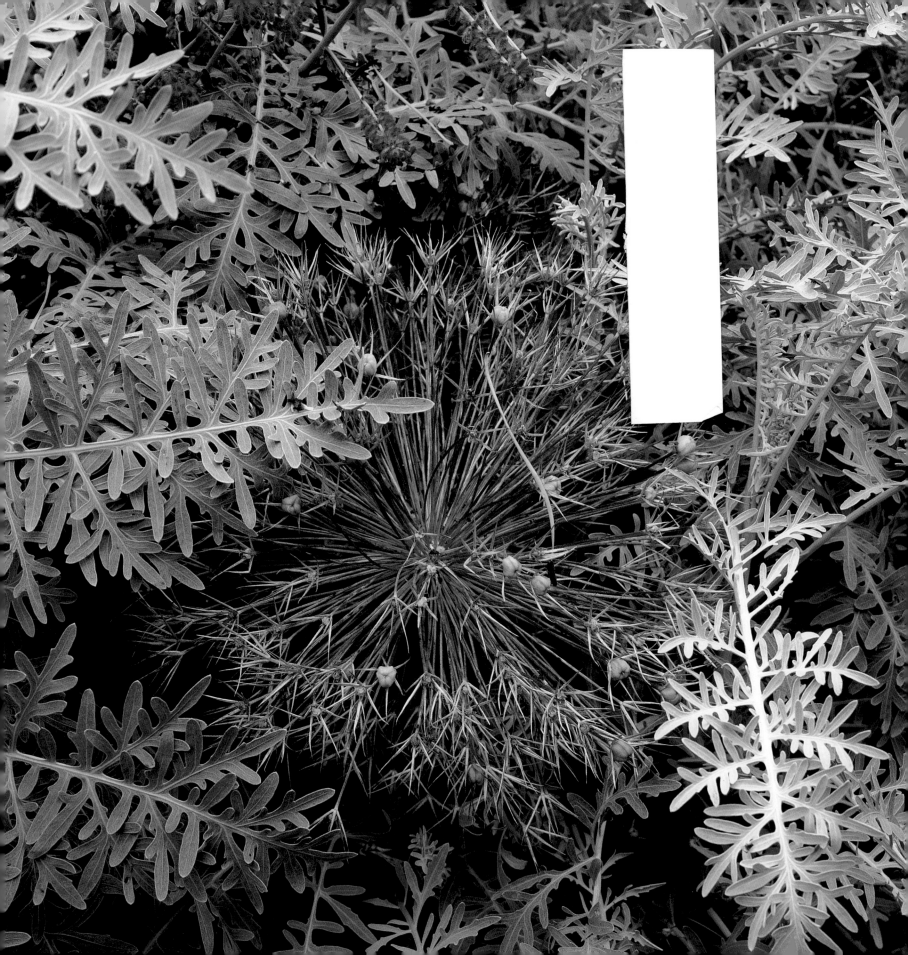

I HAVE NOTICED A SWITCH IN GARDENING, FROM "PRETTY" TO WHAT I call "The New Ugly." I find this fascinating and very, very attractive. In gardening, *ugly has been redefined* by brilliant plantsmen and -women who get absolutely no thrill from trying to make a pretty picture. By increasing the dosage of all that is weird and unexpected, these thrillseekers are creating powerful, unforgettable experiences. What was garden ornament has become *garden incident*. Adding a few lightning rods is bound to attract bonus energy to your garden.

Certain plants have the added feature of an "afterlife" — they are still of ornamental value when dead. Poppy pods appear sinister. The giant biennial thistle (**Onopordon acanthium**) dries in situ, turning into an eight-foot silvery nightmare of razor blades by July. Of the alliums, my favorite is **Allium schubertii**. With its 18-inch sparklers atop 14-inch stems, this botanical wonder dries perfectly. **Allium christophii** is more accessible but far less spectacular. **Cardiocrinum giganteum** produces fabulous stalks of white "lilies," each with a plum-red blotch in the throat. The 10-foot stalks dry perfectly and look like something left behind by Tiki warriors.

Even though it is not reliably hardy outdoors for me in winter, I grow the very odd-looking **Pseudopanax ferox** in a pot. This New Zealand native has a fascinating, dead appearance. Its very sculptural, lizard-textured leaves feel like plastic strips of bumps and notches. A dreary army green, they clasp the beanpole-like stem and hang downward. Every so often there is a "birthing" at the top and an amazing clear goo containing a new batch of baby leaves emerges. In its windy native climate, this gel allows the new foliage to photosynthesize without dessicating!

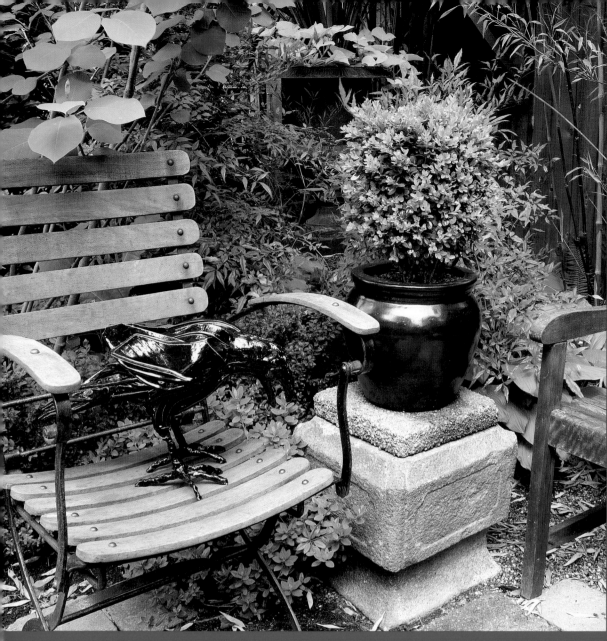

LEFT *A ceramic sculpture of a crow by artist Katherine MacLean adds tension to* JOHN RAMSAY'S *garden in* VANCOUVER, B.C. *Black accents reinforce the message that in this garden, nature meets art dealer. Designed by John Minty as an urban refuge and an extension of the house itself, this small garden succeeds as both.*

BELOW *More unsettling than cute, a baby doll head in a wreath of birch twigs "welcomes" visitors at* SHARON OSMOND'S *garden gate. I much prefer this to a "Welcome Duck" as a clue to what might lie within!*

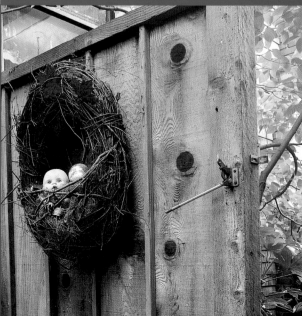

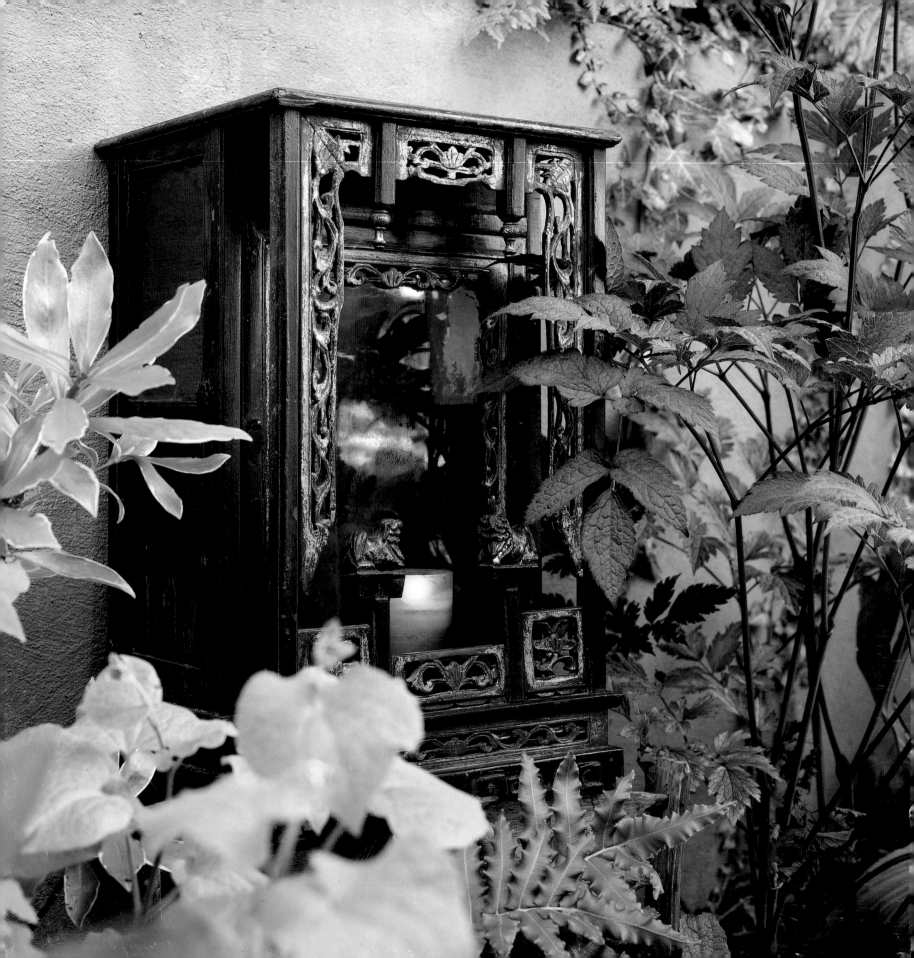

ENVISION YOUR GARDEN AS A RECEIVING DISH FOR POSITIVE energy. You don't have to tell everyone about it, but try it in secret. Wouldn't you tend an area more lovingly if your favorite pet was buried there? Extend emotional reactions to include your plants. I always tell my **Hemerocallis** 'Elusive Dream' that it's my favorite. That daylily outperforms all my others, and I have *lots* of them. Talking to plants doesn't seem so crazy if you know you are getting a reply.

Not everyone will be able to use a garden in this way. Actually, very few people do, and it shows. Just go for a drive.

In my life, many of the crinkliest eyes (always a good sign) ended up blind and dying of AIDS. This included some of the very best gardeners on the planet. I am simply unwilling to lose contact with them, and my only hope is through plants themselves. I have no proof it works, but my green thumb practically gives off sparks when I remember, "Drake gave me this plant," or "This was Gerald's **Rodgersia**."

The very '90s term "cocooning" sounds all warm and fuzzy, but the terrorist attacks of 9/11 awakened the desire in *everyone* for a safe haven. Those of us who have gardens use them as ongoing therapy. As the world gets scarier, our sessions are longer and we schedule them more often. The sensitive gardener's garden is looking better than ever!

FACING PAGE *The dark foliage of **Cimicifuga simplex** 'Brunette' brushes against an antique Asian shrine in my garden. Only used on rare occasions, and more for garden lighting than worship, I'm sure it doesn't hurt to light this candle ...*